BROMLEY COLLEGE LIBRARY
B20256

BRITISH MEDICAL BULLETIN

British Medical Bulletin is published four times each year, in January, April, July and October.
Subscriptions and single-copy orders should be sent to: Longman Group Ltd, PO Box 77, Harlow, Essex CM19 5BQ. Tel: 0279 623760
Subscription rates for 1995 are: £126 (UK, £6 postage), £126 (Europe, £8 postage), $207 (USA, $15 postage) or £126 (RoW, £11 postage)
Single copies will be available at £49.95 (UK)

NEXT ISSUE

Volume 51 *No. 2* RHEUMATOID DISEASE *April 1995*

Scientific Editors: M J Walport & J. Saklatvala

BRITISH MEDICAL BULLETIN

VOLUME FIFTY-ONE
1995

CHURCHILL LIVINGSTONE
EDINBURGH, LONDON, MADRID, MELBOURNE,
NEW YORK, TOKYO AND HONG KONG

CHURCHILL LIVINGSTONE
Medical Division of Pearson Professional Ltd

Distributed in the United States of America by Churchill Livingstone Inc., 650 Avenue of the Americas, New York, NY10011, and by associated companies, branches and representatives throughout the world.

ISSN 0007-1420
ISBN 0-443-05333-2

Published by Pearson Professional Ltd
Printed in Great Britain by Bell and Bain Ltd., Glasgow

This journal is indexed, abstracted and/or published online in the following media: Adonis, Biosis, BRS Colleague (full text), Chemical Abstracts, Colleague (Online), Current Awareness in Biological Science, Current Contents/Clinical Medicine, Current Contents/Life Science, Excerpta Medica/Embase, Index Medicus/Medline, Medical Documentation Service, Reference Update, Research Alert, Science Citation Index, Scisearch, SIIC-Database Argentina, UMI (Microfilms), USSR Academy of Sciences

British Medical Bulletin is published quarterly in January, April, July and October by Churchill Livingstone c/o Mercury Airfreight International Inc Ltd, 2323 Randolph Avenue, Avenel, New Jersey 07001. Subscription price is $222.00 per annum. Second Class Postage paid at Rahway NJ (USPS No. 011-369). Postmaster: Send address corrections to British Medical Bulletin c/o Mercury Airfreight International Inc Ltd, 2323 Randolph Avenue, Avenel, New Jersey 07001.

Gene Therapy

Scientific Editors: *A M L Lever & P Goodfellow*

1995 Vol. 51 No. 1

Professor A M L Lever chaired the committee which included Dr R Levinsky, Professor G Brownlee and Professor M Evans which planned this number of the British Medical Bulletin. We are grateful to them for their help and particularly to Professor T W Meade for his work as Scientific Editor.

British Medical Bulletin is published by Churchill Livingstone for The British Council, 10 Spring Gardens, London SW1A 2BN

British Medical Bulletin (1995) Vol.51, No.1, pp.1-11

Scope and limitations of gene therapy

D J Weatherall
Institute of Molecular Medicine, University of Oxford, John Radcliffe Hospital, Oxford, UK

Although there are still many technical difficulties to be overcome, recent advances in the molecular and cellular biology of gene transfer have made it likely that gene therapy will soon start to play an increasing role in clinical practice. It will not be restricted to the management of monogenic disorders, but will have applications across many other fields of medicine, particularly the treatment of cancer and infectious disease.

Ever since the classical studies of Avery, McLeod and McCarty on DNA-mediated genetic transformation,[1] human geneticists have toyed with the idea of gene transfer for the treatment of inherited diseases. But it is only in the last few years that remarkable advances in recombinant DNA technology and cell biology have made it likely that this pipedream will become a reality, and, furthermore, that gene therapy will not be restricted to the correction of single-gene disorders, but will have applications for many other branches of medicine.[2–5]

There are two main approaches. First, any cells other than germ cells might have their genetic make-up altered. Somatic-cell gene therapy of this kind would change an individual's genetic constitution only during their lifetime and would not affect their children. Alternatively, germline gene therapy would entail injecting 'foreign' genes into fertilised eggs; the inserted genes would be distributed among somatic and germ cells and would be transmitted to future generations. For a variety of technical and ethical reasons current research is restricted to somatic-cell gene therapy.

STRATEGIES

Ideally, gene therapy would emulate transplantation surgery and remove a mutant gene and replace it with a normal one. Another way of achieving the same end, gene correction, would entail the specific alteration of a mutant gene sequence using nature's way of exchanging genetic material, that is by site-directed recombination.

Because of the technical difficulties of these approaches much current research in gene therapy is directed towards gene augmentation, that is introducing a gene into cells in a way that will allow it to produce sufficient of its product to compensate for the lack of expression of its defective counterpart. This avenue is best suited to the treatment of recessive monogenic diseases. It will not, however, be of value for dominantly inherited disorders in which abnormal gene products interfere with cellular function. The same constraint applies to the treatment of many forms of cancer or infectious disease. In these cases it may be necessary to interfere with the expression of an abnormal or amplified gene.

REQUIREMENTS FOR GENE THERAPY

The requirements for gene therapy, while easily stated, have been extremely difficult to fulfill. First, it is necessary to isolate a particular gene together with its regulatory sequences. Second, it must be possible to obtain sufficient numbers of the cells into which the gene is to be inserted and find an effective way of returning them to the patient. Third, there must be an efficient mechanism for inserting the gene into target cells. And, finally, the inserted gene must produce sufficient amounts of its product over a reasonable length of time, and the procedure must not have any deleterious side effects.

Regulation

In the context of gene therapy it is useful to think of genes as existing in two classes. There are 'housekeeping genes', that is genes that are expressed in most tissues at all stages of development and do not require precise regulation. Alternatively, there are genes that are tissue-specific in their expression, sometimes developmentally regulated, and which require very tight control of the levels of their products. This is particularly important in the case of genes for subunits of proteins, the α and β chains of haemoglobin for example.

There are 2 main classes of regulatory sequences. First, there are those in *cis* to a particular gene, that is on the same chromosome. *Cis*-acting elements may function as promoters, regions of DNA that are involved in binding RNA polymerases to initiate transcription and that lie immediately 5′(upstream) of the initiation sequence. Alternatively, they may act as enhancers, sequences that increase the utilisation of promoters, and that can function in either orientation and in any location up- or downstream from a gene, often at a considerable distance from it. In addition, there are families of *trans*-acting regulatory proteins, that is elements which act on both of a pair of homologous genes, and that may be encoded on other chromosomes. When considering the regulation of genes that are to be inserted into 'foreign' cells, it is assumed that it will be necessary to include some or all of the *cis*-acting sequences, while the *trans*-acting regulatory proteins will be supplied by the recipient cells.

Recently a great deal has been learned about the DNA sequences required for fully regulated gene expression in vivo, mainly from transgenic mice in which 'foreign' DNA has been integrated into the genome and is present in different tissues.[6] While in some cases it may be possible to obtain adequate expression by transferring a gene and its promoters, in others it is necessary to include much larger pieces of DNA. For example, high-level developmentally-regulated expression of the human α or β globin genes in transgenic mice requires the insertion of the globin gene complexes together with regulatory regions located between 5 and 40 kilobases (kb) upstream from the gene clusters.[7,8] Similar sequences have been found near other human genes.[9] One of the major problems of gene therapy is how to transfer large DNA fragments into cells, and to ensure that they are stably expressed over a reasonable length of time.

Approaches to gene transfer or manipulation (Table 1)

While it is relatively easy to insert DNA into cells, it is what happens to it after that presents the major challenge. DNA introduced by physical methods, calcium-phosphate or cationic-lipid-mediated, or electroporation, for example, may be taken up readily but only a few cells integrate it into their genome and become stably transformed; the non-integrated DNA is degraded. Direct DNA transfer may be of value however. For example, DNA injected directly into muscle enters the cells and is expressed for up to a year.[10] DNA can be delivered to the airway epithelial cells using an aerosol; expression of inserted genes has been observed for up to several weeks.[11,12]

Because they integrate DNA into the genome much recent research in gene transfer has focused on retroviral vectors, retroviruses from which many of the viral genes have been removed or altered so that no viral proteins can be made in the cells which they infect.[13,14] Viral replication functions are provided by 'packaging' cells that contain helper viruses that produce all the viral proteins that are required, but which themselves have been altered so that they are unable to produce infectious viruses.[13] The main advantage of retroviral vectors is the high efficiency of gene transfer into replicating cells. On the other hand it is difficult to insert large pieces of DNA into these vectors and most retroviruses are unable to infect non-dividing cells. Furthermore, integration is random

Table 1 Methods for gene therapy

Methods for gene therapy
Physical
Direct injection of DNA
Calcium phosphate transfection
Electroporation
Liposome-mediated DNA transfer
Retroviral vectors
Other viral vectors
Targetted gene transfer via receptors
Artificial chromosomes
Site-directed recombination
Activation of genes of related function

and there is a danger of unwanted side-effects, insertional mutagenesis for example.

Other viral transfer systems are being explored.[3–5] Adenorivus vectors have the advantage that they can carry larger segments of DNA and infect non-replicating cells. On the other hand, they contain a number of adenovirus genes with the potential for stimulating immunity or producing other adverse effects. Another promising vector, AAV-2, is derived from a defective parvovirus.[15] In this case integration is targeted specifically to the long arm of human chromosome 19.

Several approaches are being explored for targetting genes to particular cell populations.[16] Some involve complexing plasmid DNA to proteins. For example, polylysine can be conjugated to an asialoglycoprotein; this complex is targetted to receptors on hepatocytes that internalise galactose terminal (asialo) glycoproteins. Similarly, DNA complexed with transferrin is taken up by cells which express transferrin receptors. Systems designed to direct DNA to the nucleus, rather than to lysosomes, are being explored. It is also possible to engineer tissue-specific retroviral vectors. Using streptavidin, antibodies directed against proteins that are expressed on the surface of a target cell can be coupled to antibodies specific for virus envelope proteins. Alternatively, retroviral vectors can be constructed which contain tissue-specific promoters.

The possibility of transferring and maintaining DNA by the use of extrachromosomal elements is also being explored.[17] For example, such elements are formed after fusion of mouse cells with yeast carrying a yeast artificial chromosome (YAC) containing a human gene. Unfortunately, they segregate poorly during cell division and are lost from the cells. But recent progress in defining the sequences required for both centromere and telomere function in mammalian cells may, in the long term, make it possible to construct mammalian artificial chromosomes for gene therapy. Some progress has also been made towards gene correction by site-directed recombination. Targeted sequences have been introduced into cells by physical methods and, under appropriate conditions, homologous recombination can be obtained with specific sequences.[18]

Gene therapy may not always require the transfer of DNA into cells. In some cases it may be possible to by-pass a defective gene by utilising genes of similar function. The best example is the activation of the fetal γ globin genes to correct disorders of adult β chain synthesis, β thalassaemia and sickle cell anaemia.[19] A similar principle is being explored for activating homologues of the dystrophin gene for the management of muscular dystrophy.[20]

Target Cells (Table 2)

The first gene transfer protocols involved the insertion of genes into lymphocytes.[4] Populations of T cells, isolated directly from tumours and expanded by growth in vitro, may cause regression of tumours when reinjected. Such tumour infiltrating lymphocytes (TIL) cells have been transfected with a marker gene to prove that they return to the site of the tumour. Lymphocytes obtained from patients with severe combined immunodeficiency (SCID) due to adenine deaminase (ADA) deficiency have been exposed to a retroviral vector containing a normal human ADA gene and reinjected. Preliminary results suggest that the transduced genes restore some degree of immune function during the lifespan of the lymphocyte population.

Table 2 Some target cells for gene therapy

Peripheral blood lymphocytes
Haemopoietic stem cells
Fibroblasts
Hepatocytes
Keratinocytes
Skeletal muscle myoblasts
Airway epithelial cells
Vascular endothelial cells
Tumour cells

The problem of transferring genes into haemopoietic stem cells to cure a genetic disease is much more daunting however. They constitute only a small percentage of the bone marrow and most of them are out of cycle and not susceptible to retroviral infection. Thus attempts to transfer genes into these cells, even if stimulated by cocktails of haemopoietic growth factors, have met with only limited success.[21,22] It has been found recently however that there are populations of circulating haemopoietic progenitor cells, identifiable because they express CD34 antigens, that can repopulate the bone marrow after its ablation. If prestimulated with haemopoietic growth factors they can be transduced by retroviral vectors containing marker genes that are stably expressed in vitro.[23]

Many genetic diseases involve the liver, which is comprised of quiescent, differentiated hepatocytes that are refractory to retroviral infection. However, hepatocytes are susceptible to infection during the differentiation phase of growth in vitro.[24] Several genes have been inserted into cultured hepatocytes, which, if they are reinjected via the portal vein, seed to the liver and express their gene products for long periods. The major problem is how to treat sufficient cells; gene therapy using this approach requires the removal of most of the left lobe of the liver.[25]

Keratinocytes have been used for gene therapy, although it has not been possible to target stem cell populations.[26] It is also feasible to transduce fibroblasts and vascular endothelial cells; these ubiquitous cells may provide a source of therapeutic agents for many different tissues, including the brain.[2,5]

Airway epithelial cells are of particular current interest as one of the sites of expression of the defect in cystic fibrosis. Using adenovirus vectors or plasmids complexed with cationic lipids the human cystic fibrosis transmembrane conductance regulator (CFTR) gene has been transferred by intratracheal instillation.[11,12] Expression of the transferred CFTR gene has been detected for up to six weeks, suggesting that these cells have a relatively slow turnover. Whether this will be the case in the infected airways of patients with cystic fibrosis remains to be seen.

CLINICAL APPLICATIONS (Table 3)

Monogenic disease

There are over 4000 monogenic diseases. Until the molecular pathology of dominantly-inherited diseases is understood it will be difficult to develop strategies for gene therapy and current efforts are directed at recessive disorders.

Successful delivery of genes to the epithelium of the respiratory tract of animals has generated several protocols for phase 1 clinical trials for the treatment of cystic fibrosis. Because of the slow evolution of lung damage long periods of observation may be required. Recent results, both in animals and humans, suggest that it may be possible to control monogenic hypercholesterolaemia due to mutations of the low density lipoprotein receptor (LDLR) gene, either by in vitro transfection of hepatocytes followed by their return to the patient,[25] or by targetted transfection by retroviral vectors containing LDLR genes.[16] Other im-

Table 3 Some clinical applications of gene transfer therapy

Correction of monogenic disease
Cancer therapy
Control of refractory infectious diseases
Management of degenerative neurological disease
Symptomatic control of vascular disease
Control of metabolic disease

portant monogenic diseases which are manifest mainly in the liver cell, including α1 antitrypsin deficiency and phenylketonuria, may be treated in the same way.

Over 30 genetic diseases have been corrected by bone marrow transplantation,[27] suggesting that it should also be possible to treat them by gene therapy directed at haemopoietic stem cells. As mentioned earlier, the latter are difficult to isolate but CD34 antigen-expressing cells in the peripheral blood may offer a more practical alternative. Initially, diseases are being explored in which even a low level of expression may provide a proliferative advantage to the transduced cell population, the form of severe combined immune deficiency (SCID) due to ADA deficiency for example. There have been several attempts to transfect bone marrow cells from patients with SCID with retroviruses carrying the human ADA gene but so far it has not been possible to obtain an effective level of expression over a long period. It will not be feasible to treat common disorders like sickle cell anaemia and β thalassaemia until all these criteria have been met, and this will require the development of gene transfer systems which accept much larger pieces of DNA.

Gene therapy should be applicable to muscle disease. Direct gene transfer into muscle by intramuscular injection of plasmid DNA is being augmented by a variety of pre-injection procedures to improve the distribution of the injected genes among muscle cells.[10] Furthermore, it is possible to isolate and modify myoblasts in vitro and to reimplant them into the muscle. Although these techniques are still a long way from clinical application they have shown that inserted genes can be expressed for a reasonable length of time in muscle.

Many monogenic diseases affect development or brain function. Once the current techniques of gene transfer are improved it will be necessary to evolve methods for inserting genes early during human development.

Cancer

Several approaches to cancer therapy are being explored.[28,29] First, immune responses to tumours are being enhanced. Second, genes are being inserted into tumour cells to evoke ‘cell suicide’. And, finally, methods are being developed to modify tumour suppressor or anti-oncogenes. The prime target for stimulating an immune response to a tumour is the major histocompatability complex (MHC) class 1-restricted tumour-specific cytotoxic (CD8) T cell. Two criteria must be met. First, the CD8 T cell receptors must be occupied by an MHC class 1-peptide complex. Second, a helper T cell must be activated to secrete cytokines which act on the CD8 T cell. This second signal could be bypassed by inducing CD8 cells to produce their own cytokines. With this objective, tumour tissue is grown in culture and transfected with vectors carrying different cytokines, including interleukin (IL)-2, IL-4, tumour necrosis factor, and interferon-γ, after which the cells are re-injected, usually after irradiation to ensure that they do not grow. A variation on this theme, that is the use of TIL cells, was mentioned earlier. Alternatively, an appropriate class-1 gene can be delivered by lipofection directly into tumours.

'Cell suicide' involves the insertion of a herpes simplex virus thymidine kinase (HSV-TK) gene. Mammalian cells contain a TK gene that can only phosphorylate a thymidine nucleotide but cannot add a phosphate to the nucleoside base T. On the other hand, HSV-TK can phosphorylate a nucleoside base. Thus any cell infected with HSV can be killed by exposing it to nucleoside agents such as ganciclovir which, when phosphorylated, interfere with DNA synthesis. To treat brain tumours retroviral vectors containing HSV-TK gene are injected into the vicinity of the tumour; since only the malignant cells are dividing the vector should be targeted to the tumour. Ganciclovir is then administered, which causes selective destruction of the transfected tumour cells. In animal experiments complete eradication of tumours has been observed even though only some 20% of the cells carried the HSV-TK gene. The mechanism for this valuable 'bystander' effect is unclear.

Tumour suppressor genes are being inserted into human tumours. One protocol involves inserting a normal p53 gene into non-small cell lung carcinomas that are p53 defective. In another, antisense DNA is injected to try to suppress the activity of activated oncogenes, in this case k-*ras* in lung carcinoma.

Infection

Because immunodeficiency virus 1 (HIV-1) transcribes its RNA genome and integrates it into chromosomes of host cells, AIDS is, in effect, an acquired genetic disease in which all the progeny of the infected cell population are themselves affected. A radical cure would require either the death of the entire infected cell population or selective gene excision using methods such as site-directed homologous recombination. We are a long way from achieving either of these aims. However, strategies based on gene transfer technology are being evolved to control the disease, including transdominant modifications of HIV proteins, the development of RNA decoys, antisense RNA technology, and modification of soluble CD4.[30] Several of these strategies have reached the stage of limited clinical trials.

Other applications of gene therapy

Several systems are being explored for the delivery of hormones, coagulation factors, anticoagulants, and other therapeutic agents.[2,4] When their genes are introduced into fibroblasts or vascular endothelial cells, their products can be detected in the blood for varying periods of time. Recent studies in mice suggest that myoblasts may be particularly advantageous target cells for the delivery of recombinant proteins.[31] They fuse randomly with other muscle fibres in their vicinity and become an integral part of vascularised muscle tissue; human growth hormone has been detected in the circulation of mice treated this way for up to 6 months.

In vitro gene transfer followed by cell grafting is also being explored to restore function in chronic diseases of the nervous system. If such combined gene transfer/implantation techniques prove effective they could offer a novel way of treating chronic disorders such as Parkinson's or Alzheimer's disease.

FUTURE PROBLEMS AND ETHICAL ISSUES

There are still formidable technical problems to be overcome. There is much to learn about the regulation of mammalian genes and the sequences required for their stability when introduced into foreign genomes. It is still not clear whether it is safe to incorporate genes into nuclear DNA or whether it will be possible to develop stable extrachromosomal gene transfer systems. Little is known about the antigenicity of gene products which the immune system is encountering for the first time; replacement therapy for haemophilia often evokes an immune response.

The reasons for the clinical diversity of many genetic diseases is still not clear. It is difficult to make the case for a trial of a completely new and potentially risky form of treatment for diseases like sickle cell anaemia when we still have no way of knowing whether they will run a mild or severe course in an individual patient.

The notion that it is possible to alter an individual's genetic makeup is still repugnant to many people. However, from the work of the Clothier Committee in Great Britain, and similar groups in other countries, some effective codes of practice have evolved.[32] Somatic cell gene therapy does not present any fundamentally new ethical issues; essentially it is no different to any other form of transplantation. The inserted genes will, if all goes well, simply modify the genetic makeup of one organ system. But because of the technical complexity of these new procedures most countries have established regulatory bodies that are able to assess both the clinical, ethical and technical merits of particular protocols, and advise hospital ethics committees about their suitability.

The same general principles could be applied to genetic modification of germ cells. But here we are entering uncharted areas of medical ethics. If successful, genes transferred in this way would be passed on to future generations which would have had no input into the decision. For this reason, and because of uncertainties about the safety of genetic modification of this type, most countries have banned germ cell gene therapy, at least for the foreseeable future. As the field progresses this decision may have to be revised, particularly for the management of genetically determined disorders of development. However, since it is now possible to identify genetic disease in fertilised ova it is at least theoretically possible to sort through eggs after in vitro fertilisation and to replace those which do not carry a particular defective gene. Thus for the immediate future there seems no reason to consider germline therapy.

REFERENCES

1 Avery DT, Macleod CM, McCarty M. Studies on the chemical nature of the substance inducing transformation of pneumococcal types. Induction of transformation by a deoxyribonucleic acid traction isolated from pneumococcus type III. J Exp Med 1944; 79: 137–158.
2 Friedmann T. Progress toward human gene therapy. Science 1989; 244: 1275–1281.
3 Miller AD. Human gene therapy comes of age. Nature 1992; 357: 455–460.
4 Anderson WF. Human gene therapy. Science 1992; 256: 808–813.
5 Friedmann T. A brief history of gene therapy. Nature Genet 1992; 2: 93–98.
6 Jaenisch R. Transgenic animals. Science 1988; 240: 1468–1474.
7 Grosveld F, Blom van Assendelft G, Greaves DR, Kollias G. Position-independent, high level expression of the human β globin gene in transgenic mice. Cell 1987; 51: 975–985.
8 Higgs DR, Wood WG, Jarman AP, et al. A major positive regulatory region is located far upstream of the human α globin locus. Genes Dev 1990; 4: 1588–1601.
9 Lang G, Mamalaki C, Greenberg D, Yannoutsos N, Kioussis D. Deletion analysis of the human CD2 gene locus control region in transgenic mice. Nucl Acids Res 1991; 19: 5851–5856.
10 Davis HL, Whalen RG, Demeneix BA. Direct gene transfer into skeletal muscle *in vivo*: factors affecting efficiency of transfer and stability of expression. Hum Gene Ther 1993; 4: 151–159.
11 Hyde SC, Gill DR, Higgins CF, et al. Correction of the ion transport defect in cystic fibrosis transgenic mice by gene therapy. Nature 1993; 362: 250–255.
12 Alton EWFW, Middleton PG, Caplen NJ, et al. Non-invasive liposome-mediated gene delivery can correct the ion transport defect in cystic fibrosis mutant mice. Nature Genet 1993; 5: 135–142.
13 Miller AD. Retrovirus packaging cells. Hum Gene Ther 1990; 1: 5–14.
14 Kotani H, Newton III PB, Zhang S, et al. Improved methods of retroviral vector transduction and production for gene therapy. Hum Gene Ther 1994; 5: 19–28.

15 Walsh CE, Liu JM, Xiao X, Young NS, Nienhuis AW. Regulated high level expression of a human γ-globin gene introduced into erythroid cells by an adeno-associated virus vector. Proc Natl Acad Sci USA 1992; 89: 7257–7261.
16 Salmons B, Gunzburg WH. Targeting of retroviral vectors for gene therapy. Hum Gene Ther 1993; 4: 129–141.
17 Huxley C. Mammalian artificial chromosomes: a new tool for gene therapy. Gene Ther 1994; 1: 7–12.
18 Shesely EG, Kin H-S, Shehee WR, Papayannopoulou T, Smithies O, Popovich BW. Correction of a human β^S-globin gene by gene targeting. Proc Natl Acad Sci USA 1991; 88: 4294–4298.
19 Perrine SP, Ginder GD, Faller DV, et al. A short–term trial of butyrate to stimulate fetal-globin-gene expression in the β-globin disorders. N Engl J Med 1993; 328: 81–86.
20 Tinsley JM, Blake DJ, Roche A, et al. Primary structure of dystrophin-related protein. Nature 1992; 360: 591–592.
21 Anderson WF. Prospects for human gene therapy. Science 1984; 226: 401–409.
22 Karlsson S, Bodine DM, Perry L, Papayannopoulou T, Nienhuis AW. Expression of the human β-globin gene following retroviral-mediated transfer into multipotential hematopoietic progenitors of mice. Proc Natl Acad Sci USA 1988; 85: 6062–6066.
23 Lu L, Xiao M, Clapp DW, Li Z-H, Broxmeyer HE. High efficiency retroviral mediated gene transduction into single isolated immature and replatable $CD34^{3+}$ hematopoietic stem/progenitor cells from human umbilical cord blood. J Exp Med 1993; 178: 2089–2096.
24 Wilson JM, Jefferson DM, Chowdhury JR, Novikoff RP, Johnston DE, Mulligan RC. Retrovirus-mediated transduction of adult hepatocytes. Proc Natl Acad Sci USA 1988; 85: 3014–3018.
25 Grossman M, Raper SE, Kozarsky K, et al. Successful *ex vivo* gene therapy directed to liver in a patient with familial hypercholesterolemia. Nature Genet 1994; 6: 335–341.
26 Palmer TD, Thompson AR, Miller AD. Production of human factor IX in animals by genetically modified skin fibroblasts: potential therapy for hemophilia B. Blood 1989; 73: 438–445.
27 Hobbs JR. Correction of 34 genetic diseases by displacement bone marrow transplantation. Plasma Ther Transfus Tech 1985; 6: 221–246.
28 Gutierrez AA, Lemoine NR, Sikora K. Gene therapy for cancer. Lancet 1992; 339: 715–720.
29 Anderson WF. Gene therapy for cancer. Hum Gene Ther 1994; 5: 1–2.
30 Yu M, Poeschla E, Wong-Staal F. Progress towards gene therapy for HIV infection. Gene Ther 1994; 1: 13–26.
31 Blau HM, Dhawan J, Pavlath GK. Myoblasts in pattern formation and gene therapy. TIG 1993; 9: 269–274.
32 Weatherall DJ. The New Genetics and Clinical Practice, 3rd edn. Oxford: Oxford University Press, 1991.

British Medical Bulletin (1995) Vol. 51, No. 1, pp. 12–30

Retroviruses as vectors

R G Vile
Laboratory of Cancer Gene Therapy, Imperial Cancer Research Fund Rayne Institute, St Thomas' Hospital, London, UK

S J Russell
Cambridge Centre for Protein Engineering, MRC Centre, Cambridge, UK

Recombinant retroviruses have long been used to deliver heterologous genes to mammalian cells. Convenient packaging cell lines and vector plasmids have been distributed widely and 'home-made' retroviral vectors have now become a useful research tool in many laboratories.

Compared to more traditional methods of gene transfer, retroviral vectors are extraordinarily efficient gene delivery vehicles which cause no detectable harm as they enter their target cells. In the nucleus the retroviral necleic acid becomes integrated into chromosomal DNA, ensuring its long-term persistence and stable transmission to all future progeny of the transduced cell. Up to 8 kilobases of foreign gene sequence can be packaged in a retroviral vector and this is more than enough for most gene therapy applications.

Retroviral vectors can also be manufactured in large quantities to meet very stringent safety specifications. They have therefore been selected as the vectors of choice in 80% of the clinical gene therapy trials that have been approved to date. So far there have been no reported short- or long-term toxicity problems associated with their use in human gene therapy trials, now dating back to 1989.

However, despite this impressive record, there is still great scope (and need) for the development of new, improved retroviral vectors and packaging systems to fuel further advances in the field of human gene therapy. In the following discussion, existing retroviral vectors are reviewed and current areas of technological development are emphasised.

In recent years there has been a proliferation of human gene therapy trials, most of which have employed recombinant murine C-type retroviruses for gene transfer. These retroviral vectors have been generated using primitive packaging systems, yielding viral stocks of relatively low titre and purity. Their performance has therefore been disappointing in most of the clinical protocols attempted to date. However, improved technologies for the production of retroviral vectors promise to remedy this situation.

RETROVIRUS LIFE CYCLE

Structure

A mature retrovirus comprises an inner core (nucleoid) enclosed in a phospholipid envelope. The core consists of an icosahedral protein shell, the capsid, which is separated from the envelope by matrix protein and which houses two copies of the positive sense viral mRNA genome including 5′cap and 3′poly(A) structures. Also contained within the capsid are the virally-encoded protease, reverse transcriptase and integrase enzymes. The envelope is a roughly spherical phospholipid bilayer derived from the plasma membrane of the virus-producing cell and is covered with closely packed oligomeric membrane spike glycoproteins which appear as surface projections on electron microscopy.

The arrangement of the positive-sense mRNA retrovirus genome is shown diagrammatically in Fig. 1b. It is capped at its 5′end with an m7G5′ppp5′G_{m}p group and carries a string of about 200 A residues at its 3′end. Occasional A residues throughout the genome are 6-methylated and each genome copy is base-paired to the 3′-terminal 18 nucleotides of a tRNA molecule which primes reverse transcription. All the non-coding sequences that are required *in cis* for genome synthesis, processing, encapsidation, reverse transcription and integration are located in terminal regions, with internal regions dedicated entirely to protein coding functions.

Taxonomy

The family *Retroviridae* has been divided into three subfamilies, based primarily on pathogenicity; *Spumavirinae* (or foamy viruses) such as the Simian Syncytial Virus and Human Foamy Virus (HFV); *Lentivirinae*, such as the Human Immunodeficiency Virus Types 1 and 2 and Caprine Arthritis-Encephalitis Virus (CAEV); and *Oncovirinae* which are further subclassified into 5 groups, largely on the basis of their morphology, as seen under the electron microscope during viral maturation.[1,2] The group which has been used most extensively to derive retroviral vectors are the murine C-type oncoviruses.

A

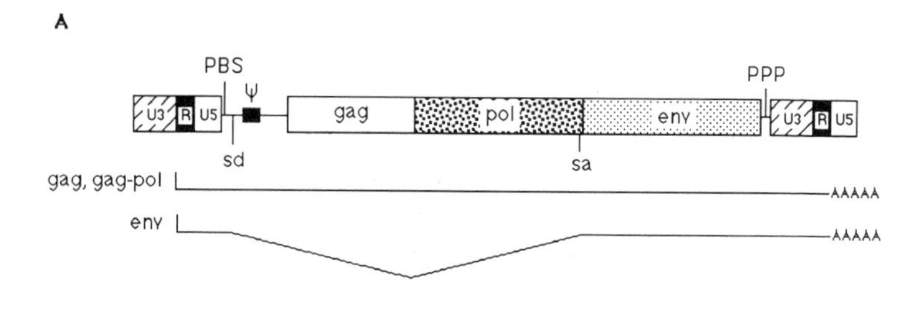

B

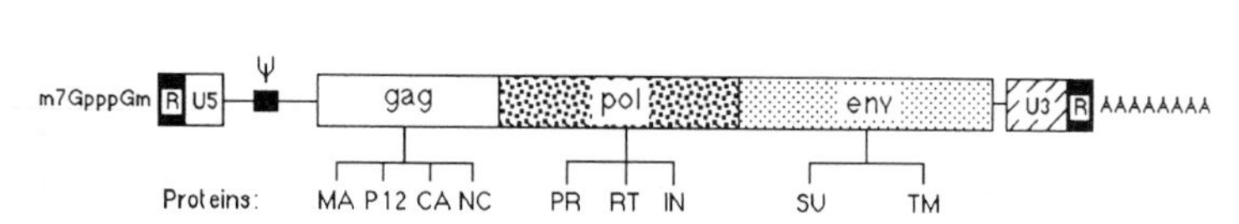

Fig. 1A Structure, transcription and splicing of Moloney MLV provirus. PBS = tRNA primer binding site; Psi = packaging signal sequence; PPP = polypurine tract or plus strand primer binding site; sd = splice donor; sa = splice acceptor. **B.** RNA genome of Moloney MLV. Also shown is the 2 letter code for the 9 virally encoded proteins.

Life cycle

The retroviral life cycle has been extensively reviewed elsewhere[2–4] and is summarised in Fig. 2. The viral envelope glycoprotein (env) attaches the virus to its cell surface receptor and catalyses a membrane fusion event which releases the viral core into the cytoplasm of the target cell. The RNA genome is converted to double-stranded (pro viral) DNA[5] as it is transported to the cell nucleus and integrates, after capsid disassembly, into a random chromosomal site. The capsids of C-type retroviruses, in contrast to those of lentiviruses, cannot traverse the intact nuclear membrane and cell mitosis is therefore required for successful progression of the viral life cycle. Retroviral integration is non-homologous with some degree of sequence specificity[6] and a preference for transcriptionally active host integration sites.[7]

After integration of the double stranded DNA provirus, regulatory promoter and enhancer elements in the U3 region of the proviral long terminal repeat (LTR) drive transcription of the viral genome (Fig. 1a). The full-length transcript encodes the gag and gag-pol polyproteins while a smaller, spliced transcript encodes the env proteins. A 10:1 ratio of gag to gag-pol is maintained by means of an amber suppressor codon at the end of gag.

Oligomerisation of the gag and gag-pol polyproteins to form budding viral core particles is central to the assembly and release of fully infectious viral progeny. Full-length (unspliced) viral mRNA binds through

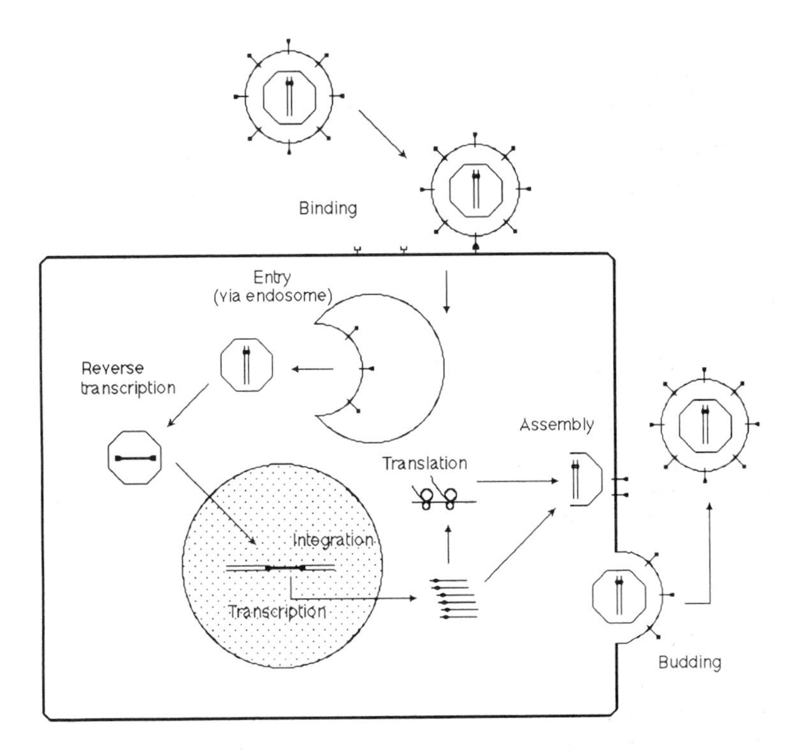

Fig. 2 The retroviral life cycle.

its packaging signal sequence (Psi) to the gag polyprotein during par ticle assembly and env glycoproteins, present at the plasma membrane, are incorporated into viral progeny as they bud from the cell surface. Newly budded virions are not infectious until the viral protease cleaves the gag and gag-pol polyproteins into their component parts.

MAKING RECOMBINANT RETROVIRUSES

Retroviruses have been engineered as vehicles for delivery, stable integration and expression of cloned genes in a wide variety of mammalian cells. Various retroviruses have been used as vectors,[8] but those based on Murine Leukaemia Viruses (MLVs) are the most advanced and have been most widely used to date. Most human gene therapy applications require replication defective retroviral vectors capable of delivering therapeutic genes to individual target cells without further replicative spread. Although replication-competent retroviral vectors have been successfully constructed, they have little relevance to human gene therapy at the present time and are therefore not discussed in this chapter.

Retroviral vector constructs

A retrovirus is essentially a small package containing nucleic acid. To ensure that it is incorporated into the package, the nucleic acid carries a packaging signal sequence which is recognised and bound by one of the package components. Additional sequences are required *in cis* for reverse transcription and integration of the viral nucleic acid (Table 1). Retroviral vectors are therefore constructed with these requirements in mind. The protein coding sequences of the retroviral genome (gag, pol and env) are discarded and replaced by heterologous coding sequences, but the essential cis-acting elements listed in the Table are retained.

Table The essential *cis*-acting sequences which must be retained within the retroviral vector genome.

1. The packaging signal sequence which ensures the encapsidation of the vector RNA into virions (Psi in murine vectors or E in avian systems). More recent vectors retain an extended Psi sequence, which incorporates the start of the gag gene (Psi+) but with the AUG start codon of the viral mutated.[62,63]

2. Elements which are necessary to direct the process of reverse transcription:
   (i) The primer binding site (PBS) which binds the tRNA primer of reverse transcription
   (ii) Terminal repeat (R) sequences that guide the 'jumping' of the reverse transcriptase between RNA strands during DNA synthesis.
   (iii) A purine-rich sequence 5′of the 3′LTR that serves as the priming site for synthesis of the second (plus) DNA strand.

3. Specific sequences near the ends of the LTRs that are necessary for the integration of the vector DNA into the host cell chromosome in the ordered and reproducible manner characteristic of retroviruses.[64]

A number of designs are possible for the genome of a retroviral vector although insertion of more than 8 kbp of foreign sequence is not possible. Above this size limit the vector-derived RNA transcript is too large to be packaged efficiently into retroviral particles. Adhering to this size constraint, it is possible to insert 1, 2 or even 3 genes into the vector genome in forward or reverse orientation, controlled by viral or non-viral promoter and enhancer sequences (Fig. 3). 2 gene constructs in which 1 of the genes encodes an antibiotic resistance marker offer the advantage that the gene-transduced target cells in a culture can be selected from a background of non-transduced cells.

Recently picornavirus sequences, known as Internal Ribosome Entry Sites (IRES), have been used within retroviral vectors to direct transla-

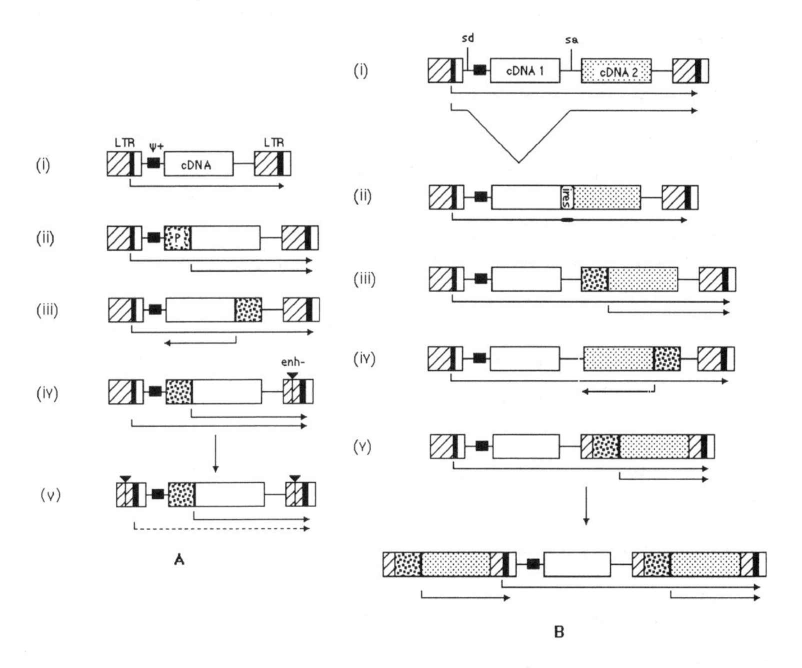

Fig. 3. Retroviral vector constructs. (A). *Single gene constructs*. Expression of the therapeutic gene is driven off the viral LTR (i) or an internal promoter which may be in forward (ii) or reverse (iii) orientation. Deletion of the 3′ LTR enhancer creates a self-inactivating vector (iv). The enhancer deletion is copied into the 5′ LTR during reverse transcription, giving rise to an enhancer deleted provirus in which the LTRs no longer influence the activity of the internal promoter (v). (B). *Two-gene constructs*. Expression of both genes may be driven off a single promoter using appropriately placed splicing signals (i) or internal ribosome entry sites (ii) to ensure that both genes are translated. Alternatively, two genes may be driven separately off the viral LTR and an internal promoter (iii). The internal promoter-driven expression cassette may be in reverse orientation (iv). Finally, a second therapeutic gene may be inserted into the 3′ LTR enhancer (double copy vector) and is duplicated into the 5′ LTR during reverse transcription to create a provirus with two copies of the gene (v) and (vi). sd = splice donor; sa = splice acceptor; ires = internal ribosome entry site.

tion of LTR-driven polycistronic RNA transcripts.[9–11] IRES can direct cap-independent initiation of translation at internal start codons on polycistronic mRNAs. Therefore, inclusion of poliovirus or encephalomyocarditids IRES sequences within the retroviral transcription unit now makes it possible to express several genes from the same promoter,[12] although retroviral vectors are still restricted to a total of 8kbp inserted DNA. This approach is particularly attractive for expression of multiple, small therapeutic genes, such as the cytokines, in which combination therapies may be more effective than single expression constructs. For a comprehensive discussion of the varied range of vector types the reader is referred to Reference 8.

Retroviral packaging cell lines

The purpose of the retroviral packaging cell line is to provide the viral 'helper' functions which have been deleted from the vector genome, namely the gag, pol and env proteins. These helper functions are stably expressed in the packaging cells from one or more helper plasmids whose RNA transcripts are not efficiently packaged into viral part icles because they lack the packaging signal sequence. When a vector genome is transfected into such packaging cells, the viral gag proteins recognise and package the vector RNA genome into viral particles which are released into the culture supernatant (Fig. 4). Packaging cell lines have been constructed using both avian and murine retroviral structural proteins and are reviewed in Reference 13.

PERFORMANCE REQUIREMENTS OF RETROVIRAL VECTORS FOR GENE THERAPY

Choosing between the various viral and non-viral gene transfer technologies can be difficult when designing a gene therapy protocol.[14] Safety is a prime consideration. Other key factors are the efficiency and accuracy of gene delivery, and the tissue-specific regulation and long-term stability of gene expression. Because of their efficient integration, retroviral vectors are most suitable for gene therapy protocols in which proliferating (stem) cells are modified ex vivo and the genetic modification is transmitted to their in vivo progeny after reimplantation.

Safety

The principal safety concerns relating to the use of retroviral vectors are the dangers of replication competent retroviruses (RCR) and the risk of vector-induced target cell transformation.

Replication competent retrovirus

It is essential that retroviral vector stocks are not contaminated with replication competent retrovirus (RCR). Between them, the helper and vector sequences introduced into a packaging cell carry all the viral genes and regulatory sequences required to reconstitute a wild type viral genome. The greater the sequence homology between helper and vector genomes, the higher is the chance that they will align and undergo homologous recombination and the risk is further increased if multiple copies of the helper and vector genomes coexist in a single packaging cell. Also, the two strands of RNA packaged into a single virus particle

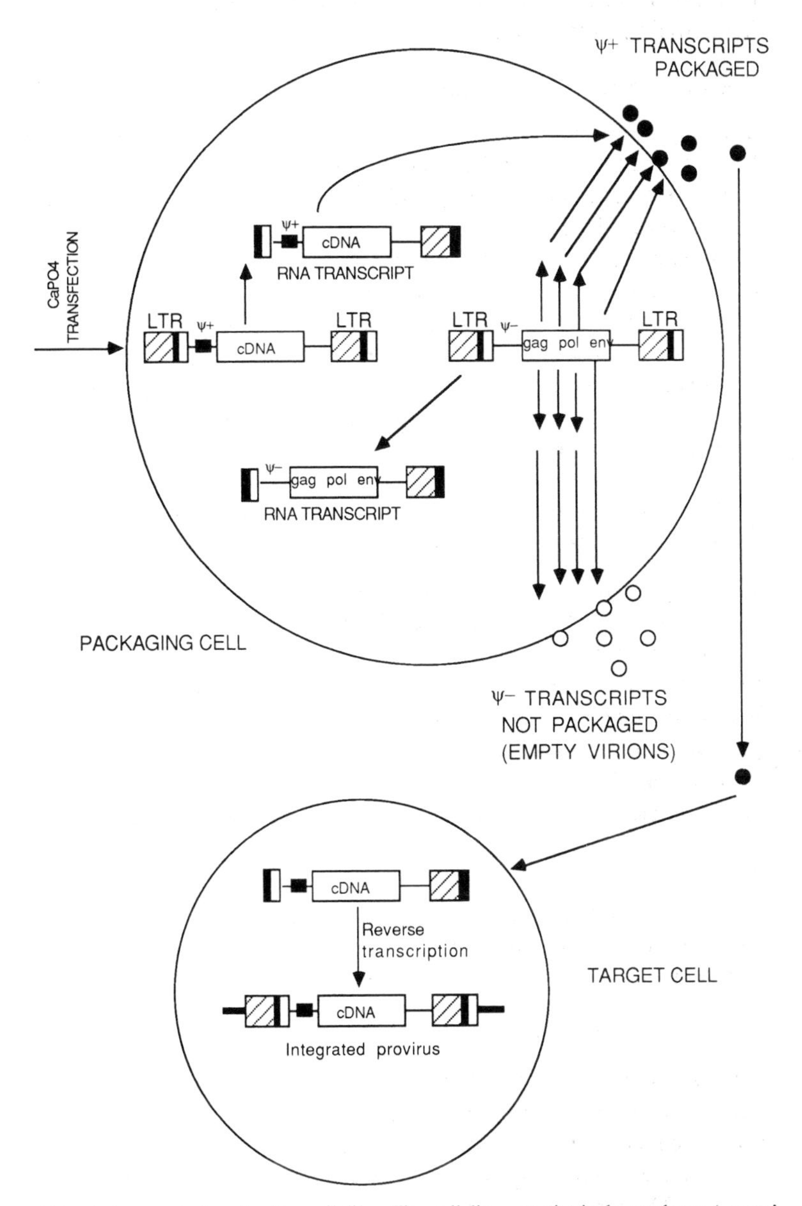

Fig. 4 A retroviral packaging cell line. The cell line constitutively produces 'empty' retroviral particles lacking an RNA genome. RNA molecules carrying the packaging signal sequence (derived from the vector contruct) are efficiently packaged.

may be derived separately from helper and vector genomes and may recombine during reverse transcription in an infected target cell.

RCR was frequently encountered with early packaging cells of the type shown in Figure 4 in which the retroviral helper functions were supplied by a retroviral genome (pMOV-Psi-) deleted only in the Psi region.[15] The Psi- RNA transcripts were shown to be co-packaged with Psi+ vector transcripts at low frequency (0.1%) into budding retroviruses and RCR most frequently arose by recombination of the co-packaged transcripts during reverse transcription. The best way to reduce the risk of RCR is to provide the helper functions on more extensively deleted helper plasmids having minimal sequence homology with the vector genome or, better still, to split them onto multiple helper plasmids. Second and third generation packaging cell lines have been developed according to these principles and are considerably safer due to the increased number of helper-vector recombination events required to generate a wild type viral genome. PA317[16], a second generation packaging cell line which has been used to produce retroviral vectors for human clinical trials (e.g. Ref 17), was generated using the plasmid pPAM3 which lacks not only the packaging sequence but also the 3′LTR and polypurine tract which have been replaced by an SV40 polyadenylation signal sequence. Two recombinations between helper and vector sequences are therefore necessary to regenerate RCR and this double recombination has proven to be a very low frequency event. Third generation packaging cells have further reduced the risk of RCR by separating the gag, pol transcription unit from the env transcription unit on different plasmids and by using packaging constructs which have minimal areas of homology with the vector genome.[13] This arrangement excludes the possibility that two co-packaged constructs can recombine to generate RCR since the entire viral genome is now split three ways onto the vector construct and the two helper constructs. However, even third generation packaging cell lines may package and transfer endogenous murine viral genomes[18] and the only solution to this problem may be to generate packaging cells based on primate, rather than murine cell lines.

Although RCR is unlikely to arise using third generation packaging cells, it is essential that every stock of retroviral vectors intended for human use should be subjected to rigorous testing to to exclude this possibility. The importance of this practice is illustrated by a recent study in which RCR-contaminated vector stocks were used to infect primate bone marrow cells which were then transplanted into monkeys. Three out of ten monkeys that received marrow treated in this way became viraemic and developed aggressive T cell lymphomas.[19] However, the titre of RCR used in these experiments was orders of magnitude higher than the detection limit of in vitro assays for RCR[20] and in another study, monkeys exposed to high levels of replicating MLV (in excess of 10^9 ffu) showed no signs of malignancy even after seven years of follow up.[21]

The murine retroviral vectors which are currently used in clinical trials are rapidly inactivated by human complement.[22] Although this is a drawback for in vivo gene delivery (see below), it can be considered a safety advantage in that it should prevent the spread of RCR inadvertantly introduced into a patient.

Target cell transformation

Retroviral vectors are theoretically capable of causing neoplastic transformation of some of the patient's cells by insertional mutagenesis.[23] However, using non-replicating retroviral vectors, cell transformation has not been observed in numerous animal experiments and human gene therapy trials and theoretical models suggest that the overall risk is very low.[24]

An additional risk of cell transformation may arise as a consequence of the high error rate of the retroviral reverse transcriptase.[25] For example, recombinant retroviruses may be used to deliver correct copies of tumour suppressor genes, such as *p53*, to tumour cells in order to reverse the malignant phenotype. However, a fraction of the cells may receive a provirus encoding a mutated *p53* gene, as a result of errant reverse transcription. If the mutation converts the normal *p53* into a transforming mutant of *p53*, the infected cells may become transformed themselves. In the absence of engineered reverse transcriptase enzymes which have a higher intrinsic fidelity, the risk of such events cannot currently be controlled, but should be considered in the use of gene therapy strategies where the introduction of mutated 'therapeutic' gene may be damaging.

Efficiency of gene delivery

For maximum efficiency of gene delivery, a retroviral vector should be available at high titre and and should have unimpeded access to its target cell population. It should bind and enter efficiently into the target cells and the target cells should be permissive to subsequent steps in the retroviral life cycle leading to proviral integration and gene expression.

Retroviral titre

Under optimal conditions, the most widely used retroviral producer cells can generate 10^6–10^7 infectious vector particles/ml of tissue culture supernatant[26] but most human trials to date have employed retroviral producers giving titres below 10^6 per ml. However, with optimisation of the technologies for retroviral vector production, storage and concentration, it is now possible to think in terms of titres as high 10^{10} per ml, free of RCR.

Retrovirus titre is limited by the rate at which infectious particles are released from the producer cells and the rate at which they lose their infectivity. To create a packaging system yielding retroviral stocks with very high titres, it is necessary to optimise the helper constructs and the vector constructs, and to optimise the independent processes contributing to the assembly and release of fully infectious virus progeny.

The concentration-driven process of gag and gag-pol polyprotein oligomerisation drives the production of new viral core particles whose release into the culture supernatant does not require the presence of viral RNA or viral envelope proteins. To maximise particle release from the packaging cells, a strong promoter should be used to drive expression of the gag-pol helper construct and a large number of transfected clones should be screened for release of reverse transcriptase into the culture supernatant. An alternative strategy is to use a plasmid incorporating sequences which lead to its episomal amplification in the packaging line so that higher levels of gag-pol proteins can be produced.[27,28]

Env glycoproteins are transported to the plasma membrane and incorporated into the envelopes of budding retroviruses. Retroviruses devoid of env glycoproteins are non-infectious so the env helper plasmid should be designed to drive high-level env expression (using strong promoters and/or episomal replication origins) and should be introduced into packaging cells previously selected for maximal expression of the gag-pol helper plasmid.

The design of the vector plasmid also has a major influence on virus titre. Depending on its abundance in the packaging cell and the length of its packaging signal sequence, the vector mRNA is incorporated into a variable proportion of the viral core particles. For maximal titres of recombinant retroviruses which are competent for gene transfer, the vector construct should therefore be designed to give abundant full-length packagable RNA transcripts. In this respect, simple single-gene vector constructs with an extended packaging signal sequence give higher titres than more complex reverse-orientation or two-gene constructs.[26]

One alternative approach that has been used successfully to increase the abundance of packagable transcripts is to use a mixed culture of producer cells releasing viruses with different tropisms. Vectors released from producer cell type A can infect producer cells of type B and vice versa (ping-pong), so that the average proviral copy number per producer cell is progressively increased.[29] This is a very effective way to increase the titre of a vector but invariably results after a variable time lag, in the emergence of RCR.

Retroviral stability

Loss of retroviral infectivity is significant during continued incubation at 37°C ($t_{1/2}$ ~ 8h), after each freeze-thaw cycle (~50%) and after virus concentration by centrifugation. This instability has been attributed to dissociation of $gp70^{SU}$ envelope protein from the particle surface. Particle stability is enhanced at 32°C compared to 37°C due to decreased SU dissociation and the titres of retroviral vector stocks can be boosted 10-fold by harvesting from producer cells cultured at 32°C.[30]

Moreover, retroviral pseudotype vectors incorporating the Vesicular Stomatitis Virus (VSV) G protein (which is not readily shed from the particle surface) in place of their natural envelope protein were sufficiently stable to allow efficient concentration to very high titre by high-speed ultracentrifugation.[31]

As mentioned previously, murine retroviral vectors are rapidly inactivated by human complement[22] and are therefore unsuitable for efficient gene delivery to human tissues in vivo. Complement-sensitive murine retroviral vectors have nevertheless been used to transfer the Herpes Simplex thymidine kinase gene to intracerebral tumour deposits in human subjects[32] with further clinical protocols planned.[33,34] So far, however, there is no direct evidence from these studies of successful in vivo gene transfer to human tissues using complement-sensitive retroviral vectors.

The sensitivity of murine retroviral vectors to human complement may be attributable to the virally-encoded env protein or to the lipid composition of the viral envelope. It might therefore be possible to engineer murine retroviral vectors resistant to human complement by modification of the envelope protein or by the use of packaging cells which provide the viruses with a more hardy lipid envelope.

An alternative solution might be to develop retroviral vectors based on different viruses. For instance, human foamy viruses (a member of the *Spumaviridae* class of retroviruses) are not clearly associated with any disease and do not appear to be so sensitive to inactivation by human complement.[35] Lentiviral vectors have also been developed based on Human Immunodeficiency Virus (HIV)[36] and have been proposed for in vivo gene transfer to CD4-positive cells to reduce their ability to support the replication and spread of wild type HIV.[36–38]

Status of target cells

Retroviral titres are usually measured under optimal in vitro conditions on highly susceptible mouse NIH 3T3 cells, and the titres of amphotropic vectors are usually lower when tested on human target cells. This might be due in part to a lower density of virus receptors on the human target cells, and one solution could be to use vectors with different envelope proteins which bind to different receptors, such as the VSV(G) retroviral pseudotype vectors mentioned above.[31]

Target cell quiescence can also limit the efficiency of gene transfer with C-type retroviral vectors since they do not enter the nucleus and integrate unless the target cell enters mitosis. Haemopoietic stem cells, for example, cannot readily be amplified ex vivo and are therefore difficult to transduce with murine retroviral vectors. Advances in the area of stem cell biology may eventually permit the efficient purification of haemopoietic stem cells and their reliable ex vivo amplification (using cocktails of growth factors) without lineage commitment and differentiation. This would allow for their more efficient transduction using murine C-type retroviral vectors.

Alternatively, lentiviral vectors, based for example on HIV or caprine arthritis-encephalitis virus (CAEV) may be of value for the efficient transduction of quiescent cells. In contrast to murine C-type retroviruses,[39] HIV can productively infect non-dividing cells.[40] This property may be due, at least in part, to a nuclear transport signal on the HIV capsid which allows transport of the reverse transcribed provirus across the intact nuclear membrane even in the absence of mitosis.[41]

Accuracy of gene delivery

In the interests of safety and efficiency, it is desirable that retroviral gene delivery should be accurate[42]: the therapeutic genes should be delivered exclusively to the target cells and should integrate into a selected chromosomal location. Mouse amphotropic retroviral vectors bind promiscuously to all human cells and integrate into random chromosomal sites. Their only intrinsic targeting property is their failure to integrate in non-dividing cells which has been exploited to target proliferating tumour cells in the brain where the surrounding neuronal tissue is quiescent.[32]

Accurate gene delivery can be achieved in vitro by placing amphotropic retroviral vectors in contact with purified human target cells. For targeted in vivo gene delivery, the vectors or vector-producing cells can be administered by a route which favours their selective interaction with the target cells. Thus, retroviral vectors have been inoculated directly into tumour deposits, they have been instilled into the bladder, the airways, the joints, the peritoneal and pleural cavities, the cerebral ventricles and the subarachnoid space, and they have been infused into the blood vessels supplying selected target organs. Although regional delivery is more accurate than systemic delivery, the efficiency of gene transfer remains low because of retroviruses binding and entering non-target cells in close proximity to the target cells. This wastage of perfectly good retroviral vector particles might be prevented if they were incapable of promiscuous binding to bystander cells.

Targeted retrovirus attachment

The tropism of a retoviral vector can be altered by the incorporation of foreign or hybrid envelope proteins.[43,44] However, there are only two naturally occurring retroviruses (HIV and HTLV-1) whose tropisms are known to be restricted to a subset of human cells by virtue of the binding specificity of the envelope protein. There has therefore been considerable interest in the possibility of constructing targeted retroviral vectors displaying envelope proteins with artificially engineered binding specificities.[45]

When monoclonal antibodies were used to crosslink mouse ecotropic retroviral particles to human cells, gene transfer was observed but the efficiency was low and not all cell surface antigens could act as surrogate receptors.[46] In another study, mouse ecotropic retroviral particles which had been chemically modified with lactose were shown to bind specifically to the asialoglycoprotein receptor on human HepG2 cells.[47] Binding was followed by retroviral infection of the human cells as indicated by transfer of a functional β-galactosidase gene. Subsequently, it was shown that functional antibody fragments expressed as a viral envelope-single chain antibody chimaeric protein could be incorporated into retroviral particles to confer a predictably altered binding specificity.[48] Further studies on ecotropic retroviruses displaying nonviral polypeptides have shown that, although they can bind efficiently to human target cells through the nonviral polypeptide moiety, this does not necessarily lead to efficient gene delivery. However, taken together these studies point to the likely development of retroviral vectors displaying engineered coat proteins which transfer genes in a target cell-selective manner.

Targeted retroviral integration

Apart from a small risk of cell transformation by insertional mutagenesis, variability of gene expression is the major problem arising from lack of site-specific retrovirus integration. In principle, the process of retroviral integration might be manipulated by appropriate modifications the sequences at the termini of the proviral LTRs or to the structure of the viral integrase protein. However, despite improved understanding of the mechanism of retroviral integration[49] and advances in the design of plasmid vectors for targeted gene insertion and replacement by homologous recombination, targeted retroviral integration remains an elusive goal.

Regulation of retroviral gene expression

Tissue specificity of gene expression

Tissue-specific or tumour-selective regulation of gene expression is likely to be a requirement for many future human gene therapy protocols. Firstly, when gene delivery is inaccurate, it avoids potentially damaging expression of the therapeutic protein in non-target tissues. This is particularly important when contemplating the use of gene therapy strategies to bring about the destruction of tumour cells. Tissue-specific gene expression may also be required for haemopoietic stem cell correction where the goal is to express the therapeutic gene exclusively in differentiated (e.g. erythroid, T-cell or macrophage) stem cell progeny.

Many retroviral vectors have been described in which tissue specific transcriptional promoters and enhancers were used to drive expression of foreign genes.[50–54] In many cases correct control of expression was maintained from the tissue specific promoter, although there have also been reports of interference between different regulatory elements within such vectors leading to partial loss of cell type-specific expression, depending on the precise design of the vector.[50]

A number of tissue-specific locus control sequences (LCRs) have been isolated and shown to modulate the level of gene expression such that it becomes independent of integration site effects.[55–57] Attempts to insert functional LCR elements into retroviral vectors have so far met with limited success, but further progress in this area is to be expected.

Stability of gene expression

Cells infected with retroviral vectors and maintained in vitro usually show constant levels of gene expression for long periods of time. However, when the cells are returned in vivo they often lose expression of the foreign gene over a period of a few weeks. This in vivo instability of gene expression may be due to methylation[58,59] or deletion[60] of the proviral DNA and hinders the development of stem cell correction protocols seeking to cure inherited metabolic disorders. One approach to the problem has been to develop vectors in which the therapeutic genes are expressed from constitutive or tissue-specific cellular promoters rather than viral promoters. There have been some encouraging results using celluar promoters to drive expression of marker genes in retroviral vectors, but others have encountered problems due to interference effects between promoters[45,50] as well as a blanket methylation shutdown of all vector-associated promoters.[58] Interference effects can be decreased by the construction of self-inactivating vectors which lack viral enhancer and promoter elements, leaving just a cellular promoter which is known to be highly active in the target tissue.[61]

PROSPECTS

Current retroviral vectors are relatively rudimentary gene delivery ve hicles which will require considerable further development and tailoring to individual applications if their full clinical potential is to be realised. To take a single illustrative example, a retroviral vector designed for the genetic correction of β-thalassaemia by direct in vivo gene transfer to haemopoietic stem cells would require the following special features:

1. The provirus should carry a functional β-globin gene.
2. It should be easy to produce at very high titre and easy to purify from producer cell culture supernatant.
3. It should be resistant to complement and other potentially virolytic factors in the blood and interstitial fluid.
4. To minimise the sequestration of the vector in non-target tissues, it should not be capable of binding to non-target cells.
5. It should bind selectively to a cell surface receptor present on HSCs but absent from non-target cells.
6. It should fuse selectively with HSCs after binding to the HSC receptor, delivering the retroviral core particle plus encapsidated nucleic acid into the cytoplasm.
7. Since most HSCs remain quiescent for long periods of time, the vector should stimulate the target cell to divide at, or shortly after the time at which the nucleic acid is delivered.
8. The provirus should integrate efficiently into a predetermined site in a host cell chromosome where it does not influence the structure or expression of the genes of the host cell by cis-acting mechanisms.
9. The transcriptional regulatory elements contained within the provirus should include erythroid-specific promoter, enhancer and locus control sequences capable of driving long-term stable expression of the β-globin gene exclusively in erythroid progeny of the HSC. The level of gene expression should be dependent on the proviral copy number and independent of the site of provirus integration.

In summary, retroviral vectors have come a long way since the first packaging system was described in 1983, but they still have a long way to go.

REFERENCES

1 Weiss RA, Teich N, Varmus HE, Coffin J. Molecular biology of RNA tumor viruses. Vol. 1,2. Cold Spring Harbor Laboratory, Cold Spring Harbor, NY. 1982, 1985.
2 Coffin JM. Retroviridae and their replication. In: Fields BN, Knipe DM et al. eds. Virology. New York; Raven Press 1990: pp1437-1500.

3 Varmus HE. Retroviruses. Science 1988; 240: 1427-1435.
4 Vile RG. The retroviral life cycle and the molecular construction of retrovirus vectors. In: Collins MKL, ed. Practical molecular virology: Viral vectors for gene expression. New Jersey Humana 1991: pp 1-16.
5 Panganiban AT, Fiore D. Ordered interstrand and intrastrand DNA transfer during reverse transcription. Science 1988; 241: 1064-1069.
6 Shih C, Stoye JP, Coffin JM. Highly preferred targets for retrovirus integration. Cell 1988; 53: 531-537.
7 Mooslehner K, Karls U, Harbers K. Retroviral integration sites in transgenic mov mice frequently map in the vicinity of transcribed DNA regions. J Virol 1990; 64: 3056-3058.
8 Miller AD. Retroviral vectors. Curr Top Microbiol Immunol 1992; 158: 1-24.
9 Morgan RA, Couture L, Elroy-Stein O, Ragheb J, Moss B, French Anderson W. Retroviral vectors containing putative internal ribosome entry sites: development of a polycistronic gene transfer system and applications to human gene therapy. Nucleic Acids Res 1992; 20: 1293-1299.
10 Adam MA, Ramesh N, Dusty Miller A, Osborne WRA. Internal initiation of translation in retroviral vectors carrying picornavirus 5′non-translated regions. J Virol 1991; 65: 4985-4990.
11 Koo H, Brown AMC, Kaufman RJ, Prorock CM, Ron Y, Dougherty JP. A spleen necrosis virus-based retroviral vector which expresses two genes from a dicistronic mRNA. Virology 1992; 186: 669-675.
12 Boris-Lawrie KA, Temin HM. Recent advances in retrovirus vector technology. Curr Opin Genet Dev 1993; 3: 102-109.
13 Miller AD. Retrovirus packaging cells. Hum Gene Ther 1990; 1: 5-14.
14 Mulligan RC. The basic science of gene therapy. Science 1993; 260: 926-931.
15 Mann RM, RC, Baltimore D. Construction of a retrovirus packaging mutant and its use to produce helper free defective retrovirus. Cell 1983; 33: 149-153.
16 Miller AD, Buttimore C. Redesign of retrovirus packaging cell line to avoid recombination leading to helper virus formation. Mol Cell Biol 1986; 6: 2895-2902.
17 Rosenberg SA, Aebersold P, Cornetta K, et al. Gene transfer into humans-immunotherapy of patients with advanced melanoma using tumor-infiltrating lymphocytes modified by retroviral gene transduction. N Engl J Med 1990; 323: 570-578.
18 Scadden DT, Fuller B, Cunningham JM. Human cells infected with retrovirus vectors acquire an endogenous murine provirus. J Virol 1990; 64: 424-427.
19 Donahue RE, Kessler SW, Bodine D et al. Helper virus induced T cell lymphoma in non human primates after retroviral mediated gene transfer. J Exp Med 1992; 176: 1125-1135.
20 Anderson WF. What about those monkeys that got T-cell lymphoma? Hum Gene Ther 1993; 4: 1-2.
21 Cornetta K, Morgan RA, Gillio A, et al. No retroviremia or pathology in long-term follow up of monkeys exposed to a murine amphotropic retrovirus. Hum Gene Ther 1991; 2: 215-219.
22 Welsh RM, Cooper NR, Jensen FC, Oldstone MBA. Human serum lyses RNA tumour viruses. Nature 1975; 257: 612-614.
23 Cornetta K. Safety aspects of gene therapy. Br J Haematol 1992; 80: 421-426.
24 Moolten FL, Cupples LA. A model for predicting the risk of cancer consequent to retroviral gene therapy. Hum Gene Ther 1992; 3: 479-486.
25 Varela-Echavarria A, Prorock CM, Ron Y, Dougherty JP. High rate of genetic rearrangement during replication of a Moloney Murine Leukemia virus-based vector. J Virol 1993; 67: 6357-6364.
26 Russell SJ. Making high titre retroviral producer cells. Methods Mol Biol 1991; 8: 29-60.
27 Takahara Y, Hamada K, Housman DE. A new retrovirus packaging cell for gene transfer constructed from amplified long terminal repeat-free chimeric proviral genes. J Virol 1992; 66: 3725-3732.

28 Landau NR, Littman DR. Packaging system for rapid production of murine leukemia virus vectors with variable tropism. J Virol 1992; 66: 5110-5113.
29 Bestwick RK, Kozak SL, Kabat D. Overcoming interference to retroviral super infection results in amplified expression and transmission of cloned genes. Proc Nat Acad Sci USA 1988; 85: 5404-5408.
30 Kotani H, Newton III PB, Zhang S et al. Improved methods of retroviral vector transduction and production for gene therapy. Hum Gene Ther 1994; 5: 19-28.
31 Burns JC, Friedmann T, Driever W, Burrascano M, Yee JK. Vesicular stomatitis virus G glycoprotein pseudotyped retroviral vectors: concentration to very high titer and efficient gene transfer into mammalian and nonmammalian cells. Proc Nat Acad Sci USA 1993; 90: 8033-8037.
32 Oldfield EH, Ram Z, Culver KW, Blaese RM, DeVroom HL, Anderson WF. Clinical Protocol: Gene therapy for the treatment of brain tumors using intra-tumoral transduction with the thymidine kinase gene and intravenous ganciclovir. Hum Gene Ther 1993; 4: 39-69.
33 Georges RN, Mukhopadhyay T, Zhang Y, Yen N, Roth JA. Prevention of orthotopic human lung cancer growth by intratracheal instillation of a retroviral antisense K-ras construct. Cancer Res 1993; 53: 1743-1746.
34 Fujiwara T, Grimm EA, Mukhopadhyay T, Cai DE, Owen-Schaub LB, Roth JA. A retroviral wild-type *p53* expression vector penetrates human lung cancer spheroids and inhibits growth by inducing apoptosis. Cancer Res 1993; 53: 4129-4133.
35 Flugel RM. Spumaviruses: A group of complex retroviruses. J Acquired Immune Defic Syndr 1991; 4: 739-750.
36 Buchschacher GL, Panganiban AT. Human immunodeficiency virus vectors for inducible expression of foreign genes. J Virol 1992; 66: 2731-2739.
37 Gilboa E, Smith C. Gene therapy for infectious diseases: the AIDS model. Trends Genet 1994; 10: 109-114.
38 Brady HJM, Miles CG, Pennington DJ, Dzierzak EA. Specific ablation of human immunodeficiency virus Tat-expressing cells by conditionally toxic retroviruses. Proc Nat Acad Sci USA 1994; 91: 365-369.
39 Miller DG, Adam MA, Miller AD. Gene transfer by retrovirus vectors occurs only in cells that are actively replicating at the time of infection. Mol Cell Biol 1990; 10: 4239-4242.
40 Lewis PF, Emerman M. Passage through mitosis is required for oncoretroviruses but not for the human immunodeficiency virus. J Virol 1993; 68: 510-516.
41 Bukrinsky MI, Haggerty S, Dempsey MP, et al. A nuclear localisation signal within HIV-1 matrix protein that governs infection of non-dividing cells. Nature 1993; 365: 666-669.
42 Vile RG, Russell SJ. Gene transfer technologies for the gene therapy of cancer. Gene Ther 1994; 1: 88-98.
43 Battini JL, Heard JM, Danos O. Receptor choice determinants in the envelope glycoproteins of amphotropic, xenotropic and polytropic murine leukemia viruses. J Virol 1992; 66: 1468-1475.
44 Cosset FL, Ronfort C, Molina RM, et al. Packaging cells for avian leukosis virus-based vectors with various host ranges. J Virol 1992; 66: 5671-5676.
45 Salmons B, Gunzburg WH. Targeting of retroviral vectors for gene therapy. Hum Gene Ther 1993; 4: 129-141.
46 Roux P, Jeanteur P, Piechaczyk M. A versatile and potentially general approach to the targeting of specific cell types by retroviruses: Application to the infection of human cells by means of major histocompatibility complex class I and class II antigens by mouse ecotropic murine leukemia virus. Proc Natl Acad Sci USA 1989; 86: 9079-9083.
47 Neda H, Wu CH, Wu GY. Chemical modification of an ecotropic murine leukaemia virus results in redirection of its target cell specificity. J Biol Chem 1991; 266: 14143-14146.
48 Russell SJ, Hawkins RE, Winter G. Retroviral vectors displaying functional antibody fragments. Nucleic Acids Res 1993; 21: 1081-1085.

49 Whitcomb JM, Hughes SH. Retroviral reverse transcription and integration: progress and problems Annu Rev Cell Biol 1992; 8: 275-306.
50 Vile RG, Miller N, Hart IR. A comparison of the properties of different retroviral vectors containing the murine tyrosinase promoter to achieve transcriptionally targeted expression of the HSVtk or IL-2 genes. Gene Ther 1994; (In Press).
51 Huber BE, Richards CA, Krenitsky TA. Retroviral-mediated gene therapy for the treatment of hepatocellular carcinoma: An innovative approach for cancer therapy. Proc Nat Acad Sci USA 1991; 88: 8039-8043.
52 Dillon N. Regulating gene expression in gene therapy. Trends Biotechnol 1993; 11: 167-173.
53 Hatzoglou M, Lamers W, Bosch F, Wynshaw-Boris A, Clapp DW, Hanson RW. Hepatic gene transfer in animals using retroviruses containing the promoter from the gene for phosphoenolpyruvate carboxykinase. J Biol Chem 1990; 265: 17285-17293.
54 Harris JD, Guttierez AA, Hurst HC, Sikora K, Lemoine NR. Gene therapy for cancer using tumour-specific prodrug activation. Gene Ther 1994; 1: 170-175.
55 Grosveld F, van Assendelft GB, Greaves DR, Kollias G. Position-independent, high-level expression of the human β-globin gene in transgenic mice. Cell 1987; 51: 975-985.
56 Greaves DR, Wilson FD, Lang G, Kioussos D. Human CD2 3′-flanking sequences confer high-level, T cell-specific, position-independent gene expression in transgenic mice. Cell 1989; 56: 979-986.
57 Bonifer C, Vidal M, Grosveld F, Sippel AE. Tissue specific and position independent expression of the complete gene domain for chicken lysozyme in transgenic mice. EMBO J 1990; 9: 2843-2848.
58 Richards CA, Huber BE. Generation of a transgenic model for retrovirus-mediated gene therapy for hepatocellular carcinoma is thwarted by the lack of transgene expression. Hum Gene Ther 1993; 4: 143-150.
59 Palmer TD, Rosman GJ, Osborne WRA, Miller AD. Genetically modified skin fibroblasts persist long after transplantation but gradually inactivate introduced genes. Proc Nat Acad Sci USA 1991; 88: 1330-1334.
60 Russell SJ, Eccles SA, Flemming CL, Johnson CA, Collins MKL. Decreased tumorigenicity of a transplantable rat sarcoma following transfer and expression of an IL-2 cDNA. Int J Cancer 1991; 47: 244-251.
61 Yee JK, Moores JC, Jolly DJ, Wolff JA, Respress JG, Friedmann T. Gene expression from transcriptionally disabled retroviral vectors. Proc Nat Academy Sci USA 1987; 84: 5197-5201.
62 Bender MA, Palmer TD, Gelinas RE, Miller AD. Evidence that the packaging sequence of Moloney murine leukemia virus extends into the gag region. J Virol 1987; 61: 1639-1646.
63 Morgenstern JP, Land H. Advanced mammalian gene transfer: high titre retroviral vectors with multiple drug selection markers and a complementary helper-free packaging cell line. Nucleic Acids Res 1990; 18: 3587-3596.
64 Panganiban AT, Varmus HM. The terminal nucleotides of retrovirus DNA are required for integration but not virus production. Nature 1983; 306: 155-160.

British Medical Bulletin (1995) Vol.51, No.1, pp.31-44

Adenovirus and adeno-associated virus mediated gene transfer

E J Kremer and M Perricaudet

Laboratoire de Génétique de Virus Oncogènes, Institut Gustave Roussy, Villejuif, France

In this review we describe current strategies for adenoviral mediated gene transfer (AMGT) and adeno-associated viral mediated gene transfer (AAVMGT). We consider the structure and molecular biology of adenoviruses and adeno-associated viruses and detail the current advantages and disadvantages of AMGT and AAVMGT. Potential solutions to some of the specific drawbacks to AMGT, including the development of new vectors, addition of gp19k, organoides, and the use of non-human adenoviral vectors, are discussed.

As you may have read many times before, the burgeoning field of gene therapy is still very much in its infancy. Enormous progress has been made, but a sound scientific base for understanding and harnessing all the nuances in each DNA-based delivery system is still lacking.

This review will present current strategies for adenoviral mediated gene transfer (AMGT) and adeno-associated viral mediated gene transfer (AAVMGT) and address the possible future direction of AMGT vectorology. It will address the basic scientific issues limiting AMGT and AAVMGT methods and will complement the detailed uses described later in this issue.

Before addressing the present situation and future work in this field, it is necessary to review briefly the basic features and molecular biology of adenoviruses and adeno-associated viruses.

ADENOVIRIDAE AND *PARVOVIRIDAE*

Adenoviruses (Ads) belong to the family *Adenoviridae* and the human Ads belong to the genera *Mastadenovirus*. Human Ad infections are found worldwide. Ads were initially characterised in 1953 by Rowe et al.[1] when trying to cultivate epithelial cells from the adenoids. The

47 different serotypes are grouped (A–F) according to their ability to cause tumours in newborn hamsters.[2,3] Respiratory epithelial cells are the primary target for Ads in vivo. 5% of the acute respiratory diseases in children under the age of 5 are due to Ads. Other sites of infection include the eye, the gastro-intestinal tract and the urinary tract. Many Ad infections are subclinical and only result in antibody formation.[4]

Adeno-associated viruses (AAVs), characterised in 1966,[5] belong to the family *Parvoviridae* and genera *Dependovirus*. AAVs are widely prevalent and infect >90% of human adults. AAVs are unique among animal viruses in that they normally require coinfection with an unrelated helper virus for productive infection in cell culture. There are 5 human serotypes (AAV1–5). Their natural tropism is presumably the respiratory and gastro-intestinal tract, but all human cells tested in vitro have been successfully transduced. AAVs have not been associated with any clinical symptoms in any host and are not known to be tumourgenic.[6]

VIRUS STRUCTURE

Adenovirus

Three loosely defined sets of protein exist in the mature Ad: proteins that form the outer coat of the capsid, scaffolding proteins that hold the capsid together and DNA-binding proteins. The diameter of the icosahedral-shaped capsid various from 65 to 80 nm depending on the serotype. The capsid is composed of a total of 720 hexon and 60 penton subunit proteins, 360 monomers of polypeptide VI, 240 monomers of polypeptide IX, and 60 trimeric fibre proteins.

Bound to the penton subunits and protruding from the capsid is the fibre protein which mediates the initial attachment of the virus to a target cell. Polypeptides IX, IIIa, and VI form the scaffolding which holds the capsid together. Polypeptide IX stabilises the packing of adjacent hexons in the capsid, polypeptide IIIa spans the capsid to link hexons of adjacent faces, and polypeptide VI connects the structural proteins to the core. The core consists of DNA associated with polypeptides V, VII, μ and the terminal protein.

Ads contain double stranded DNA as their genetic material. The base composition of the 47 characterised serotypes (Ad1–Ad47) varies in the % G+C content, and the lengths of the genome (≈36 kb) and inverted terminal repeats (100–140 bp). The genome is covalently linked at each 5′ end to individual 55 kd terminal proteins and they associate with each other to circularise the DNA upon lysis of the virion. It is not known if the genome exists in a circular form inside the capsid, however a circular form is an intermediate in viral DNA synthesis.

Adeno-associated virus

The 18–26 nm icosahedral virion of AAV has a more simple structure. It is composed of 3 unglycosylated proteins of 87 (≈90%), 73 (≈5%) and 62 (≈5%) kd which have similar tryptic digestion patterns, consistent with them being derived from splice variants of a single RNA transcript.[7] The AAV genome is a linear single-stranded DNA molecule. The AAV2 genome has been sequenced and is 4680 nt long with 145 nt inverted terminal repeats (ITR).[8]

MOLECULAR BIOLOGY

Adenovirus

The Ad genome is functionally divided into 2 major non contiguous overlapping regions, **early** and **late**, based on the time of transcription after infection. The **early** regions are defined as those that are transcribed before the onset of viral DNA synthesis. The switch from **early** to **late** gene expression takes places about ≈7 h after infection. The terms **early** and **late** are not to be taken too literally as some early regions are still transcribed after DNA synthesis has begun.

There are 6 distinct **early** regions; E1A, E1B, E2A, E2B, E3, and E4, each (except for the E2A–B region) with individual promoters, and one **late** region, which is under the control of the major late promoter, with 5 well characterised coding units (L1–L5)[3] (Fig. A). There are also other minor intermediate and/or **late** transcriptional regions that are less well characterised, including the region encoding the viral-associated (*VA*) RNAs. Each **early** and **late** region appears to contain a cassette of genes coding for polypeptides with related functions. Each region is transcribed initially as a single RNA which is then spliced into the mature mRNAs. More than 30 different mature RNA transcripts have been identified in Ad2, one of the most studied serotypes.

Once the viral DNA is inside the nucleus (*see*[9] for description of mechanism of viral entry) transcription is initiated from the viral E1 promoters. This is the only viral region that **must** be transcribed without the aid of viral-encoded *trans*-activators. There are other regions that are also transcribed immediately after cell infection but to a lesser extent, suggesting that the E1 region is not the only region **capable** of being transcribed without viral-encoded transcription factors. The E1A region codes for more than six polypeptides. One of the polypeptides from this region, a 51 kd protein, transactivates transcription of the other **early** regions and amplifies viral gene expression. The E1B region codes for three polypeptides. The large E1B protein (55 kd), in association with the E4 34 kd protein, forms a nuclear complex and quickly halts cellular protein synthesis during lytic infections.[10] This 55 kd polypeptide also interacts with p53 and directly inhibits its function.[11] A 19 kd *trans*-activating protein encoded by the E1B region is essential to transform primary cultures. The oncogenicity of Ads in new-born rodents requires the E1 region.[10] Similarly when the E1 region is transfected into primary cell cultures, cell transformation occurs. Only the E1A region gene product is needed to immortalise cell cultures.

The E2A and E2B regions code for proteins directly involved in replication, i.e. the viral DNA polymerase, the pre-terminal protein and DNA binding proteins. In the E3 region, the 9 predicted proteins are not required for Ad replication in cultured cells.[12] Of the 6 identified proteins, 4 partially characterised ones are involved in counteracting the immune system; a 19 kd glycoprotein, gp19k, prevents cytolysis by cytotoxic T lymphocytes (CTL); and a 14.7 kd and a 10.4 kd/14.5 kd complex prevent, by different methods, E1A induced tumour necrosis factor cytolysis.[13] The E4 region appears to contain a cassette of genes whose products act to shutdown endogenous host gene expression and upregulate transcription from the E2 and **late** regions.[3]

Once viral DNA synthesis begins the **late** region genes, coding mainly for proteins involved in the structure and assembly of the virus particle, are expressed.

Adeno-associated virus

The complex expression and function of the AAV genes and gene products are less well characterised.[6] For AAV to replicate, it requires coinfection with a helper virus. Without a helper virus, AAVs integrate into the host genome and remain as a provirus. Ad helper functions are the most well characterised for AAV replication and AAVs appear to require the Ad E1A 51 kd, E1B 55 kd, E4 35 kd polypeptides, the E2A DNA binding-protein and the *VA* RNAs. The polypeptides that act as intracellular helper of gene expression do not interact directly with the viral genome, but enhance expression of certain types of genes (viral or cellular-encoded). AAV replication is not solely dependent on a helper virus, but can also be induced by carcinogens and chemical agents that disrupt the cell cycle.[14]

The AAV2 genetic map is the most extensively analysed. The viral genome is transcribed in 3 overlapping regions producing 7 primary transcripts (Fig. B). Differential splicing of these transcripts account for the coding regions of the 7 characterised polypeptides.

One or all of the 4 *rep* gene products are required for replication during coinfection with Ad. Without helper virus coinfection, one of the *rep* gene products appears to act as a transcriptional repressor of some promoters,[15] including its own.[16] This positive and negative autoregulation allows tight transcriptional control.

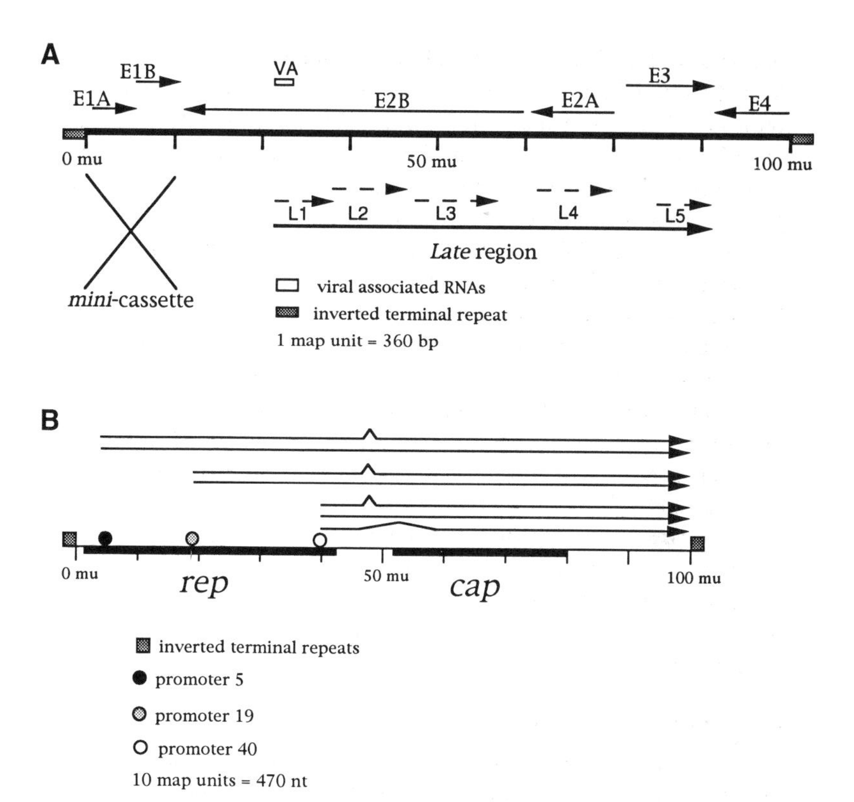

Fig. Schematic diagram of the genomes and major transcripts from Ad5 and AVV2 (A) The 36 kb AD5 genome with: 6 **early** region primary transcripts E1A, E1B, E2A, E2B, E3, and E4 (thin lines); the single **late** (thick line) and its spliced transcripts, L1–L5 (dashed lines); and the viral associated (opened box) transcriptional region. The Ad5 genome is thought to code for at least 2700 polypeptides. The E1 region is deleted in rAds and replaced by a *mini*-cassette that usually contains a promoter, cDNA, and polyadenylation signal. (B) The 4680 nt AAV2 genome with the 7 primary transcripts (solid lines – including intron) from the three major promoters (p5, p19, p40). The coding regions *rep*, which codes for at least 4 polypeptides involved in replication with at least one of these a multifunctional transcription factor, and *cap*, which codes for at least the 3 capsid polypeptides, are represented as solid boxes. Both genomes are divided into 100 map units, and arrowed lines indicate the direction of transcription. For a more detailed description for adenovirus and adeno-associated virus genomes *see* reviews by Horwitz[3,4] and Berns,[6] respectively.

ADVANTAGES FOR GENE THERAPY

Adenoviral mediated gene therapy

The most highly touted advantage of AMGT is that *wt*Ads are safe. Millions of North American army recruits have been vaccinated by oral administration of enteric-coated capsules containing unattenuated Ad and have rarely displayed adverse side effects. Furthermore, the Ads that are modified to make the current lines of vectors (Ad2 and Ad5) do not cause tumours in rodents and appear to cause only mild respiratory problems in humans.[4]

Human *wt*Ads readily infect almost all cell types in vitro and in vivo, and infect dividing as well as quiescent cells, with high efficiency. In comparison retroviruses require actively dividing cells to integrate the recombinant viral genome and many retroviral mediated gene transfer (RMGT) protocols call for an ex vivo approach to gene therapy, although in vivo RMGT has been partially successful following a partial hepatectomy.[18] An ex vivo approach may limit the potential applicability of this technology to a small number of patients because of cost and the demand for considerable technical expertise. Furthermore, some diseases can not be treated by this approach (such as cystic fibrosis – *see* Evans, this issue). An ex vivo approach may be able to help thousands but certainly not millions of patients with today's technology. Direct intravenous injection, or as in the case of cystic fibrosis trials, aerosolisation or fiberoptic bronchoscopic administration of a recombinant Ad (rAd) – *see* ref. 19 for a description of rAd synthesis – may be the only possible method of delivering the vector to quiescent cells or tissues that cannot be treated ex vivo.

Current Ad vectors can accept large foreign DNA inserts. They have deletions in the E1 and E3 regions and can safely package 5% more DNA than the *wt*Ad,[20] putting the theoretical limit at 7–8 kb. Deletion of the E1 region also renders Ad vectors replication deficient.

Ads are relatively stable and amenable to purification and concentration. Titres as high as 5×10^{11} plaque forming units (pfu)/ml can be obtained and we routinely obtain purified stocks at 2×10^{11} pfu/ml.

Ads rarely integrate into host genome and therefore have little chance to activate a dormant oncogene or interrupt a tumour suppressor gene. The rAd vector, once inside the nucleus, remains as a nonreplicating extrachromosomal entity (often mislabelled as an episome).

We have shown that long-term expression in mice is possible with intravenous[21,22] and stereotaxic[23] administration of a rAd (AdRSVβ-gal) expressing the reporter gene β-galactosidase. *In situ* histochemical staining revealed blue nuclei in smooth muscle more than one year after a single intravenous injection. Although short-term expression of the *mini*-cassette in rAds after in vivo delivery in adult animals, is also possible.[24]

Adeno-associated virus mediated gene transfer

There are many attractive advantages of AAVMGT. *wt*AAVs have not been associated with the cause of a disease or tumour in humans. AAVs can infect all cultured cells that have been tested. *rep*$^+$AAV vectors have a preferred site of integration into the human genome (at 19q13.4)[25] and can exist as a latent infection for the life of the cell, if free from complementing viral infections.[6] Furthermore, an AAV *rep* gene product(s) exhibits inhibitory effects on tumour formation by oncogenic Ads and oncogenes as well as gene amplification induced by carcinogens.[26]

In addition, *rep*$^-$AAV vectors have high transduction frequency, and cannot be rescued by Ad challenge alone (i.e. they require *wt*AAV coinfection also).[27] The sole sequence needed for AAV vector integration is in the terminal 145 nt ITR making the cloning capacity of the *rep*$^-$AAV vector 4.7 kb.[8]

Finally, it appears that there is no superinfection immunity for AAV vectors, i.e. cultured cells can be consecutively transduced with different recombinant AAVs without affecting cell viability.[26]

THE DRAWBACKS FOR GENE THERAPY

Adenoviruses

Replication-deficient adenoviral vectors are deleted in the E1A region coding for a transactivator that dramatically upregulates transcription from the other early regions. Although designed to be replication-deficient, there is the potential for replication in vivo secondary to *trans*-complementation by 'E1a-like' factors due to pre-existing or acquired Ad sequences, other viruses and/or host cellular transcription factors. Low level replication of rAd has occurred at high multiplicity of infection (moi) in Hela cells.[28] (Moi is used loosely in this context, it is not meant as the number of viral particles absorbed/cell but as the number of pfu/cell during transduction.) This suggested that requirement of the E1A gene product is not absolute. There is a caveat to these results by Shenk and his colleagues. Hela cells are highly differentiated cervical carcinoma cells that express an 'E1a-like' viral transcription factor. It has never been demonstrated that E1$^-$Ads can replicate in any primary cultures. However, we have been able to demonstrate that in primary human fibroblasts transduced with a rAd containing a supposedly E1A 51 kd *trans*-activator dependent promoter (the E4 promoter from Ad5) driving transcription of the β-galactosidase gene, there is enough transcriptional activity to detect low-level β-galactosidase activity (N Hanania, personal communication). The transcription from an E1a 'dependent' promoter in transduced cells does not necessarily mean that replication can occur. Continued work will be needed to determine if low level gene expression can lead to low level replication.

Another possible problem is the creation of a replication competent virus by recombination with viral or cellular sequence. Recombination with cellular E1A sequences is considered the culprit when supposedly *wt*Ads contaminate rAd stocks. rAds are capable of recombining with *wt*Ads of the same group[3] (i.e. Ad1, 2, 5, and 6) and Ad antibodies are present in 50% of the 2-year-olds and 95% of the 16–34 year-olds in the Washington DC area.[29] With only a single debilitating deletion in one end of the rAd vector (the E1 region where the *mini*-cassette is usually placed) recombination is a possibility. This scenario seems most likely for cells along the respiratory tract because of the high number of adventitious viral particles capable of infecting this tissue and because it is the natural tropism for Ad2 and Ad5.

Despite the fact that expression for >1 year has been observed, duration of expression from the *mini*-cassette is normally short (≈8 weeks) in adult animals. Therefore, repeated administration may be necessary. The fact that Ads do not integrate into the host genome, may not only be a blessing but a bane and limit some of their potential uses in AMGT. When a retrovirus randomly integrates into a genome it is there for the life of the cell and its daughter cells. However, copies of the Ad genome are lost or reduced during each subsequent cell cycle. For long-term treatment of genetic defects in dividing cells this scenario is not acceptable.

A number of other hypotheses have been proposed to explain the short duration of expression in adult animals. There is no doubt an immune response to capsid polypeptides and overexpression of gene products from the *mini*-cassette (M Lee, personal communication) may target the cell for destruction by a cytotoxic T cell response. A slow accumulation of toxic viral-encoded-proteins may eventually kill the cell, and extinction of the viral promoter in the *mini*-cassette by an intracellular mechanism (probably methylation) may also reduce the duration of expression.[30]

Other potential problems that must be addressed include: shedding of a rAd and contaminating the environment, anaphylactic shock due to an overload of the immune system from a therapeutic dose of a rAd, the immune response to a second administration if needed and the possibility that in vivo test in laboratory animals may not be applicable to humans.

AAV drawbacks

Integration of AAV into the host genome at 19q13.4 occurs only if the AAV vector is *rep*$^{+}$, while *rep*$^{-}$AAV vectors appear to integrate randomly.[8] This raises the same worries as RMGT with respect to activation of a dormant oncogene or inactivation of a tumour suppressor gene. Furthermore, there is no guarantee that site-specific integration is any more advantageous than a random pattern. Fluorescent in situ hybridisation results, with *rep*+AAV vector transduced cell lines, show integration into only one chromosome 19/cell vectors (even at high infectious units/cell).[25] This suggests a potential lethal condition when both copies of chromosome 19 have an integrated copy. Data also suggest a deletion/substitution mechanism during viral integration, and the AAV genome is prone to rearrangement during integration. Also, AAVs tend to integrate in multiple copies in the genome (average 2–4 copies). Finally, viral stocks of 1×10^8–10^9 infectious units/ml are feasible, but difficult to prepare and are easily contaminated with *wt*AAV and helper virus.

POTENTIAL SOLUTIONS

A major aim in our laboratory is to make AMGT safer and better.

Minimum vectors

We are taking a number of complementary approaches to achieve the goal of producing better vectors. The human 293 cell line is used to amplify the rAd because it has been transfected with a fragment from the E1 region and can complement deleted functions in $E1^-$Ad vectors. This cell line may be transfected with fragments from other regions of the Ad genome (e.g. the E4 and the **late** region). This classic approach of making a complementing cell line has a few drawbacks. The *trans*-activating E4 proteins and some of the structural proteins, such as the penton base polypeptide, are cytotoxic to cells. Constructing a cell line expressing all or parts of the E4 region, and some of the structural proteins may only be possible with an inducible system. We are testing several inducible promoters that can be activated during amplification of a rAd. We have produced subclones from the human 293 cell line that are able to replicate an $E1^-E4^-$Ad but at a slower than normal rate (P Yeh, personal communication).

The second approach is to create a helper virus system that will provide all the gene functions from the deleted region. This 'one-cell two-virus' approach has the potential to delete all sequences except for *cis* acting elements that are necessary to package the rAd. This could allow inserts of up to 37 kb because only a few sequences from the genome (the 100–140 bp ITR and the packaging signal) appear to be necessary to package the DNA. Initial efforts are restricted to removing the entire E4 region and expressing the replication dependant polypeptides by a helper virus. The major drawback to this approach (similar to that in other viral systems) is separating the rAd from the helper virus. Preliminary studies suggest that it will be possible to separate the rAd from the helper virus on a continuous isopycnic CsCl gradient (E Vigne, personal communication).

Creation of the complementing cell line and/or a helper virus system will improve a number of safety features **and** increase the cloning capacity in the vector in order to insert '*midi-*' or '*maxi*-cassettes'. Safer, because the more that is deleted from the *wt*Ad to create a rAd, the lower the probability of a functional recombinant virus being produced and of in vivo replication. Recombination between the $E1^{-}$Ad and a *wt*Ad is possible, but with deletions in each end ($E1^{-}E4^{-}$Ad) a double recombination would have to occur to produce a viable virus. *Maxi*-cassettes may allow controlled expression of the gene if its endogenous *cis* regulatory factors (enhancers, promoters, polyadenylation signals, etc) are present **as well as** the whole genomic fragment encompassing the gene. This may be possible if either of these approaches, or a combination of the two, is successful. Any system which would allow 'normal' gene regulation, or maybe even a future technology to induce homologous recombination with the DNA insert[31] in order to replace the faulty gene in affected tissue, would be an ideal situation.

Organoides

Although the ex vivo approach appears to be a drawback of RMGT, it does provide an advantage in some instances. This advantage can be exploited and enhanced using AMGT. We are currently modifying a technique[32] for making neo-organs or 'organoides' from fibroblasts which are encapsulated in a collagen and polytetrafluoroethylene lattice and re-implanted in the host. This approach is attractive since skin grafting is well established, and fibroblasts do not readily transform into cancer cells in culture. An advantage of AMGT, as previously mentioned, is that Ads do not integrate into the genome, and there is a potential for a high copy numbers of the *mini*-cassette, and long-lasting expression using AMGT.

Long-term stable expression from rAds seems to require fully differentiated quiescent cells. This, we believe, can be achieved by experimenting with other cell types in the organoides. Myoblasts are good candidates because expression has been detected in these cells for up to 15 months after an intravenous injection of AdRSVβ-gal.[21] Organoides can be used for a range of conditions that require secreted gene products or gene products that are not normally secreted but can be endocytosed by tissues displaying the adverse phenotype. The organoide may then act as a small pump continually producing a therapeutic polypeptide. We are exploring this technology for the treatment of haematopoietic disorders, thalassemia, lysosomal storage diseases, cardiovascular diseases, etc.

The safely features of AMGT are augmented when using organoides because it is possible to: (1) assay the level of expression of the *mini*-cassette before implantation and hence have a greater degree of control; (2) use 10–100 fold less rAd in an organoide versus intravenous injection, for the same physiological response; (3) avoid expression and transduction in undesirable tissues; (4) remove the organoide and transduced cells if needed; and (5) implant the organoide subcutaneously or intraperitoneally with similar efficiency (E Kremer, unpublished observation).

Short-term expression: blessing and bane

It is pertinent to AMGT that the *mini*-cassette, delivered via the rAd vector, is delivered to the nucleus and exists as an extrachromosomal entity. This advantage/disadvantage is an oxymoron. Functional in vivo tests of expression from rAds have shown a half life of about 6 weeks when administered intravenously, intramuscularly and via organoides into adult animals. These data are consistently reproduced in animal models in our laboratory and others. The long term (>1 year) expression seen in mouse smooth muscle and presumably mouse hepatocytes[22] may have been due to administering the rAd to newborns and thereby circumventing the immune response. There is insufficient data at the present time to determine if the duration of expression in humans will be the same as that in adult animals. It has been reported that *wt*Ad infections can persist for up to 2 years in humans.[4]

Many of the current first-generation vectors have 2 kb deleted from the central part of the E3 region. This region is non-essential for replication in cell culture and is removed to increase the cloning capacity. The second-generation vectors have added back the gene coding for gp19K which is in this deleted region. This protein prevents transport of MHC polypeptides to the cell surface by anchoring the complex to the endoplasmic reticulum membrane. The MHC presents potential antigens to cytotoxic T lymphocytes which then, in turn, may target the cells for destruction. Usually diminished expression of the gene product from the *mini*-cassette correlates with loss of the vector from tissue.[24] This is possibly due to the loss of transduced cells. Re-incorporation of the gp19K gene into the vector may help to mask the cells from this part of the host's immune surveillance system and, perhaps prolong the life of the cell that has been transduced by a rAd.

Surprisingly, in nude mice (which lack a cytotoxic T cell (CTL) response) we have found a similar short length of expression from a *mini*-cassette. Using organoides, made with human fibroblasts transduced and expressing erythropoetin, expression persisted at a detectable level for only 6–8 weeks (E Kremer, unpublished observation). This is similar to the duration found in other strains of mice who have a CTL response, implying that the CTL response is not the only factor affecting the duration of in vivo expression.

On the other hand, short-term expression from the *mini*-cassette in the rAd may be an advantageous characteristic for some applications of AMGT (as in vaccines, AIDS or acquired genetic diseases, i.e. cancer[33]).

Alternative non-human Ads

Another approach that we are exploring is the use of non-human Ads as potential vectors. Most human serotypes are not pathogenic to animals, and animal Ads are only pathogenic within the species of origin. Asymptomatic infections of bovine, canine and simian Ad have been documented in human sera by antibody determination and neutralisation tests.[4] Furthermore, there is less than 20% homology at the nucleotide level among different human Ad groups, suggesting that a non-human Ad would have at least a similar variability. Also, Ads of different groups in humans do not recombine but can show complementation of gene function. The use of non-human Ads may allow an extra safety factor if it can be shown that the *cis/trans* acting elements are not complemented by the human cellular factors and that non-human Ads cannot recombine with human Ads even at optimal conditions. A series of tests to develop this system is underway (B Klonjkowski, personal communication). The first step is to make a recombinant non-human Ad and then, to check its potential safety as far as complementation, recombination and viability are concerned. Although new to AMGT, this approach is not novel. The commonly used retrovirus vector in gene transfer protocols is derived from a virus that naturally infects mice (i.e. murine leukaemia virus, MLV).

An enormous amount of work will be needed to develop non-human Ad vectors. As has been accomplished with the human Ad vectors now in use, it will be necessary to make a stable transfected cell line that can complement the deleted function in the potential non-human vector and ultimately make minimum vectors similar to the one we, and others, are currently developing.

CONCLUSION

Recall the first computers, motion picture, or ultrasound. It is unlikely that any single method of gene transfer (based on today's technology) will be recognisable in 15 years. No single system is perfect or even adequate. Most, if not all, of the advances will be made at the basic scientific level, which underlies many of the problems in gene therapy. Each gene transfer technique (retrovirus, Ad, AAV, herpes, liposome, plasmid, receptor-mediated, etc) will continue to evolve and will certainly incorporate the advantages of many gene transfer systems. Many different DNA based delivery systems will find niches in the field of gene/cell therapy. DNA as a drug is now a reality but its full potential is yet to be exploited.

ACKNOWLEDGEMENTS

EJK souhaite remercier T Hecht, V Kalatzis, et les membres du laboratoire pour leurs commentaires et leurs discussions utiles.

REFERENCES

1 Rowe WP, Huebner RJ, Gilmore LK, Parrott RH, Ward TG. Isolation of a cytopathogenic agent from human adenoids undergoing spontaneous degeneration in tissue culture. Proc Soc Exp Biol Med 1953; 84: 570–573.
2 Ginsberg HS, Pereira HG, Valentine RC, Wilcox WC. A proposed terminology for the adenovirus antigens and virion morphology. Virology 1966; 28: 782–783.
3 Horwitz MS. Adenoviridae and their replication. In: Fields BN, Knipe DM, et al, eds. Virology, 2nd edn. New York: Raven Press, 1990: 1679–1723.
4 Horwitz MS. Adenoviruses. In: Fields BN, Knipe DM, et al, eds. Virology, 2nd edn. New York: Raven Press, 1990: 1723–1741.
5 Hoggan M, Blacklow N, Rowe W. Studies of small DNA virus found in various Ad preparations: physical, biological, and immunological characterization. Proc Natl Acad Sci USA 1966; 55: 1457.
6 Berns KI. Parvovirus replication. Microbiol Rev 1990; 54(3): 316–329.
7 Siegl G, Bates RC, Berns KI, et al. Characteristics and taxonomy of Parvoviridae. Intervirology 1985; 23(2): 61–73.
8 Muzyczka N. Use of adeno-associated virus as a general transduction vector for mammalian cells. Curr Top Microbiol Immunol 1992; 158(97): 97–129.
9 Greber UF, Willetts M, Webster P, Helenius A. Stepwise dismantling of adenovirus 2 during entry into cells. Cell 1993; 75: 477–486.
10 Bernards R, Van dEA. Adenovirus: transformation and oncogenicity. Biochim Biophys Acta 1984; 783(3): 187–204.
11 Moran E. Interaction of adenoviral proteins with pRB and p53. FASEB J 1993; 7(10): 880–885.
12 Wold WSM, Goodling LR. Region E3 of adenovirus: a cassette of genes involved in host immunosurveillance and virus-cell interactions. Virology 1991; 184: 1–8.
13 Goodling LR, Ranheim TS, Tollefson AE, Brady HA, Wold WSM. The 10,400- and 14,500-dalton proteins encoded by region E3 of adenovirus function together to protect many but not all mouse cell lines against lysis by tumor necrosis factor. J Virol 1991; 65(8): 4114–4123.
14 Schlehofer JR, Ehrbar M, Zur HH. Vaccinia virus, herpes simplex virus, and carcinogens induce DNA amplification in a human cell line and support replication of a helpervirus dependent parvovirus. Virology 1986; 152(1): 110–117.
15 Labow M, Graf L, Berns K. Adeno-associated virus gene expression inhibits cellular transformation by heterologous genes. Mol Cell Biol 1987; 7(4): 1320.
16 Tratschin J, Tal J, Carter B. Negative and positive regulation in trans of gene expression from AAV vectors in mammalian cells by a rep gene product. Mol Cell Biol 1986; 6: 2884.
17 Cotten M, Wagner E, Zatloukal K, Phillips S, Curiel DT, Birnstiel ML. High-efficiency receptor-mediated delivery of small large (48 kilobase) gene constructs using the endosome-disruption activity of defective or chemically inactivated adenovirus particles. Proc Natl Acad Sci USA 1992; 89: 6094–6098.

18 Kay MA, Rothenberg S, Landen CN, et al. In vivo gene therapy of hemophilia B: sustained partial correction in factor IX-deficient dogs [*see* comments]. Science 1993; 262(5130): 117–119.
19 Stratford-Perricaudet L, Stratford-Perricaudet M. Adenovirus-mediated in vivo gene therapy. In: Vos J, ed. Viruses in human gene therapy. Durham, N.C.: Carolina Academic Press, 1994.
20 Bett AJ, Prevec L, Graham FL. Packaging capacity and stability of human adenovirus type 5 vectors. J Virol 1993; 67:; 5911–5921.
21 Stratford-Perricaudet LD, Makeh I, Perricaudet M. Briand P. Widespread long-term gene transfer of mouse skeletal muscles and heart. J Clin Invest 1992; 90: 626–630.
22 Stratford-Perricaudet LD, Levrero M, Chasse J-F, Perricaudet M, Briand P. Evaluation of the transfer and expression in mice of an enzyme encoding gene using a human adenovirus vector. Hum Gene Ther 1990; 1: 241–256.
23 Akli S, Caillaud C, Vigne E, et al. Transfer of a foreign gene into the brain using adenovirus vectors. Nature Genet 1993; 3: 224–234.
24 Smith TA, Mehaffey MG, Kayda DB, et al. Adenovirus mediated expression of therapeutic plasma levels of human factor IX in mice. Nature Genet 1993; 5(4): 397–402.
25 Samulski RJ, Zhu X, Xiao X, et al. Targeted integration of adeno-associated virus (AAV) into human chromosome 19 [published erratum appears in EMBO J 1992; 11(3): 1228]. EMBO J 1991; 10(12): 3941–50.
26 Lebkowski JS, McNally MM, Okarma TB, Lerch LB. Adeno-associated virus: a vector system for efficient introduction and integration of DNA into a variety of mammalian cell types. Mol Cell Biol 1988; 8(10): 3988–96.
27 McLaughlin SK, Collis P, Hermonat PL, Muzyczka N. Adeno-associated virus general transduction vectors: analysis of proviral structures. J Virol 1988; 62(6): 1963–1973.
28 Jones N, Shenk T. Isolation of adenovirus type 5 host range deletion mutants defective for transformation of rat embryo cells. Cell 1979; 17(3): 683–689.
29 Huebner JR, Rowe WP, Ward TG, Parrott RH, Bell JA. Adenoidal-pharyngeal conjuctival agents. N Engl J Med 1954; 251: 1077–1086.
30 Doerfler W. Patterns of de novo DNA methylation and promoter inhibition: studies on the adenovirus and the human genomes. Exs 1993; 64(262): 262–299.
31 Wan Q, Taylor MW. Correction of a deletion mutant by gene targeting with an adenovirus vector. Mol Cell Biol 1993; 13(2): 918–927.
32 Moullier P, Marechal V, Danos O, Heard JM. Continuous systemic secretion of a lysosomal enzyme by genetically modified mouse skin fibroblasts. Transplantation 1993; 56(2): 427–432.
33 Haddada H, Cordier L, Perricaudet M. Applications of adenovirus towards gene therapy. In: Doerfler W, Boehm P, ed. Curr Top Microbiol Immunol. Berlin: Springer Verlag 1994.

British Medical Bulletin (1995) Vol.51, No.1, pp.45–55

Herpes virus-based vectors

S Efstathiou and A C Minson

Division of Virology, Department of Pathology, University of Cambridge, Cambridge, UK

Herpesviruses are a diverse family of large DNA viruses, all of which have the capacity to establish lifelong latent infections. Many different herpesviruses may have potential as gene delivery vehicles, but exploitation of this potential has, to date, been explored only using Herpes simplex virus (HSV), a virus which naturally establishes a silent, latent infection of neurones in man and in a number of experimental animal models. Delivery of reporter genes in vitro and in vivo has been demonstrated using a variety of replication competent and replication defective vectors, and significant physiological modification in the CNS has been achieved by HSV-mediated gene delivery. Much remains to be done using animal models and, in particular, the requirements for long-term gene expression from latent virus genomes needs to be defined in different cell types in vivo.

Herpesviruses are nuclear DNA viruses with large genomes of ≈100–250 kbp. The potential of these viruses as gene vectors lies in their ability to carry large foreign DNA inserts and their ability to establish lifelong latent infections in which the virus genome exists as a stable episome with no apparent effect on the host cell. Herpesviruses are, however, enormously diverse, varying in their genome size, genome organisation, genetic content, cell tropism and pathogenesis,[1] and in consequence different herpesviruses have very different potential uses in gene delivery. The nature of viral latency is of particular relevance. Epstein Barr virus and other members of the gamma-herpesviruses can establish latent infection in dividing cells; the viral episome replicates co-ordinately with cell division and is inherited by all progeny cells. Like retroviruses, this group of herpesviruses has the potential for gene delivery to stem cells and to their differentiated progeny. A major drawback to the use of these viruses in gene therapy, however, is the fact that gamma-herpesviruses are associated with lymphoproliferative disease and in some instances with malignancy. The use of gamma-herpesviruses will require the identification and elimination of those genes involved in cell transformation while retaining those functions necessary for viral replication and viral plasmid maintenance. Considerable progress has been made in this area.[2]

In contrast to gamma-herpesviruses, herpes simplex virus (HSV), and other members of the alpha-herpesvirus subfamily, cannot maintain latent infection in dividing cells. The viral genome contains no 'latent origin' of DNA replication and the virus persists in the host by establishing latent infection in long-lived cells – sensory neurons in the case of HSV. Genes delivered using a herpes simplex virus vector can therefore be maintained indefinitely as a component of the latent viral episome in long-lived cells, but inheritance of the delivered gene by daughter cells following division would occur only as a result of fortuitous non-specific integration. A third group of herpesviruses, the beta-herpesviruses or cytomegaloviruses, may have potential as gene vectors for therapy, but our knowledge of the biology of these viruses, and in particular the nature of latent infection, is meagre and there are no immediate prospects of exploiting this potential.

Although many herpesviruses may ultimately prove of value in foreign gene delivery and gene therapy, to date only herpes simplex virus has been used in vivo and the remainder of this article will be limited to a review of the progress made with this virus. The topic has also been reviewed recently by Glorioso et al[3] and Breakefield and DeLuca[4].

THE BIOLOGY OF HERPES SIMPLEX VIRUS

HSV has a very broad cell tropism and is probably capable of infecting virtually any human cell type. Natural infection in man, which can be mimicked experimentally in several animal species including the mouse, is however very restricted, virus spread being limited by specific and non-specific defence mechanisms and by intracellular requirements for virus growth. HSV infects epithelial cells of the skin or mucosa. Productive, cytolyic infection of these cells is followed by virus entry into sensory nerve endings and transmission by fast retrograde flow to the neuronal body where limited virus replication occurs; a life-long latent infection is established in a proportion of infected neurons. Productive infection of a neuron may result in transneuronal transmission, and HSV has been used as a neuronal tracer to map motor and sensory neuronal networks.[5] Potentially, then, HSV has the ability to deliver foreign genes to CNS networks from peripheral sites. We must assume however, that productive infection of neurons, like that of other cell types, is cytopathic, and that acceptable HSV vectors must be incapable of replication in neurons. While there is some evidence to suggest that neurons survive productive infection,[6] it is certain that the levels of virus replication required in order to trace neuronal pathways results in extensive neuropathology and usually in fatal encephalitis, and in practise HSV gene delivery is likely to be limited to cells that can be accessed directly. Given its very broad cellular host range it is apparent that HSV could be used to deliver foreign genes to a variety of tissues or cell types. Nevertheless, the ability of the virus to establish latent infection in long-lived cells and its efficient transmission from axons and nerve endings to the neuronal nucleus has focused attention on the potential of HSV for gene delivery to the CNS.

PRODUCTIVE INFECTION AND THE LATENT STATE

The nucleotide sequence of HSV has been determined, nearly all the gene products have been identified[7] and the function of the majority of gene products is understood at least at the superficial level. Productive infection involves the expression of all known genes in a temporal cascade in three phases. Immediate-early (IE) genes encode regulatory proteins some of which are essential for initiation of the cycle; early genes encode enzymes required for viral DNA synthesis and proteins involved in a variety of host cell modifications; late genes encode virion proteins. The productive cycle results in cell death following infection in vivo. The events leading to latent infection are uncertain, but mutant viruses incapable of initiating the productive cycle are able to establish neuronal latency, and latent infection can be established in other wise permissive cells provided that the productive cycle is suppressed, suggesting that latency is a default pathway resulting from failure of the productive cycle. Latently infected neurons express a family of transcripts (the latency-associated transcripts or LATs) (Fig. 1) from the LAT promoter but the function of these transcripts is unknown and interruption of the LATs or deletion of the LAT promoter do not prevent latent infection.[8] The conclusion pertinent to vector construction is that no viral gene function appears to be required for the establishment or maintenance of the latent state.

HSV VECTORS

Replication competent vectors

Of the approximately 70 genes of HSV about half are dispensable for growth in cell culture. The dispensable gene products include transcriptional activators, nucleoside and nucleotide modifying enzymes, a protein kinase and several membrane proteins of unknown function. These genes represent multiple convenient sites for the insertion of foreign sequences and their deletion results in varying levels of attenuation. It has been shown for many years, for example, that thymidine kinase negative mutants are incapable of growth in neurons and are entirely

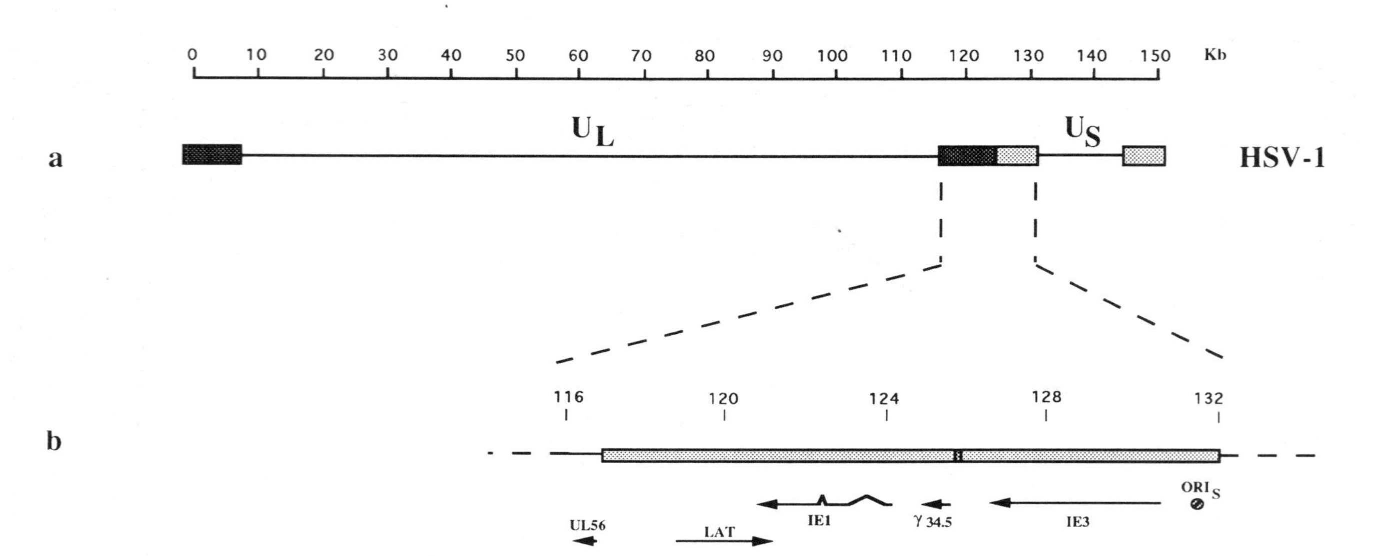

Fig. 1 (a) The HSV genome consists of 152 kbp of double stranded DNA comprising of unique long (U_L) and a unique short (U_S) region each of which are flanked by inverted repeats. (b) An expanded view of the fused internal repeats showing the location of the latency associated transcripts (LATs) and their relationship to other lytic virus transcripts discussed in the text. The LATs are encoded by diploid genes located in the repeats flanking the $U_L$region. The low abundance 8kb putative primary transcript designated minor (m)LAT and the stable 2.0 kb LAT transcript which are synthesised in the opposite direction and overlapping the IE1 gene are shown.

non-neurovirulent. More recent studies have identified a specific neurovirulence function encoded by HSV designated ICP34.5 which is required for productive infection both of CNS and PNS neurons.[9] Many other genes have been identified whose deletion results in dramatic attenuation and it is possible to engineer replication competent vectors that are entirely apathogenic. While these vectors are useful in investigating the problems of gene delivery and long term gene expression, it is unlikely that replication competent vectors will be acceptable for clinical use. In particular, attenuation through the deletion of multiple genes might result in the generation of viruses that are only partially attenuated if recombination were to occur with HSV resident in the recipient.

Replication defective vectors

The function of many HSV genes is absolutely required for virus replication and deletion of these genes necessitates provision of the corresponding function *in trans* from a helper cell. HSV mutant-helper cell combinations based on a number of gene functions have been described including mutants lacking the IE-3 transcriptional regulator,[10] the virion transactivator Vmw65 (VP16)[11] and a number of essential surface glycoproteins.[12] Attention has focused on vectors lacking the IE-3 gene because the gene function is required throughout the productive cycle, but other IE genes are expressed, indeed over-expressed, in the absence of IE-3, and it appears that some of these IE gene products are cytotoxic.[13] Vectors lacking the virion transactivator (VP16) offer the potential advantage that this protein functions to activate transcription of all immediate early genes and is also an essential structural component of the virion.

Amplicon vectors

HSV DNA replicates by a rolling circle mechanism and plasmids containing an HSV origin of replication will act as a template for DNA synthesis in cells co-infected with HSV. If the plasmid also contains an HSV packaging signal then the linear concatamer will be packaged into virus particles. The principle is illustrated in Figure 2. Plasmids of this type have been called ‘amplicons’ and their properties are reviewed by Frenkel et al.[14] As shown in Figure 2, amplicon replication and packaging is helper-virus dependent and infection progeny is a mixture of packaged amplicon and helper virus that cannot be physically distinguished or separated. Provided that the helper virus is itself replication defective, such that propagation of the amplicon-helper virus mixture requires a complementing cell line, then the helper virus component of the mixture represents no risk and can be ignored for the purpose of gene transfer. The advantage of this system, which has received considerable attention,[15,16] is that the amplicon will accommodate a foreign sequence that approximates to the packaging limit of HSV – approximately 150 kb. Thus packaged amplicons can deliver very large genes or many copies per particle of small genes. The disadvantage common to all helper-dependent systems, is that the helper-amplicon ratio varies considerably on passage and reproducible vector populations are therefore difficult to prepare.

IN VIVO GENE DELIVERY USING HSV VECTORS

In addition to the design and construction of disabled HSV vectors the choice of promoters which will result in the stable long-term expression of a transduced gene in the desired cell type is an area of active investigation. To date studies have focused largely on the expression of the reporter gene lacZ which has been placed under the control of various cellular or viral promoters with the aim of defining those cis-acting elements sufficient to confer long-term neuronal gene expression. Our current poor knowledge of those cis- and trans-acting factors important in the control of neuronal gene expression in vivo coupled with the possible inactivation of heterologous promoters in the context of the histone-associated latent virus genome has led to the empirical testing of a number of viral and cellular regulatory elements.

Transient expression has been observed with the majority of promoters tested to date including lytic cycle HSV promoters, the RSV LTR, the HCMV IE promoter and the, neurofilament and phosphoglycerol kinase promoters.[3,17] Long-term expression of the lacZ gene under the control of the Moloney murine leukaemia virus LTR (MoMuLV LTR) inserted into the HSV IE3 gene locus has been reported in sensory but not motor neurons,[18] and expression from this promoter appears to be facilitated by the proximity of HSV LAT promoter regulatory elements.[17] The MoMuLV LTR therefore appears to operate during latency when placed within the repeats sequences adjacent to the LAT transcription unit but when inserted at other locations it functions only when fused to LAT promoter elements.[17] Similarly placing the HCMV IE promoter in the proximity of the HSV LAT promoter appears to confer long-term activity to this promoter which is otherwise quiescent in the context of the virus genome during latent infection (Efstathiou et al. unpublished observations). Studies utilising the rat neuron-specific enolase promoter inserted into the HSV thymidine kinase gene indicate that this mammalian promoter can give stable neuronal expression of lacZ for at least 30 days following sterotactic injection into the adult rat caudate nucleus although long term expression from this promoter also appears to be influenced by its site of insertion into the virus genome.[19]

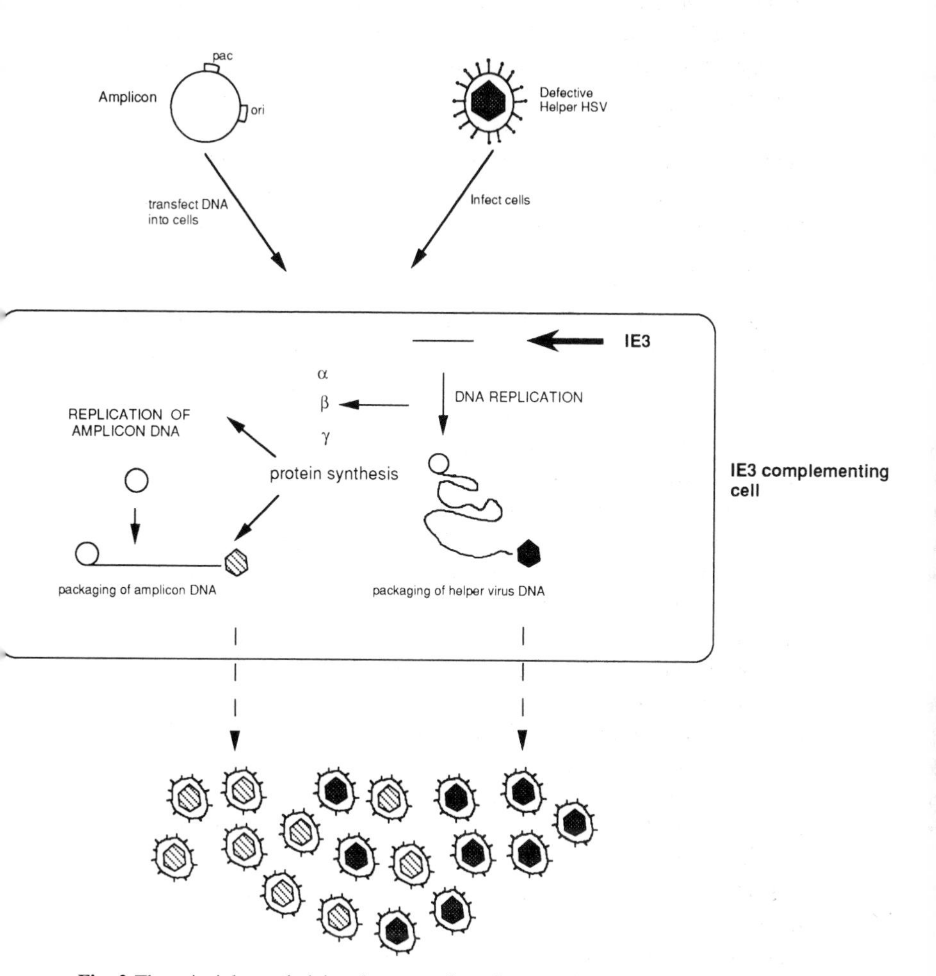

Fig. 2 The principles underlying the generation of an amplicon virus vector are shown. Amplicon vector DNA containing an origin of virus DNA replication, packaging signal and the gene of interest is transfected into cells. Cells are then superinfected with a defective helper virus which, in this example, lacks the essential IE3 transactivator. The IE3 gene product is provided *in trans* by an engineered complementing cell line which initiates the lytic cascade of gene expression from the defective virus genome. These gene products replicate and package both amplicon and defective virus DNA resulting in the release of a mixed virus population. Subsequent infection of a non-complementing cell line will result in the efficient delivery of both amplicon and defective helper virus DNA to the cell but helper virus gene expression is not initiated due to the absence of a functional IE3 gene product.

This it appears that the site of insertion of heterologous promoters in the HSV genome and/or the proximity of LAT promoter regulatory sequences can significantly influence their activity during latency.

Since the virus encoded LATs are transcribed indefinitely during neuronal latency considerable effort has been made to define those elements of the LAT promoter important for long-term neuronal gene expression and to determine whether this promoter can be used to drive foreign gene expression. It has been demonstrated that replication competent HSV vectors are capable of the stable expression of β-globin[20] and β-galactosidase[21] in a proportion of murine sensory neurons when these reporter genes were placed at different localities downstream of the TATA box-containing LAT promoter termed LAP1. Recent data has highlighted the complexity of the LAT promoter regulatory region[22,23] and has indicated that long-term expression is likely to be facilitated by elements contained with a second promoter region, termed LAP2, which resides downstream of LAP1 and has features common to eukaryotic housekeeping gene promoters. The LAP2 promoter has been shown to drive expression of the reporter gene lacZ in trigeminal neurons for up to 300 days post-infection, independently of LAP1 when inserted into an ectopic genomic location.[22] Thus the increasingly complex HSV LAT promoter region offers considerable promise as an element sufficient to confer long-term gene expression in neuronal cells in vivo and it is now important to determine the level of expression that can be achieved from this promoter region in different neuronal cell types since early studies suggested that the activity of this promoter in neurons of the CNS is considerably less than that observed in the PNS.[24]

Table Examples of biologically active genes delivered in vivo using HSV vectors

Vector	Target	Foreign gene	Promoter	Expression	Ref
Amplicon	Rat hippocampal neurons	Glucose transporter	HCMV IE	Transient	26
Amplicon	Rat sympathetic neurons	Nerve growth factor	HSV IE 4/5	Transient	25
Replication competent LAT$^-$	Mouse trigeminal & CNS neurons	β-glucoronidase	HSV LAT	18 weeks	27
Replication incompetent IE3$^-$	Mouse liver, hepatocytes	Canine factor IX	HCMV IE	Transient	29
Replication incompetent IE3$^-$	Mouse liver hepatocytes	Canine factor IX	HSV LAT	3–5 weeks	29
Attenuated TK$^-$	Mouse CNS	HPRT	HSV TK	Tansient	30

The potential of HSV mediated gene delivery to neurons within discrete regions of the nervous system in vivo relies on the stereotactic injection of a replication defective or amplicon vector carrying a physiologically relevant gene (Table). The observation that direct injection of an amplicon vector transiently expressing nerve growth factor into the superior cervical ganglia or rats prevented the decline of tyrosine hydroxylase levels after axotomy[25] was the first demonstration that an HSV vector could modify neuronal physiology in vivo. Using a similar approach Ho et al[26] have shown that an amplicon vector encoding the brain type glucose transporter gene injected directly into the rat hippocampus enhanced glucose transport at the injection site thus demonstrating that such a strategy can be used to alter central nervous system physiology. The genetic deficiency of β-glucoronidase, which results in a lysosomal storage disease affecting a number of organs including the CNS, has been a target for HSV mediated gene transfer.[27] In this study a replication competent HSV vector containing the β-glucoronidase gene placed under the control of the LAT promoter was used to infect a strain of mice lacking this enzyme. Although the lysosomal storage disease phenotype of infected mice was not altered in these experiments, β-glucoronidase gene expression was detected within a small number of neurons, both in the peripheral and central nervous system, for up to four months post-infection demonstrating the feasibility of the approach. In this instance, it will be of great interest to determine whether an increase in the level of transgene expression in addition to an increase in the number of transduced cells will be sufficient to observe a beneficial clinical effect.

The ability of HSV to latently infect non-neuronal cells in vitro[28] indicates that replication defective HSV vectors may also be useful in the stable transduction of other non-proliferating cell types in addition to post-mitotic neurons in vivo. Utilising a replication defective virus lacking the essential IE3 gene Miyanohara et al.[29] have successfully delivered genes encoding the Hepatitis B surface antigen or canine factor IX to murine liver and achieved high levels of foreign protein in the circulation. In this study more prolonged transgene expression was observed using the HSV LAT promoter in comparison to the HCMV IE promoter, a surprising result in view of the observation that the HCMV IE promoter has a very broad cell specificity whereas the LAT promoter appears to be neuron-specific in transient assays. This highlights the general problem of promoter selection.

It is clear that although HSV gene delivery vectors are in their early stages of development significant progress has been made with respect to the development of apathogenic replication defective and amplicon based systems. A major obstacle which has yet to be overcome, and remains problematic with all currently employed vector systems, is that of long-term expression. Thus although transient expression can be achieved readily with many well characterised promoters our understanding of the precise requirements which facilitate stable gene expression is poor and the influence of factors such as chromatin organisation, methylation and RNA stability have yet to be fully explored.

REFERENCES

1 Honess RW. Herpes simplex virus and 'the herpes complex': Diverse observations and a unifying hypothesis. J Gen Virol 1984; 65: 2077–2107.
2 Kieff E, Izumi K, Kaye K et al. Specifically mutated Epstein Barr virus recombinants: Defining the minimal genome for primary B lymphocyte transformation. In: Minson A, Neil J, McCrae M, eds. Viruses and cancer, Society for General Microbiology Symposium 51, Cambridge: Cambridge University Press, 1994; 123–146.
3 Glorioso J, Goins WF, Fink DJ. Herpes simplex virus-based vectors. Semin Virol 1992; 3: 265–276.
4 Breakefield OX, DeLuca NA. Herpes simplex virus for gene delivery to neurons. New Biol 1991; 3: 203–218.
5 Ugolini G, Kuypers HGJM, Strick PL. Transneuronal transfer of herpes virus from peripheral nerves to cortex and brainstem. Science 1989; 243: 89–91.
6 Simmons A, Tscharke DC. Anti-CD8 impairs clearance of herpes simplex virus from the nervous system: implications for the fate of virally infected neurons. J Exp Med 1992; 175: 1337–1344.
7 McGeoch DJ, Barnett BC, MacLean CA. Emerging functions of alphaherpesvirus genes. Semin Virol 1993; 4: 125–134.
8 Ho DY. Herpes simplex virus latency: Molecular aspects. Prog Med Virol 1992; 39: 76–115.
9 Chou J, Kern ER, Whitley RJ, Roizman B. Mapping of herpes simplex virus-1 neurovirulence to γ_1 34.5, a gene non-essential for growth in culture. Science 1990; 250: 1262–1265.
10 DeLuca NA, McCarthy A, Schaffer PA. Isolation and characterization of deletion mutants of herpes simplex virus type 1 in the gene encoding immediate-early regulatory protein ICP4. J Virol 1985; 56: 558–570.
11 Weinheimer SP, Boyd BA, Durham SK, Resnick JL, O'Boyle II DR. Deletion of the VP16 open reading frame of herpes simplex virus type 1. J Virol 1992; 66: 258–269.
12 Forrester A, Farrell H, Wilkinson G, Kaye J, Davis-Poynter N, Minson T. Construction and properties of a mutant of herpes simplex virus type 1 with glycoprotein H coding sequences deleted. J Virol 1992; 66: 341–348.
13 Johnson PA, Yoshida K, Gage FH, Friedmann T. Effects of gene transfer into cultured CNS neurons with a replication-defective herpes simplex virus type 1 vector. Mol Brain Res 1992; 12: 95–102.
14 Frenkel N, Singer O, Kwong AD. Minireview: The herpes simplex virus amplicon – a versatile defective virus vector. Gene Ther 1994; 1: S40–S46.
15 Geller AI, Breakefield XO. A defective HSV-1 vector expresses *Escherichia coli* β-galactosidase in cultured peripheral neurons. Science 1988; 241: 1667–1669.
16 Geller AI, Freese A. Infection of cultured central nervous system neurons with a defective herpes simplex virus 1 vector results in stable expression of *Escherichia coli* β-galactosidase. Proc Natl Acad Sci USA 1990; 87: 1149–1153.
17 Bloom DC, Lokensgard JR, Maidment NT, Feldman LT, Stevens JG. Long-term expression of genes *in vivo* using non-replicating HSV vectors. Gene Ther 1994; 1: S36–S38.
18 Dobson AT, Margolis TP, Sedarati F, Stevens JG, Feldman LT. A latent, nonpathogenic HSV-1 derived vector stably expresses β-galactosidase in mouse neurons. Neuron 1990; 5: 353–360.
19 Andersen JK, Garber DA, Meaney CA, Breakefield XO. Gene transfer into mammalian central nervous system using herpes virus vectors: extended expression

of bacterial *lacZ* in neurons using the neuron-specific enolase promoter. Hum Gene Ther 1992; 3: 487–499.

20 Dobson AT, Sedarati F, Devi-Rao G et al. Identification of the latency associated transcript promoter by expression of rabbit beta-globin mRNA in mouse sensory nerve ganglia latently infected with a recombinant herpes simplex virus. J Virol 1989; 63: 3844–3851.

21 Ho DY, Mocarski ES. Herpes simplex virus latent RNA (LAT) is not required for latent infection in the mouse. Proc Natl Acad Sci USA 1989; 86: 7596–7600.

22 Goins WF, Sternberg LR, Croen KD et al. A novel latency-active promoter is contained within the herpes simplex virus type 1 U_L flanking repeats. J Virol 1994; 68: 2239–2252.

23 Marglois TP, Bloom DC, Dobson AT, Feldman LT, Stevens JG. Decreased reporter gene expression during latent infection with HSV LAT promoter constructs. Virol 1993; 197: 585–592.

24 Deatly AM, Spivack JG, Lavi E, O'Boyle II DR, Fraser NW. Latent herpes simplex virus type 1 transcripts in peripheral and central nervous system tissues of mice map to similar regions of the virus genome. J Virol 1988; 62: 749–756.

25 Federoff HJ, Geschwind MD, Geller AI, Kessler JA. Expression of nerve growth factor in vivo from a defective herpes simplex virus 1 vector prevents effects of axotomy on sympathetic ganglia. Proc Natl Acad Sci USA 1992; 89: 1636–1640.

26 Ho DY, Mocarski ES, Sapolsky RM. Altering central nervous system physiology with a defective herpes simplex virus vector expressing the glucose transporter gene. Proc Natl Acad Sci USA 1993; 90: 3655–3659.

27 Wolf JH, Deshmane SL, Fraser NW. Herpesvirus vector gene transfer and expression of β-glucoronidase in the central nervous system of MPS VII mice. Nature Genet 1992; 1: 379–384.

28 Harris RA, Preston CM. Establishment of latency (*in vitro*) by the herpes simplex virus type 1 mutant *in* 1814. J Gen Virol 1991; 72: 907–913.

29 Miyanohara A, Johnson PA, Elam RL et al. Direct gene transfer to the liver with herpes simplex virus type 1 vectors: transient production of physiologically relevant levels of circulating factor IX. New Biol 1992; 4: 238–246.

30 Palella TD, Hidaki Y, Silverman LJ, Levine M, Glorioso J, Kelly WN. Expression of human HPRT mRNA in brains of mice with a recombinant herpes virus-1 vector. Gene 1989; 80: 137–144.

British Medical Bulletin (1995) Vol.51, No.1, pp.56–71

Non-viral approaches to gene therapy

J P Schofield[1] and C T Caskey[1,2]

[1]Department of Molecular and Human Genetics and [2] Howard Hughes Medical Institute, Baylor College of Medicine, Houston, Texas USA

There have been rapid advances in the development of non-viral techniques for gene transfer. Although viruses are highly evolved to infect mammalian cells, they have several limitations. The general theme is to mimic the advantageous components of viral systems whilst separating them from their limiting functions. The systems described here are broadly divided into true non-viral techniques and viral-assisted technologies. The merits and limitations of each method are presented, and examples of their application to current developments in gene therapy are discussed. At present no preferred technique has emerged as a clear favourite for non-viral delivery. Further refinement of the technology with particular emphasis on achieving long-term gene expression is required before initiating clinical trials of non-viral gene delivery.

Viruses infecting mammalian cells have evolved sophisticated and specific mechanisms for cell attachment, penetration, survival and replication. However, limitations of the relatively low titres and oncogenic potential of integrating retroviruses, as well as their requirement for active cell division,[1] has led to a recent research shift to explore alternative viruses for gene transfer. Adenoviruses can be recovered in high titres, are trophic for many cell types, and can transduce non-dividing cells.[2] However, major limitations of currently available adenoviral vectors include a packaging constraint of around 7.5 kb, and host immune rejection leading to destruction of transduced cells. These limitations provide an impetus to the development of alternative non-viral modes of DNA delivery. The ultimate goal is to imitate desirable features of viruses whilst avoiding their inherent limitations.

The aim of any gene therapy is to achieve an easy, safe, non-toxic delivery of DNA to a specified target tissue. On arrival at the tissue the DNA should be rapidly and efficiently endocytosed across the lipid bilayer, and directed to the host cell nucleus. Sequences encoded by the foreign DNA interacting with regulatory host factors should achieve long-term expression. This may require targeted integration into the host genomic DNA[3] existence as a stable episome,[4] or survival and propagation as a 'mini-chromosome'.[5] As with viral systems, there are several questions relating to non-viral gene transfer still to be overcome before in vivo human gene therapy is incorporated into daily clinical practice. *En route* to this goal fundamental scientific issues must be addressed, including a more detailed understanding of endocytosis, endosome destabilisation, nuclear transfer, and regulated long-term gene expression in transduced cells (Fig. 1).

Non-viral gene therapy can be broadly divided into truly non-viral methods, and virally-enhanced modes of delivery. We begin this chapter by reviewing the non-viral methods of DNA-coated particle bombardment, direct plasmid injection and cationic liposomes. This is followed by consideration of virally-enhanced methods including receptor-mediated transfer and the inactivated haemagglutinating virus of Japan (HVJ)-neutral liposome complex. Wherever possible, examples are given of applications of the techniques to deliver DNA to cells in tissue culture (i.e. in vitro), or by delivery to tissues in animals (i.e. in vivo). In general, a new gene transfer method is tested in vitro before proceeding to in vivo delivery. Several animal methods of human diseases have been genetically engineered to facilitate in vivo studies. [6–10] Pre-clinical trials investigate the most effective route of delivery, e.g. inhalation or injection into peripheral or central blood vessels. Questions of biological efficacy and toxicity are addressed by phase I clinical trials. If the data acquired from these studies support progression to testing in humans, approval is sought from governmental agencies (the Recombinant DNA Advisory Committee [RAC] of the National Institutes of Health [NIH], and The Food and Drug Administration [FDA], in the USA). Figures from the data management report of the RAC in June 1993 show 58 approved gene therapy clinical trials in USA, and a further 5 international trials.[11] Of these, only 3 trials use non-viral approaches to deliver DNA. This is a reflection of the more extensive experience using viral systems relative to the more recent developments described here.

NON-VIRAL GENE TRANSFER

Particle bombardment

It has been shown that particle bombardment is an effective means of gene transfer both in vitro and in vivo.[12] In this physical method plasmid DNA is first coated onto the surface of 1–3 micron diameter gold or

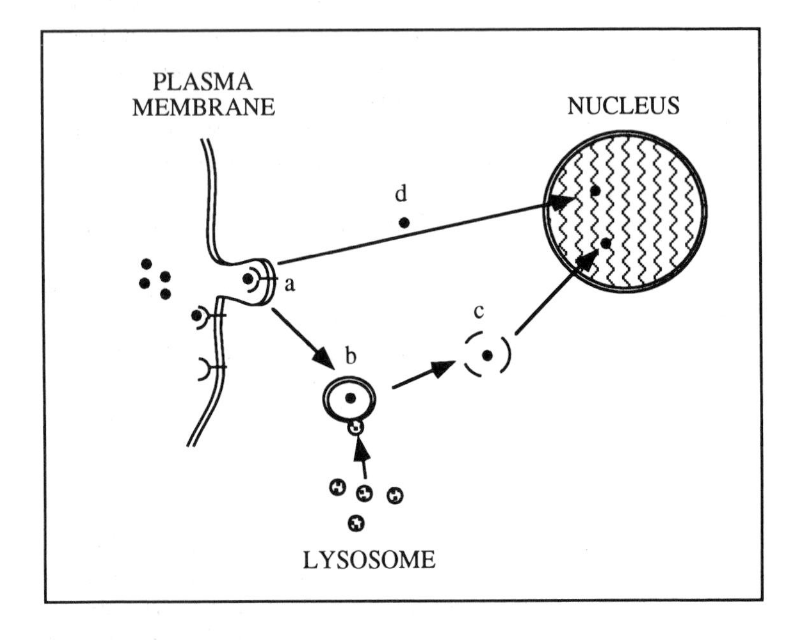

Fig. 1 Gene transfer and intracellular transport. Following arrival at the target tissue, there are several obstacles to be overcome before the DNA can reach the nucleus. The gene-delivery complex binds to the cell surface, and is endocytosed (a). Intracellular lysosomes fuse with the endocytic vesicle to form an endosome (b). To prevent nuclease degradation of the DNA, adenovirus penton base protein disrupts the endosome (c), releasing DNA into the cytoplasm. The DNA can then pass to the nucleus, aided by a nuclear localisation signal encoded within its sequence. Cationic liposomes and the HVJ-liposome complex fuse directly with the cell membrane, and release DNA into the cytoplasm (d), facilitating rapid gene transfer to the host cell nucleus.

tungsten beads. These particles are accelerated by an electric discharge device, or gas pulse (e.g. Accell® gene delivery system, Agracetus, Middleton, Wisconsin, USA, Fig. 2), and 'fired' at the tissue. A less invasive approach is by direct particle bombardment of the skin.[13] The physical force of impact overcomes the cell membrane barrier. However, the variable tissue characteristics of rigidity, foreign DNA processing, and intrinsic transcriptional capacity lead to wide variations in the efficiency of overall gene expression. For example a 1000-fold higher expression of an identical luciferase (*luc*) reporter gene was observed for bombarded rat epidermis in comparison to muscle tissues.[14] The level of expression in treated rat epidermis, liver and pancreas peaked within 3 days and rapidly declined to between 1–5% of peak levels after

1 week.[14] Analysis have shown that once inside the cell the foreign DNA does not integrate into the host cell genome, and exists as a relatively unstable episome. This would suggest a limited application of this technology for gene therapy, but could be useful for rapid screening of tissue-specific DNA expression constructs.

The requirement for a surgical procedure has also been cited as a major limitation in transferring this technology to human subjects. However, endoscopic surgical techniques could make this less of an objection. Finally, a more feasible development is the use of direct particle bombardment as part of a vaccination protocol. Ulmer and colleagues[15] demonstrated a protective immune response in mice following direct muscle injection of the gene encoding influenza A matrix protein. The mice were resistant to future challenge with influenza virus. Similar vaccination results have been obtained by DNA-coated particle bombardment of mouse ear epidermis, which is more accessible than muscle tissue.[16]

Direct DNA injection

In this method pure closed-circular plasmid DNA or RNA is directly injected into the desired tissue. Using direct skeletal muscle injection Wolff et al[17] showed significant levels of expression of the reporter gene constructs within mouse skeletal muscle cells. The longevity of expression showed persistence of injected DNA for at least 60 days, although the RNA transcript and protein had a half-life of less than 24 h. Southern blot DNA analysis suggested that the DNA exists as a non-replicating closed circular episome. The precise mechanism of nucleic acid uptake across the cell membrane into the muscle cell was postulated to be a result of the favourable structural features of multinucleate cells, sarcoplasmic reticulum, and extensive transverse tubular system. The latter contains extracellular fluid, and deeply penetrates the muscle cells, facilitating DNA transfer. Cell regeneration has been demonstrated to stimulate increased uptake of plasmid DNA injected into the tibialis anterior skeletal muscle of mice.[18] The muscle was treated with a snake (*Niga nigricollis*) cardiotoxic venom followed by a comparison of reporter gene expression, either luciferase or bacterial (*Escherichia coli*) β-galactosidase (*lac*Z). The former is assayed by luminescent emission, whilst the latter is detected by a colorimetric assay. A colourless chromogenic substrate X-gal is converted to a blue compound by *lac*Z. The *lac*Z reporter plasmid studies demonstrated that the increased expression in regenerating muscle was due to a greater cellular uptake and expression rather than increased expression levels in immature and growing cells. Finally, this study compared injection of plasmids with reporter adenoviral and retroviral constructs. Histology

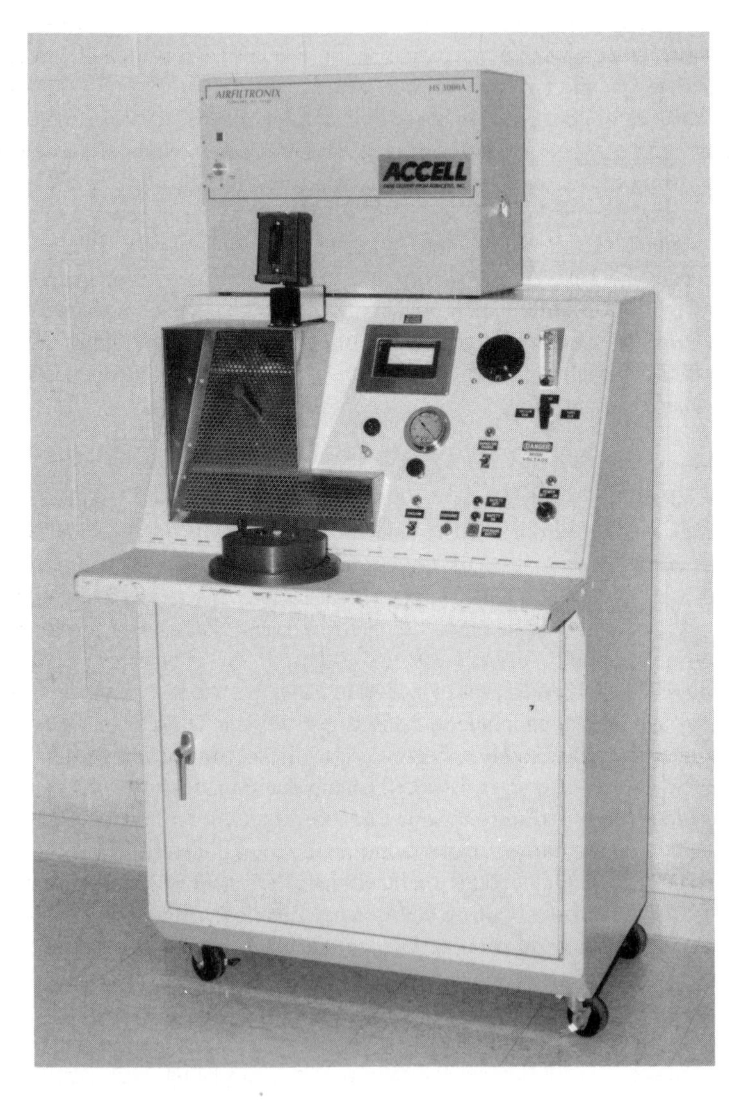

Fig. 2 The Accell® gene delivery device. The particle bombardment instrument acts as a shock wave generator. DNA coated gold beads are accelerated to any desired velocity by varying the input voltage. This large instrument was originally developed for gene delivery to cell cultures, and as a power supply for early hand-held devices. More recent hand-held devices that deliver a gas pulse are now used in surgical settings and vaccine applications (K Barton, personal communication).

indicated that expression of adenoviral and retroviral DNA was less than for pure plasmid. There was also a marked inflammatory response with adenovirus, with a mononuclear endomysial space infiltrate and little myofibre staining. As expected, retroviral transfection and expression were limited to actively regenerating cells, and again there was extensive endomysial cellular infiltration. The method of direct plasmid DNA injection is a simple, inexpensive, and non-toxic procedure when compared to viral delivery. The potential to carry large DNA constructs is also advantageous. However, the levels and persistence of gene expression is probably too short (days). This technology may, however, have potential as a vaccination procedure, as low level gene expression is often sufficient to achieve an immunological response. In contrast, it would be unacceptable to consider correction of widespread myopathic diseases such as Duchenne muscular dystrophy by multiple injections of many muscle groups on repeated occasions.

Cationic liposomes

This technique relies upon the electrical charge properties of DNA (negative due to the phosphate backbone of the double-helix), cationic lipids (positive), and cell surfaces (net negative due to sialic acid residues).

Monocationic lipids such as DOTMA[19] (*N*[1-(2,3-dioleyloxy)-propyl]-*NNN*-trimethylammonium chloride) and the second generation polycationic lipid DOPSA[20] (2,3-dioleyloxy-*N*-[2(sperminecarboxamido)ethyl]-*NN*-dimethyl-l-propanaminiumtrifluoroacetate (Fig. 3) form liposomes which spontaneously bind polyanionic DNA or RNA. The resulting complex stably captures 100% of the polynucleotide, and by charge attraction and fusion properties, the lipids can adsorb to the cell membrane and deliver the nucleic acid directly into the cytoplasm, bypassing the lysosomal degradation pathway. The ratio of lipid to DNA/RNA, as well as the total concentration has to be carefully optimised to avoid toxicity observed with high doses. This method is in widespread use as an efficient means of transfecting DNA into a wide variety of cell lines grown in tissue culture. Commercial kits are now available (e.g. LipofectAMINE® reagent, GIBCO BRL, Gaithersburg, Maryland, USA). The spermine head group of DOSPA confers an approximately 30-fold higher transfection efficiency of up to 90% in vitro in comparison to the monocationic DOTMA.[20]

Several studies have shown the effectiveness of polycationic liposome delivery of DNA in vivo. This method is an attractive alternative to viral transfer methods due to the no DNA size constraints, lower immunogenicity, and easier bulk preparation. Alton et al[21] delivered cDNA encoding the human cystic fibrosis transmembrane conductance regulator (CFTR) to the lungs of cystic fibrosis mutant mice. This was

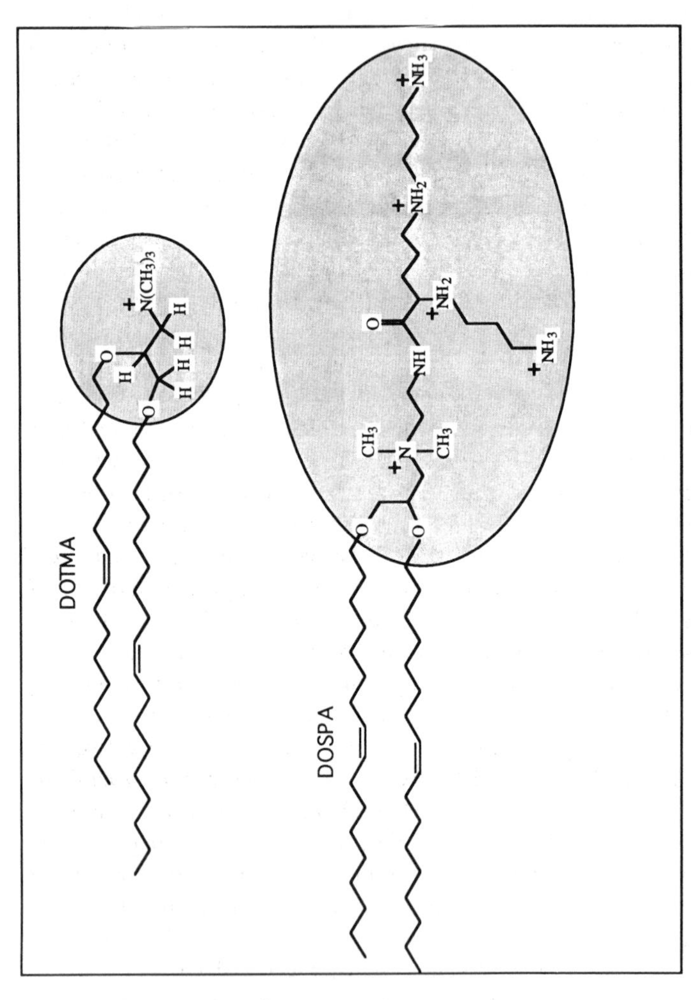

Fig. 3 Structure of lipids used to form cationic liposomes. The monocationic lipid DOTMA (*N*[1-)2,3-*dio*leyloxy)propyl]-*NNN-tri*methyl*am*monium chloride) has a single positively charged head-group. The second generation lipid DOSPA (2,3-*dio*eyloxy-*N*-[2(*s*perminecarboxyamido)ethyl]-*NN*-dimethyl-1-*p*ropanaminiumtrifluoroacetate, has a polycationic spermine head-group, conferring a charge of +5 at neutral pH.

as a nebulised preparation complexed with the cationic liposome formulation DC-chol/DOPE (3β-N-N′,N′-dimethylamino ethanecarbamoyl] cholesterol/dioleoyl phosphatidylethanolamine). This lipid combination was used as it has received approval for human trials, and has been shown by in vitro studies to be at least as effective as DOTAP (N-[1-(2,3-dioleoyloxy) propyl]-N,N,N,-trimethylammoniummethyl-sulphate) or DOTAP/DOPE. Initial studies using a β-galactosidase reporter gene showed that up to 40% of surface epithelial cells in the trachea and extrapulmonary bronchi stained blue to X-gal. There was no evidence of significant inflammation or tissue necrosis. Expression of CFTR mRNA was demonstrated by qualitative RNA reverse-transcriptase polymerase chain reaction (RT-PCR). The investigators concluded that some mice demonstrated complete correction, whilst others showed only partial correction, as judged by CFTR mRNA expression and electrophysiological studies. However, there were significant variations between animals, and only limited conclusions could be drawn which may be applied to treatment of humans. Perhaps the most intensively studied tissue for cationic liposome delivery in vivo is the arterial vessel wall. Cardiovascular disease is the commonest cause of morbidity and mortality in industrialised societies. DNA-liposome catheter delivery systems are feasible, but are limited by low transfection efficiencies and toxicity regardless of the vector DNA-liposome system used. Nabel et al[22] estimated that fewer than 1% of cells were successfully transduced when using a double-balloon catheter to transfect porcine ilio-femoral arteries with a liposome-β-galactosidase gene complex. An ability to increase the dose of cationic liposome would be predicted to increase the transfection efficiency, although this has proved to be limited by the cell toxicity at increased concentrations. To address this problem a novel cationic liposome formulation has been recently reported, consisting of DMRIE[23] (dimyristyloxy-propyl-3-dimethyl-hydroxyetyl ammonium/DOPE. Doses of up to 1000-fold higher than those used previously were injected into mice and pigs. Histopathology of major organs, together with serum biochemistry of enzymes from heart, liver, kidney and bone showed no significant abnormalities compared with control animals. There was also a slight (2- to 7-fold) increase in transfection efficiency of DMRIE/DOPE compared to DC-chol/DOPE.

As discussed earlier for direct injection of DNA into muscle cells, the proliferative state of the cell population targeted by cationic liposomes has a profound effect on transfection efficiency. Miller et al[1] showed a 100-fold inhibition of gene transfer in stationary versus replicating cells. Takeshita et al[24] have demonstrated a greater than 10-fold increase in gene expression after cationic liposome-mediated arterial transfer. This was achieved through stimulation of intimal smooth muscle cell proliferation by balloon angioplasty damage. The mechanism(s) of how cell proliferation augments liposome-mediated DNA transfer and expression is speculative. One proposed hypothesis is that the disruption of the nuclear membrane of the targeted cell which occurs during mitosis may release into the cytoplasm DNA-stabilising nuclear factors. The transfected DNA may then be protected by these factors from host cell nuclease digestion by a combination of structural and/or intracellular partitioning. One prediction resulting from this study is that gene transfer directed to prevent vessel restenosis could be favoured by delivery to this actively proliferating tissue rather than targetting quiescent primary atherosclerotic plaques. The future of cationic liposome-mediated gene delivery to the cardiovascular system looks promising in the light of these recent developments.

VIRUS-ENHANCED GENE DELIVERY

Receptor-mediated gene transfer

In this method DNA is conjugated with a cell-specific carrier molecule which is the ligand for a surface receptor. Most research has targeted the hepatocyte-specific asialoglycoprotein receptor[25] (ASGPr, approximately 500 000 per cell). Transferrin-polylysine/DNA conjugates have also been used, which bind transferrin receptors.[26] The liver is of central importance to metabolism, and is an obvious target for gene therapy, as many human metabolic disorders are secondary to hepatic enzyme deficiencies. As described previously for cationic liposomes, DNA is 'packaged' in an electrostatic complex, here using asialoorosmucoid-polylysine (ASOR-PL) in place of lipid (Fig. 4). This covalently cross-linked receptor ligand-polycation conjugate interacts with polyanionic DNA, and efficiently binds to ASGPrs on the hepatocyte surface. Careful purification of the ASOR-PL conjugates is essential, as is optimisation of the ratio of conjugate to DNA. Once this has been achieved it is a relatively inexpensive and simple procedure to perform a peripheral venous injection, avoiding the need for selective vessel catheterisation, as there is an inbuilt tissue targeting signal. Two further significant advantages are the low immunogenicity of the complex, and the ability to transfer large fragments of DNA (up to 48 kb). This is in direct contrast to current viral transfer methods. The low immunogenicity should enable multiple injections, which would almost certainly be necessary for currently available DNA constructs, as the in vivo efficiency of gene expression is relatively low, and rapidly declines with time (*see* below). Investigations of the efficiency and specificity of this system have shown that 85% of intravenously injected ASOR-PL-DNA complexes are taken up by the liver within 10 min.[27] An example of the application of this system has been the lowering of serum cholestrerol following delivery of the gene encoding the low density lipoprotein receptor (LDLr) to the hyperlipidaemic Watanabe rabbit.[28]

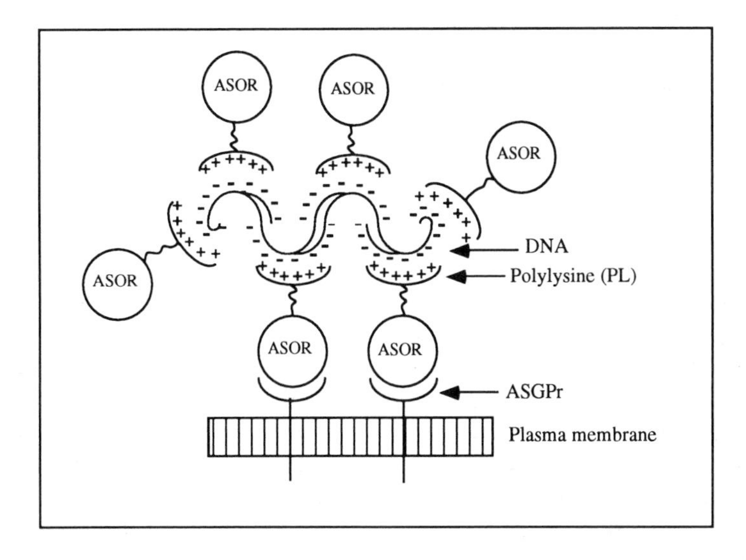

Fig. 4 Receptor-mediated gene delivery. The ASOR-PL-DNA electrostatic complex delivers DNA to the surface of cells bearing asialoglycoprotein receptors (ASGPr). Asialoorosomucoid (ASOR) is prepared by desialation of orosomucoid, using either acid or neuraminidase enzyme. ASOR-PL is formed by cross-linkage between ASOR and polylysine (PL) using carbodiimide or thiol chemistry.

Following hepatocyte receptor-mediated endocytosis (via ASGPrs), DNA is trapped within intracellular vesicles. It is at this stage that this otherwise elegant system encounters a significant limitation. Cytoplasmic liposomes fuse with the DNA-containing vesicles, forming endosomes. The DNA is largely degraded by the action of liposomal nucleases within the acidified endosome. The addition of the anti-malarial drug, chloroquine has been one method employed to increase DNA survival by inhibition of endosomal acidification.[29] Human adenovirus also enters the cell by receptor-mediated endocytosis, followed by movement into clathrin-coated pits and eventually into endosomes. At the body-temperature optimum of 37°C, and at an acidic pH 5.5–6.0, the virus disrupts the endosome membrane, allowing escape into the cytoplasm and translocation to the host cell nucleus. Adenovirus particles devoid of DNA (i.e. empty capsids) are also endosomolytic, although the efficiency is reduced relative to intact adenovirus. The adenovirus capsid has 3 major proteins: the hexon-, the fiber- and the penton base proteins. To investigate which of these proteins is involved in plasma membrane disruption, Seth[30] has shown that only antibodies to the penton base protein prevented the release of [^{3}H] choline from plasma membrane vesicles at an acidic pH. The precise mechanism of how this occurs is still uncertain. Several research groups have utilised the endosmolytic properties of adenovirus by coupling them to polylysine/DNA complexes.[31–33] Using this approach the cytoplasmic delivery and expression of transfected genes increases by as much as 1000-fold. Chemical or antibody-mediated coupling between adenovirus and the ASOR-PL-DNA complex ensures co-localisation within the endosome. In an attempt to simplify the system further, and to avoid the use of the intact virus, researchers are now characterising individual viral proteins and synthetic peptides that have demonstrated endosmolytic properties. One well studied system is the fusogenic influenza virus membrane glycoprotein, haemagglutinin. Synthetic peptides (HA-2) have been characterised, which undergo fusion with the endosomal membrane at acidic pH. Conjugation of HA-2 peptides with transferrin-polylysine-DNA conjugates considerably enhance gene delivery into the cytoplasm and then the host cell nucleus.[34] Rapid advances are being made to further develop the in vivo utility of these artificial viral complexes. In the near future the ultimate goal of a simple intravenous injection of a targeted non-viral delivery system may reach clinical application.

The inactivated Sendai virus-liposome complex

Delivery of active transgenes to the host cell nucleus could be enhanced if shuttling through the endosome is avoided. The haemagglutinating virus of Japan (HVJ; also called Sendai virus) is non-pathogenic in humans, although it causes a severe pneumonia in mice. Following attachment to the plasma membrane at the cell surface (via the spike coat glycoprotein HN), membrane fusion occurs, releasing the viral contents at neutral pH directly into the host cell cytoplasm. Kaneda et al[35] have developed a system which combines the advantages of liposome carrying capacity for large DNA fragments with the fusion properties of HVJ virus. A further advantage is the ability to deliver protein as well as

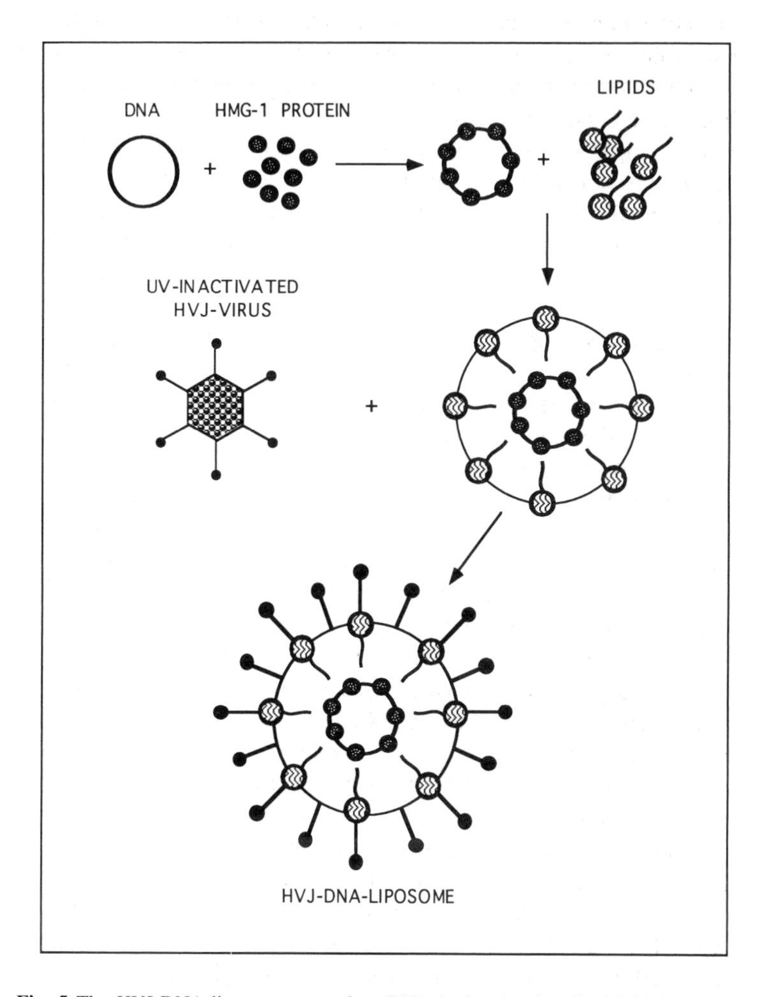

Fig. 5 The HVJ-DNA-lipsosome complex. DNA is first incubated with high mobility group-1 (HMG-1) protein. Liposomes are formed by reverse-evaporation of neutral lipids. The DNA-HMG-1 is packaged into liposomes by repeated vortexing then sonication. Finally HVJ-liposomes are prepared by mixing, incubation at 37°C for 1h, and concentration by sucrose density gradient centrifugation.

DNA in the HVJ-liposome complex. DNA is condensed by mixing with a non-histone chromosomal high mobility group-1 protein (HMG-1).[36] This protein appears to increase the efficiency of nuclear translocation and expression following cell surface fusion. Neutral lipids (cholesterol, phosphatidyl choline and phosphatidyl serine) are then mixed with the DNA-HMG-1 complex. Liposomes are formed by the chemical method of reverse-phase evaporation, and the precise ratio of components is critical to the formation of good liposomes. The HVJ virus is inactivated by brief exposure to ultraviolet irradiation, then mixed with the DNA-HMG-1 loaded liposomes to facilitate HVJ-mediated membrane fusion (Fig. 5). The HVJ-liposome is efficient in gene delivery for both in vitro and in vivo applications. This method has been used for gene delivery to vascular walls,[37] liver[38] and kidney.[39] This method is efficient, easy to perform, requires short incubation times for transfection, and theoretically has an unlimited DNA fragment size capacity. However, following peripheral vein injection the majority of the HVJ-liposomes are concentrated in the reticulo-endothelial system, with little organ uptake. Specific organ uptake requires catheterisation of vessels, e.g. renal artery, hepatic portal vein, or coronary arteries. The precise amount of HVJ-liposome complex which binds to red cell membranes is unknown, though it is estimated to be low. The main disadvantages are concerns regarding the use of intact HVJ virus, despite assurances of its non-pathogenicity in humans, and the short duration of expression of delivered transgenes. For example, expression of a human insulin gene delivered to rat liver decreased rapidly after only 7–8 days.[38] The delivered DNA is not integrated into the host genomic DNA, and exists as an (unstable) episome. Research in this field has logically switched to the development of mechanisms to increase DNA stability and/or integration to improve the prospects for long-term expression. Herein lies an advantage of this system in having the ability to co-deliver DNA with any protein in the HVJ-liposome complex. It is naive to expect that the delivery of naked plasmid expression constructs to the non-dividing host cell nucleus will achieve long-term expression. Genomic DNA is a complex structure, whose stability is the result of supercoiling into nucleosomes (involving histone and non-histone proteins) and then chromosomes. Attachment to the nuclear membrane and matrix is also required. It could be predicted that DNA stability may be increased by 'coating' the DNA with chromosomal proteins, and/or other nuclear proteins. Although HMG-1 may be partially effective, further research is continuing to improve DNA stability using chromosomal binding proteins. Integration may be possible in future by the co-delivery of DNA recombinase enzymes within the HVJ-liposome. The commercially available bacterial recombinase, *rec*A has been tried without success in non-dividing mammalian cells (Y Kaneda, personal communication). However, a structural comparison between *rec*A and recently discovered yeast, mouse and human recombinases[40] shows significant amino-terminus differences, which may partially explain this failure.

Although transient expression is a major disadvantage of the HVJ-liposome system at present, it has shown utility as an alternative to transgenic animal models of disease. Animal models of human diseases are fundamental to the development of gene therapy strategies. As an example, glomerulosclerosis is a final common lesion in several renal glomerular diseases. Isaka et al[39] selectively injected DNA plasmid vectors expressing transforming growth factor β(TGF-β) and platelet-derived growth factor-B (PDGF-B) into rat renal arteries via encapsulation in HVJ-liposomes. Using this method, glomerulosclerosis was induced. The TGF-β led to an increased extracellular matrix production, and PDGF-B stimulated mesangial cell proliferation. In future, a greater understanding of the involvement of growth factors in glomerulosclerosis may facilitate new treatments, e.g. by renal delivery of HVJ-liposomes containing anti-sense RNAs against selective growth factors to inhibit this scarring process.

CONCLUSION

The techniques for gene transfer in vivo are in a rapid phase of development. The ultimate goal is simple, non-invasive, safe and efficient gene delivery which can be incorporated into clinical practice. The challenge is long-term expression of the transferred genes, so that ideally , a single life-time treatment can be possible. In order for this to be achieved, answers to many fundamental biological questions of gene expression must be addressed. A summary that still applies today was made in 1992 by the gene therapist W French Anderson, who stated that: 'Gene therapy will have a major impact on the health care of our population only when vectors are developed that can safely and efficiently be injected into patients as drugs like insulin are now.'

ACKNOWLEDGEMENTS

JPS is supported by The Wellcome Trust. CTC is an Investigator of the Howard Hughes Medical Institute.

REFERENCES

1 Miller DG, Adam MA, Miller AD. Gene transfer by retroviral vectors occurs only in cells that are actively dividing at the time of infection. Mol Cell Biol 1990; 10: 4239–4242.
2 Berkner KL. Development of adenovirus vectors for the expression of heterologous genes. Biotechniques 1988; 6: 616–629.
3 Arbonés ML, Austin HA, Capon DJ, Greenburg G. Gene targeting in normal somatic cells: inactivation of the interferon-γ receptor in myoblasts. Nature Genet 1994; 6: 90–96.
4 Cooper MJ, Miron S. Efficient episomal expression vector for human transitional carcinoma cells. Hum Gene Ther 1993; 4: 557–566.
5 Huxley C. Mammalian artifical chromosomes: a new tool for gene therapy. Gene Ther 1994; 1: 7–12.
6 Dorin JR, Dickinson P, Alton EWFW et al. Cystic fibrosis in the mouse by targeted insertional mutagenesis. Nature 1992; 359: 211–215.

7 Ferrari G, Rossini S, Giavazzi R et al. An in vivo model of somatic cell gene therapy for human severe combined immunodeficiency. Science 1991; 251: 1363–1366.
8 Jones SN, Grompe M, Munir MI et al. Ectopic correction of ornithine transcarbamylase deficiency in sparse fur mice. J Biol Chem 1990; 265: 14684–14690.
9 Lawn RM, Wade DP, Hammer RE, Chiesa G, Verstuyft JG, Rubin EM. Atherogenesis in transgenic mice expressing human apolipoprotein(a). Nature 1993; 360: 670–672.
10 Wilson JM, Johnston DE, Jefferson DM, Mulligan RC. Correction of the genetic defect in hepatocytes from the Watanabe heritable hyperlipidaemic rabbit. Proc Natl Acad Sci USA 1988; 85: 4421–4425.
11 Human gene marker/therapy clinical protocols. In: Anderson WF, ed. Hum Gene Ther 1993; 4: 847–856.
12 Yang N-S, Burkholder J, Roberts B, Martinell B, McCabe D. In vivo and in vitro gene transfer to mammalian somatic cells by particle bombardment. Proc Natl Acad Sci USA 1991: 88 2726–2730.
13 Williams RS, Johnston SA, Riedy M, DeVit JM, McElligott SG, Sanford JC. Introduction of foreign genes into tissues of living mice by DNA-coated microprojectiles. Proc Natl Acad Sci USA 1991; 88: 2726–2730.
14 Cheng L, Ziegelhoffer PR, Yang N-S. In vivo promoter activity and transgene expression in mammalian somatic tisues evaluated by using particle bombardment. Proc Natl Acad Sci USA 1993; 90: 4455–4459.
15 Ulmer J, Donnelly J, Parker S, et al. Heterologous protection against influenza by injection of DNA encoding a viral protein. Science 1993; 259: 1745–1749.
16 Tang D, DeVit M, Johnston SA. Genetic immunisation is a simple method for eliciting an immune response. Nature 1992; 356: 152–154.
17 Wolff JA, Malone RW, Williams P, et al. Direct gene transfer into mouse muscle in vivo. Science 1990; 247: 1465–1468.
18 Davis HL, Demeneix BA, Quantin B, Coulombe J, Whalen RG. Plasmid DNA is superior to viral vectors for direct gene transfer into adult mouse skeletal muscle. Hum Gene Ther 1993; 4: 733–740.
19 Felgner PL, Gadek TR, Holm M, et al. Lipofection: A highly efficient, lipid-mediated DNA transfection procedure. Proc Natl Acad Sci USA 1987; 84: 7413–7417.
20 Hawley-Nelson P, Ciccarone V, Gebeyehu G, Jessee J, Felgner PL. Lipofectamine® reagent: a new, higher efficiency polycationic liposome transfection reagent. Focus 1993; 15: 73–78.
21 Alton EWFW, Middleton PG, Caplen NJ, et al. Non-invasive liposome-mediated gene delivery can correct the ion transport defect in cystic fibrosis mutant mice. Nature Genet 1993; 5: 135–142.
22 Nabel EG, Plautz G, Nabel GJ. Site-specific gene expression in vivo by direct gene transfer into arterial wall. Science 1990; 249: 1285–1288.
23 San H, Yang Z-Y, Pompli VJ, et al. Safety and short-term toxicity of a novel cationic lipid formulation for human gene therapy. Hum Gene Ther 1993; 4: 781–788.
24 Takeshita S, Gal D, Leclerc G, et al. Increased gene expression after liposome-mediated arterial transfer associated with intimal smooth muscle cell proliferation. J Clin Invest 1994; 93: 652–661.
25 Wu, CH, Wilson JM, Wu GY. Targetting genes: delivery and persistent expression of a foreign gene driven by mammalian regulatory elements in vivo. J Biol Chem 1989; 269: 16985–16987.
26 Wagner E, Zatloukal K, Cotten M, et al. Coupling of adenovirus to transferrin-polylysine/DNA complexes greatly enhances receptor-mediated gene delivery and expression of transfected genes. Proc Natl Acad Sci USA 1992; 89: 6099–6103.
27 Wu GY, Wu CH. Receptor-mediated gene delivery and expression in vivo. J Biol Chem 1988; 263: 14621–14624.
28 Wilson JM, Grossman M, Cabrera JA, et al. Hepatocyte-directed gene transfer in vivo leads to transient improvement of hypercholesterolemia in low density lipoprotein-deficient rabbits. J Biol Chem 1992; 267: 963–967.
29 Tietz PS, Yamazaki K, LaRusso NF. Time-dependent effects of chloroquine on pH of hepatocyte lysosomes. Biochem Pharmacol 1990; 40: 1419–1421.

30 Seth P. Adenovirus-dependent release of choline from plasma membrane vesicles at an acidic pH is mediated by the penton base protein. J Virol 1994; 68: 1204–1206.
31 Cristiano RJ, Smith LC, Woo SLC. Hepatic gene therapy: Adenovirus enhancement of receptor-mediated gene delivery and expression in primary hepatocytes. Proc Natl Acad Sci USA 1993; 90: 2122–2126.
32 Curiel DT, Agarwal S, Wagner E, Cotten M. Adenovirus enhancement of transferrin-polylysine mediated gene delivery. Proc Natl Acad Sci USA 1991; 88: 8850–8854.
33 Cotten M, Wagner E, Zatloukal K, Phillips S, Curiel D, Birnstiel J. High-efficiency receptor-mediated delivery of small and large (48kb) gene constructs using the endosome-disruption activity of defective or chemically-inactivated adenovirus particles. Proc Natl Acad Sci USA 1992; 89: 6094–6098.
34 Wagner E, Plank C, Zatloukal K, Cotten M, Birnstiel ML. Influenza virus haemagglutinin HA-2 N-terminal fusogenic peptides augment gene transfer by transferrin-polylysine-DNA complexes: towards a synthetic virus-like gene-transfer vehicle. Proc Natl Acad Sci USA 1992; 89: 7934–7938.
35 Kaneda Y, Iwai K, Uchida T. Increased expression of DNA cointroduced with nuclear protein in adult rat liver. Science 1989; 243: 375–378.
36 Kato K, Nakanishi M, Kaneda Y, Uchida T, Okada Y. Expression of hepatitis B virus surface antigen in adult rat liver: co-introduction of DNA and nuclear protein by a simplified liposome method. J Biol Chem 1991; 266: 3361–3364.
37 Dzau VJ, Morishita R, Gibbons GH. Gene therapy for cardiovascular disease. Trends Biotechnol 1993; 11: 205–210.
38 Kaneda Y, Iwai K, Uchida T. Introduction and expression of the human insulin gene in adult rat liver. J Biol Chem 1989; 264: 12126–12129.
39 Isaka Y, Fujiwara Y, Ueda N, Kaneda Y, Kamada T, Imai E. Glomerulosclerosis induced by in vivo transfection of transforming growth factor-β or platelet-derived growth factor gene into the rat kidney. J Clin Invest 1993; 92: 2597–2601.
40 Shinohara A, Ogawa H, Matsuda Y, Ushio N, Ikeo K, Ogawa T. Cloning of human, mouse, and fission yeast recombination genes homologous to RAD51 and *rec*A. Nature Genet 1993; 4: 239–243.
41 Anderson WF. Human gene therapy. Science 1992; 256: 808–813.

British Medical Bulletin (1995) Vol. 51, No. 1 pp.72–81

Gene therapy for adenosine deaminase deficiency

P M Hoogerbrugge[1,2], V W v Beusechem[3], L C M Kaptein[1], M P W Einerhand[1] and D Valerio[1,3]

[3]Department of Medical Biochemistry and [2]Department of Pediatrics, [3]University of Leiden, IntroGene B.V., Rijswijk The Netherlands

In the last decade, gene transfer into hematopoietic cells has evolved from an experimental procedure which resulted in successfully transduced in vitro hematopoietic colonies to the first clinical trials in patients suffering from severe combined immunodeficiency disease caused by the absence of functional adenosine deaminase. Significant in vivo expression of the newly introduced gene encoding human adenosine deaminase has been observed in descendents of murine and rhesus monkey hematopoietic stem cells following retrovirus mediated gene transfer. So far, 10 patients have received genetically repaired T-cells, hematopoietic stem cells or both without the appearance of any side effect. The clinical bone marrow gene transfer studies differ largely from the monkey studies with respect to myeloablation, which was applied in the monkey studies, but not in the patient studies. Ongoing studies in patients show that the introduced gene is present in circulating blood cells. In the initial phase of the trial, the frequency of transduced circulating blood cells is lower than in rhesus monkey studies. This difference may be contributed to the fact that conditioning was not performed in the patients.

Adenosine deaminase (ADA) is an enzyme involved in the purine salvage pathway. Absence of the enzyme leads to accumulation of one of its substrates, deoxyadenosine, which is primarily cytotoxic for T-cells, and, to a lesser extend, B-cells, resulting in the absence of adequate numbers of functioning T- and B-cells. In affected individuals, this leads to a severe combined immunodeficiency disease (SCID), which is usually fatal within 1 to 2 years. The affected children suffer from frequent, severe infections, which generally are the cause of death in these patients. Additional features of the disease are skeletal abnormalities, including cupping and flaring of the costochondral junctions and growth delay. A minority of patients suffer from a less severe form of the disease, resulting in late onset immunodeficiency disease.[1]

Allogeneic bone marrow transplantation (BMT) is the treatment of choice for children with SCID due to ADA deficiency (ADA-SCID). If an HLA-identical sibling is available as bone marrow donor, the cure rate of allogeneic BMT for SCID, including ADA-SCID, has increased from approximately 60% one decade ago to 90–100% at present. A successful BMT results in the occurrence of donor derived T-cells, even in children who were not pretreated with myelo-ablative chemotherapy prior to BMT. Interestingly, following BMT in non-conditioned patients, the myelopoietic lineages remain of recipient type, in contrast to the T-cells, resulting in so-called mixed chimerism. The occurrence of mixed chimerism suggests that phenotypically competent T-cells have a selective growth advantage over the defective T-cells of the recipient. The B-cells may be of either donor or recipient origin. Survival in patients transplanted with marrow from a non-HLA-identical sibling donor is around 50%. In this group of patients, immune recovery of both T- or B-cell lineage may be absent after BMT, and, little improvement in the outcome of BMT has been seen over the past 10 years. Successful engraftment of T-cells in these children can only be obtained after pretreatment with high dose chemotherapy prior to BMT.[2] For children with ADA-SCID, weekly injection of bovine ADA conjugated to polyethylene glycol (PEG-ADA) has been used as an alternative therapy, resulting in immune recovery in at least 35 children with a follow-up up to 6 years. [3]

In the last decade, techniques to stably introduce genes into bone marrow and blood cells have been developed. So far, stable expression of the introduced gene in blood cells has only been obtained following retrovirus-mediated gene transfer (for reviews *see:* Valerio[4] and Russell, this issue). Since the ADA-gene was cloned,[5] ADA-SCID is regarded as one of the first target diseases for gene therapy trials for various reasons. In the first place, ADA-SCID is a fatal disease for which the current treatment of choice, HLA-identical allogeneic BMT, is only applicable in 25–30% of the patients. In patients lacking an HLA-identical bone marrow donor, BMT is counterbalanced by high mortality and morbidity. In the second place, based on the results following allogeneic BMT, it is expected that the genetically modified cells reinfused in the patient following successful gene transfer will have a selective growth advantage over the afflicted cells of the patient. In the third place, the expression of the ADA gene does not necessarily have to be precisely regulated.

As the defect responsible for the clinical disease in ADA-SCID is in the T-cells, which are derived from the hematopoietic stem cell, gene therapy approaches in ADA deficiency have been performed, aiming at the introduction of the ADA gene in T-lymphocytes or hematopoietic stem cells (HSCs). Both approaches and the preclinical studies preceding these clinical trials will be reviewed.

GENE TRANSFER INTO ADA DEFICIENT T-CELLS

Kantoff et al [6] showed that transfer of a functional human ADA (hADA) gene into immortalized T-cells from patients with ADA deficiency results in increased ADA expression of the transduced T-cells. We used the virus producing cell line entitled POC-1[7] for gene transfer studies into freshly isolated ADA deficient Tcells. This cell line sheds a retroviral vector designated L*g*AL(ΔMo+PyF101). In this vector, the hADA gene is placed under transcriptional control of a hybrid long terminal repeat (LTR), in which the enhancer of the wild-type Moloney murine leukemia virus was replaced by a mutant polyoma virus enhancer (PyF101). [8] This LTR was chosen as it helped to overcome the expression block in the progeny of transduced hematopoietic stem cells.[9] Following co-cultivation of T-cells from an ADA deficient patient, approximately 3–5% of the T-cells were stably transduced. Following selection for T-cells expressing hADA by xylofuranosyl-adenine and 2′-deoxycoformicin, the resulting T-cells showed ADA activity comparable to that of normal T-cells.[10] These data show that complete metabolic correction of ADA-deficient T-cells can be obtained by retrovirus mediated gene transfer. In the same period, Rosenberg and co-workers showed that tumor-infiltrating T-cells transduced with a marker gene (neomycin resistance gene) could be re-infused safely into patients suffering from solid tumors, and still expressed the gene after infiltration in the tumors. [11] Based on the in vitro data on ADA-gene transfer into T-cells and the successful studies by Rosenberg et al, Blaese and his colleagues from the NIH started the first clinical trial on gene therapy for ADA deficiency, aiming at metabolic correction of circulating T-cells, in September 1990. So far, two children who were in clinical decline despite PEG-ADA, have been treated with repeated infusions of genetically modified T-cells; both children continued to receive PEG-ADA while being given gene therapy, and have continued their PEG-ADA treatment thereafter. It has been reported that the children are in good clinical condition, with significant improvement of many parameters of immune function. The gene could be detected in circulating lymphocytes of both patients, even in one of them who had not received transduced T-cells for more than year.

ADA GENE TRANSFER INTO HEMATOPOIETIC STEM CELLS

Preclinical studies

One cannot expect that ADA gene transfer into mature T-cells will result in correction of all circulating T-cells and a complete T-cell repertoire. Therefore, the transfer of a functional gene into HSC that can repopulate the hematopoietic system in vivo remains one of the most important goals to be pursued for gene therapy in general and for the treatment of ADA-SCID in particular. As retrovirus vectors are able to transduce dividing cells only, a major challenge for gene transfer into HSC, is to generate a system in which pluripotent HSC are able to divide, without differentiating into lineage-restricted progenitor cells. Hematopoietic growth factors are used to reach this goal. Transfer of the gene encoding ADA has been applied with success into human hematopoietic progenitor cells which give rise to in vitro colonies (CFU-Cs). [12–14] However, prior to clinical application of genetically transduced HSC, long-lasting in vivo expression of the introduced genes in all blood cell lineages had to be established after autologous transplantation of transduced HSC in mice and non-human primates.

ADA gene transfer into murine HSC

Efficient gene transfer via retroviral-vector technology into long-term repopulating HSC in mice was first reported approximately 10 years ago for example.[15,16] However, a drawback of retrovirus-mediated gene transfer has been that several vectors were found to be incapable of directing sustained expression in hematopoietic cells in vivo for example.[17–19] To overcome this repression in the hematopoietic system, most investigators introduced additional promoters into the viral transcription unit (reviewed by Valerio[4]). In addition, it was observed that 'simple, one-gene only' vectors, in which no selectable markers were present, were more active than more complex vectors. These findings resulted in the generation of ecotropic and amphotropic retroviral vectors which were able to efficiently transduce the long-term repopulating murine HSC followed by stable expression of the hADA gene in the blood cells of long-term repopulated mice. [7,20–22] In addition, a second transplant using bone marrow from mice repopulated with genetically modified HSC showed that the gene was integrated at the same site in the genome of the secondary recipients, indicating that a 'true' HSC was initially modified.[7] In studies to improve the gene transfer efficiency into murine HSC, we and others showed that co-culturing the murine bone marrow with the virus-producing cell line resulted in higher gene transfer efficiency than supernatant infection. The efficiency of the gene transfer procedure largely depended on the combination of hematopoietic growth factors added to the co-cultures, with the addition of IL-1 and IL-3 as most efficient combination in our experiments. [23] In this respect, it is relevant that all packaging cell lines tested in our laboratory produced large quantities of murine IL-6;[24] it might well be that other, species specific, factors are excreted as well by the virus producing cell lines.

ADA-gene transfer into non-human primate HSC

Based on the encouraging results obtained in mice, pre-clinical studies in non-human primates were initiated to study the feasibility of clinical gene transfer studies. In initial studies of gene transfer into rhesus monkey HSC, we co-cultured rhesus monkey HSC with the virus-producing cell line POC-1 in the presence of human IL-1 and rhesus monkey IL-3, as these conditions had previously been shown to be optimal for gene transfer into murine HSC. Surprisingly, engraftment of the cultured HSC resulted in the presence of the hADA gene in circulating blood cells in the monkeys for approximately 100 days only. In contrast, stable integration and expression of the gene in 0.1–1% of the peripheral blood mononuclear cells and granulocytes was observed for a period of more than 2 years if the transduction was performed in the presence of recombinant rhesus monkey IL-3 as sole growth factor.[25–27] These studies were followed by similar gene transfer studies using purified rhesus monkey HSC.

Purification of HSC reduced the number of cells added to the co-culture procedure to 0.6–1.1% of the original cell number, with obvious logistic advantages. In addition, the use of purified HSC for gene transfer studies allowed more precise assessment of the added growth factors on the gene transfer efficiency, as accessory cells (e.g. monocytes, T-cells) present in whole marrow grafts may secrete growth factors influencing gene transfer efficiency in an uncontrolled way. Co-cultivation of the enriched rhesus monkey HSC with the POC-1 cell line in the presence of IL-3 as the sole growth factor, revealed similar results in terms of regeneration rate and gene transfer efficiency as co-cultivation of unfractionated bone marrow.[25] Based on these data, initial studies on clinical gene therapy in ADA deficiency by our group used purified HSC as target cells (see later). Recently, similar results showing expression of the hADA gene in rhesus monkey blood cells was reported by Bodine et al [28] following transduction in the presence of a mouse stromal cell line producing membrane-bound stem cell factor.

Cultivation of HSC over a layer of irradiated marrow stromal cells, which provide the factors necessary for efficient gene transfer into CFU-C's, in the presence of virus containing supernatant produced promising results. [29] This experimental set-up obviates the need to co-culture the HSC with virus-producing cells, which necessarily results in infusion of irradiated virus-producing cells following harvesting of the transduced marrow cells, (the majority of the long-term repopulating cells adhered to the virus producing fibroblasts during the co-culture, necessitating trypsinization of the transduced marrow cells prior to infusion). [23] We applied the stromal layer culture method to perform gene transfer into HSC of two rhesus monkeys, which were subsequently infused in the monkeys. Despite efficient transduction of in vitro CFU-Cs, the presence of the gene was only observed during the first weeks after gene transfer and later disappeared. An additional disadvantage of this method was that engraftment was very slow, indicating that loss of HSC occurred during the culture procedure (Kaptein et al, in preparation).

So far, no side effects have been seen related to the gene transfer procedures using retroviral vectors derived from cell lines that were free of helper virus.[4] However, after exposure to murine amphotropic helper virus in immunosuppressed rhesus monkeys, lymphomas have occurred, [30] stressing the relevance of using **helper-free** virus producing cell lines for gene transfer studies.

Clinical studies

So far, the data reported on gene therapy trials in children with ADA deficiency are preliminary, as most children have been engrafted for less than 1 year at present (March, 1994) and are derived from meeting reports and personal communication with the investigators.

Based on the successful engraftment of the genetically modified cells in our rhesus monkey experiments, we performed, in collaboration with the groups headed by Fischer (Hopital Necker, Paris), Levinsky (Great Ormond Street, London) and Moseley (Applied Immune Sciences, USA), ADA gene transfer into purified HSC of 3 ADA deficient children (2 from France, and 1 from the UK) in March and April 1993. The gene transfer procedures were adapted from the monkey procedure. At serial intervals after gene transfer, the presence of the gene was seen in mono-nuclear cells and granulocytes. PCR analysis of the marrow of the children at 6 months after gene transfer showed the presence of the gene in one child, the marrow of the two other children was negative.[31]

Kohn's group (Childrens Hospital, Los Angeles, USA) treated 3 neonates with ADA deficiency in May and June 1993, in collaboration with Blaese (NIH). In these children, umbilical cord blood was used as a source of HSC. Follow-up at 6 months after gene transfer showed the presence of the gene in peripheral blood mononuclear cells; bone marrow analysis has not yet been reported.

Two patients treated from Bordignon's group (Milan, Italy) received transduced T-cells and, later on, increasing numbers of transduced HSCs. The two cell types were transduced with different retroviral vectors, allowing the determination of the contribution of both vectors separately. Both the presence of descendents of transduced T-cells and HSCs have been reported in the initial phase of the experiments.

One of the two children treated at NIH with T-cell gene therapy received in the summer of 1993 transduced HSC which were obtained from GCSF mobilized peripheral blood cells. Results of this treatment have not been reported yet.

So far, toxic side effects due to the gene transfer procedures have not been reported in any of the patients. In none of the patients has helper virus been detected. All children are in good health at present, and all children receive PEG-ADA therapy.

Table Surviving number of stem cells in rhesus monkeys after total body irradiation

Dose TBI	SF	HSC/kg surviving
0	1.000	3×10^5
2	0.209	6.3×10^4
4	0.0245	7.4×10^3
6	0.0027	8.1×10^2
8	0.0003	91
10	0.00003	10

SF: Surviving fraction. In these calculations, the relationship between radiation dose and cell survival is based on the Poisson distribution of the probability of lethal lesions: $SF=1-(1-e^{-D/DO})^2$, in which DO is 0.91.[32]

None of the children received myeloablative therapy prior to gene transfer. Instead, it is hoped that the selective advantage of the genetically repaired cells will let them outgrow the non-repaired cells. It is not clear whether the selective advantage will still be present in these patients, as they all receive PEG-ADA which reduces the levels of the toxic deoxyadenosine metabolite. In this respect, it is important that in all above mentioned rhesus monkey experiments, the monkeys received lethal myeloablative conditioning which consisted of 10–15 Gy total body irradiation (TBI). It can be calculated that the amount of stem cells surviving 10 Gy TBI is approximately 10 per kg body weight (Table). A rhesus monkey bone marrow graft of 2×10^8 bone marrow cells per kg contains approximately 2×10^3HSC per kg. This indicates that if the efficiency of the gene transfer procedure is 1%, the number of transduced stem cells infused into the monkeys is approximately 10–20 per kg, equivalent to the number of residual, unmodified stem cells after 10 Gy TBI. The percentage of transduced stem cells infused in **non-conditioned** monkeys, however, would only be approximately 0.003% (Table) of the total number of stem cells present. If these calculations can be extrapolated to human patients, it can be concluded that only a very low number of transduced cells is infused as compared to the endogenous, non-transduced cells. Whether this will be enough to influence the disease pattern in these patients will hopefully be revealed by these initial trials.

CONCLUSION

Transfer of the hADA gene has been performed efficiently into murine hematopoietic stem cells. The gene transfer frequency into stem cells of non-human primates has recently been reported as well, although the frequency of transduced blood cells is only 0.1–2%. Based on these data, initial studies to gene transfer into T-cells and hematopoietic stem cells of patients with ADA deficiency have been performed in the last years. No side effects were seen in these patients. The gene could be detected in circulating blood cells after gene transfer. In contrast to the animal models used for gene transfer studies, the patients did not receive myelo-ablative therapy prior to reinfusion of the transduced marrow, which may result in a slower appearance of circulating transduced blood cells than after comparable gene transfer procedures in non-human primates.

REFERENCES

1 Santisteban I, Arredonto-Vega FX, Kelly S et al. Novel splicing, missence and deletion mutations in seven adenosine deaminase deficient patients with late/delayed onset of combined immunodeficiency disease. J Clin Invest 1993; 92: 2291–2302.
2 Fischer A, Landais P, Friedrich W et al. European experience of bone-marrow transplantation for severe combined immunodeficiency. Lancet 1990; 336: 850–854.
3 Hersfield MS. The role of polyethylene glycol adenosine deaminase in the evolution of therapy for adenosine deaminase deficiency. In: Gupta S, Griscelli C, eds. New concepts in immunodeficiency diseases. Chichester: Wiley, 1993: 417–426.
4 Valerio D. Retrovirus vectors and their use in gene therapy protocols. In: Grosveld F, Kollias G, eds. Transgenic mice in biology and medicine. New York: Academic Press, 1992: 211–246.
5 Valerio D, McIvor RS, Williams SR et al. Cloning of human adenosine deaminase cDNA and expression in mouse cells. Gene 1984; 31: 147–153.
6 Kantoff PW, Kohn DB, Mitsuya H et al. Correction of adenosine deaminase deficiency in cultured human T and B cells by retrovirus-mediated gene transfer. Proc Natl Acad Sci USA 1986; 83: 6563–6567.
7 Beusechem VWv, Kukler A, Einerhand MPW et al. Expression of human adenosine deaminase in mice transplanted with hemopoietic stem cells infected with amphotropic retroviruses. J Exp Med 1990; 172: 729–736.

8 Linney E, Davis B, Overhauser J, Chao E, Fan H. Non-function of a Moloney Murine Leukaemia Virus regulatory sequence in F9 embryonal carcinoma cells. Nature 1984; 308: 470– 472.
9 Valerio D, Einerhand MPW, Wamsley PM, Bakx TA, Li CL, Verma IM. Retrovirus-mediated gene transfer into embryonal carcinoma cells and hemopoietic stem cells: expression from a hybrid long terminal repeat. Gene 1989; 84: 419–427.
10 Braakman E, Van Beusechem VW, Van Krimpen BA, Fischer A, Bolhuis RLH, Valerio D. Genetic correction of cultured T cells from an adenosine deaminase deficient patient: characteristics of non-transduced and transduced T cells. Eur J Immunol 1992; 22: 63–69.
11 Rosenberg SA, Aebersold P, Cornetta K et al. Immunotherapy of patients with advanced melanoma using tumor infiltrating lymphocytes modified by retroviral gene transduction. N Engl J Med 1990; 323: 570–578.
12 Hock RA, Miller AD, Osborne WRA. Expression of human adenosine deaminase from various strong promoters after gene transfer into human hematopoietic cell lines. Blood 1989; 74(2): 876–881.
13 Bordignon C, Yu SF, Smith CA et al. Retroviral vector-mediated high-efficiency expression of adenosine deaminase (ADA) in hematopoietic long-term cultures of ADA-deficient marrow cells. Proc Natl Acad Sci USA 1989; 86: 6748–6752.
14 Cournoyer D, Scarpa M, Mitani K et al. Gene transfer of adenosine deaminase into primitive human hematopoietic progenitor cells. Hum Gene Ther 1991; 2: 203–213.
15 Keller G, Paige C, Gilboa E, Wagner EF. Expression of a foreign gene in myeloid and lymphoid cells derived from multipotent haematopoietic precursors. Nature 1985; 318: 149–154.
16 Williams DA, Lemischka IR, Nathan DG, Mulligan RC. Introduction of new genetic material into pluripotent haematopoietic stem cells of the mouse. Nature 1984; 310: 476–480.
17 Valerio D, Visser TP, Wagemaker G, Van der Eb AJ, Van Bekkum DW. The introduction of human ADA sequences into mouse hematopoietic stem cells. In: Vossen J, Griscelli C, eds. Progress in immunodeficiency research and therapy. Amsterdam: Elsevier, 1986: 335–355.
18 Williams DA, Orkin SH, Mulligan RC. Retrovirus-mediated transfer of human adenosine deaminase gene sequences into cells in culture and into murine hematopoietic cells in vivo. Proc Natl Acad Sci USA 1986; 83: 2566–2570.
19 McIvor RS, Pitts S, Martin DW. Gene transfer and expression of human purine nucleoside phosphorylase and adenosine deaminase: possibilities for therapeutic application. In: Sasazuki T, ed. New approach to genetic diseases. New York: Academic Press, 1987: 231–244.
20 Wilson JM, Danos O, Grossman M, Raulet DH, Mulligan RC. Expression of human adenosine deaminase in mice reconstituted with retrovirus-transduced hematopoietic stem cells. Proc Natl Acad Sci USA 1990; 87: 439–443.
21 Moore KA, Fletcher FA, Villalon DK, Utter AE, Belmont JW. Human adenosine deaminase expression in mice. Blood 1990; 75: 2085–2092.
22 Lim B, Williams DA, Orkin SH. Retrovirus-mediated gene transfer of human adenosine deaminase: expression of functional enzyme in murine hematopoietic stem cells in vivo. Mol Cell Biol 1987; 7: 3459–3465.
23 Einerhand MPW, Bakx TA, Kukler A, Valerio D. Factors affecting the transduction of pluripotent hemopoietic stem cells: long term expression of a human adenosine deaminase gene in mice. Blood 1993; 81: 254–263.
24 Einerhand MPW, Bakx TA, Valerio D. Il-6 production by retrovirus packaging cells and cultured bone marrow cells. Hum. Gene Ther 1991; 2: 301–306.
25 Beusechem VWv, Bart-Baumeister JAK, Bakx TA, Kaptein LCM, Levinsky RJ, Valerio D. Gene transfer into non-human primate CD34+CD11b- bone marrow progenitor cells capable of repopulating lymphoid and myeloid lineages. Hum Gene Ther 1994; 5: 295–305.

26 Beusechem VWv, Kukler A, Heidt PJ, Valerio D. Long-term expression of human adenosine deaminase in rhesus monkeys transplanted with retrovirus-infected bone marrow cells. Proc Natl Acad Sci USA 1992; : 7640–7644.
27 Beusechem VWv, Bakx TA, Kaptein LCM, et al. Retrovirus-mediated gene transfer studies into rhesus monkey hematopoietic stem cells: teh effect of viral titers on transduction efficiency. Hum Gene Ther 1993; 4: 239–247.
28 Bodine DM, Moritz T, Donahue RE et al. Long-term in vivo expression of a murine ADA gene in rhesus monkey hematopoietic cells of multiple lineages after retroviral mediated gene transfer into CD34+ bone marrow cells. Blood 1993; 82: 1975–1980.
29 Moore KA, Deisseroth AB, Reading CL, Williams DE, Belmont JW. Stromal support enhances cell-free retroviral vector transduction of human bone marrow long-term culture initiating cells. Blood 1992; 79: 1393–1399.
30 Donahue RE, Kessler SW, Bodine D et al. Helper virus induced T-cell lymphoma in nonhuman primates after retroviral mediated gene transfer. J Exp Med 1992; 176: 1125–1135.
31 Hoogerbrugge PM, Beusechem VWv, et al Gene therapy in 3 children with ADA deficiency. Blood 1993; 82s: 315a (abstract).
32 Wielenga JJ. Hemopoietic stem cells in rhesus monkeys. Thesis, Rotterdam, 1990: 208.

British Medical Bulletin (1995) Vol. 51, No. 1, pp.82–90

Cystic fibrosis gene therapy

W H Colledge and M J Evans

Wellcome/CRC Institute of Cancer and Developmental Biology and Department of Genetics, University of Cambridge, Cambridge, UK

Cystic fibrosis is a common severe autosomal recessive genetic disease which is caused by dysfunction of an epithelial cell surface cAMP activated Cl^- channel. The effects of this dysfunction are pleoitropic but the human morbidity results from the effects in the respiratory epithelium. Gene therapy is an attractive possible treatment, the gene required is well characterised and only low-level expression is required. The cellular target is accessible and the clinical effects of treatment should be readily assayable. This chapter reviews current proposals for suitable gene delivery mechanisms and vectors and discusses the clinical trials, the results from the first of which are now becoming available.

Cystic Fibrosis (CF), which is one of the most common autosomal recessive genetic disorders, is caused by dysfunction of a cAMP (cyclic adenosine monophosphate) regulated chloride channel located in the apical membrane of airway and other epithelial cells. A rise in cAMP levels within the cells causes an increased chloride secretion through the CFTR (cystic fibrosis transmembrane conductance regulator) channel into the lumen. Loss of function of this channel leads to abnormal salt and water transport which causes a variety of effects including hyper-accumulation of mucus in the lungs and gastrointestinal tract, reduced ability to digest and absorb duodenal contents because of pancreatic enzyme insufficiency, male sterility and elevated salt levels in the sweat. Despite the widespread involvement of the CFTR chloride channel in normal physiological processes, the main cause of human morbidity and mortality in CF results from gradual lung destruction by progressive damage of the respiratory epithelium following chronic infection and inflammation (for reviews see [1,2]).

Cystic fibrosis is an attractive target for gene therapy. It is a severe syndrome and the present treatments are largely palliative, and eventually ineffective. CF patients have a current life expectancy of approximately 30 years and the majority of the mortality is the result of recurrent respiratory infections. This may itself be caused by changes in water absorption leading to increased mucus viscosity and lack of impaired mucociliary clearance.[3] Correction requires restoration of the cAMP activated chloride channel which acts in the epithelium. It is therefore unlikely that systemic replacement would be appropriate, but the respiratory epithelium is essentially accessible for topical treatment. There is a knowledgeable and committed patient base well able to give informed consent and ultimately a very reasonable hope for a successful therapy. With both the demand and the anticipated possibility of success, there is rapid progress in this field. A number of Phase I clinical trials have already been carried out and there is very active research and development using animal model systems.

Initial testing in animal model systems should be used to develop and improve gene delivery methods for use in clinical trials. As this treatment will ultimately be used on thousands of patients and should allow many extra decades of life, safety as well as efficiency is paramount.

ANIMAL MODELS

Animal models are playing an important role in the development of gene therapies. This includes the use of both normal animals, where studies of transfection efficiency and safety may be carried out, and the use of the cystic fibrosis transgenic mice (CF-mice). To date the CF-mice analysed in detail fall into 2 categories:

(a) null mutations where there is no CFTR function[4–8] and

(b) a hypomorph mutation where there is a partial expression of CFTR.[9]

The CF-mice show characteristics of cystic fibrosis. These include the absence or reduction of a cAMP activated chloride channel and hyper-accumulation of mucus in the gastrointestinal tract which causes intestinal obstructions both in newborn and adult animals similar to the fetal blockages, (meconium ileus) and meconium ileus equivalent, found in some adult CF patients. Although the CF-mice that completely lack a functional CFTR chloride channel do not show secondary pulmonary complications, equivalent to those in the human patients, they can be used as a sensitive electro-physiological assay for the effectiveness of a gene therapy strategy.

One mouse model which is not a null mutation but a hypomorph leading to a reduced level of CFTR expression[10] and which consequently has a much reduced pathology in the gut is more viable. This has recently been shown to have a reduced mucociliary clearance of *Staphylococcus aureus* following lung infection and also to develop a major lung pathology after a chronic exposure to *Pseudomonas aeroginosa* or *P. cepacia*.[11] These mice may therefore provide models for the secondary pathological effects consequent on CFTR deficiency in humans and a test for the ability of gene therapy to reverse this.

As well as these genetic models, a xenograph system has also been developed based upon epithelial recolonisation of a denuded trachea implanted subcutaneously in an immuno-tolerant host.[12] This system is particularly useful for studying the effect of epithelial cell proliferation on gene therapy delivery and expression. In addition to these artificial animal models, trials of gene therapy with mice, rats, cotton rats, rabbits and primates is proving useful.

GENE THERAPY VECTORS

A number of vector systems have been proposed for CF gene therapy and they broadly fall into 2 groups; viral and non-viral.

Viral

Adenoviruses

Adenoviruses have many characteristics that make them suitable for cystic fibrosis gene therapy.[13,14] They are trophic for the respiratory epithelium and can be produced in high titres which will very efficiently infect non-replicating epithelial cells. There is only a small level of integration with the attendant risks of insertional mutagenesis. They do however represent a defective form of a naturally occurring pathogenic virus. There is the possibility of both allergic and immune reaction, particularly with repeated treatment, and of a rare but potentially dangerous recombination to generate replication competent viruses.

Retroviruses

Retroviruses are not yet considered as suitable vectors for CF gene therapy because they require cell proliferation to allow proviral integration and expression. As lung epithelial cells are terminally differentiated and predominantly post-mitotic they represent an inappropriate target for retroviral infection.[12] The ability of retroviruses to integrate into the host genome, however, means that they might be suitable for targeting epithelial stem cells to give long-term expression of CFTR in daughter cells. Attempts are now being made in mice to virally infect fetal pulmonary epithelia *in utero* where the number of stem cells progenitors is fewer and also perhaps more accessible to infection. These experiments would be helped by the isolation of lung epithelial stem cells to test retroviral expression parameters.

Adeno-associated virus (AAV)

A recombinant CFTR AAV has been shown to complement the CF defect in a human bronchial epithelial line[15] and animal trials have now been initiated to assess the effectiveness of this vector in vivo.[16] Initial reports are favourable; an AAV lacZ vector gave β-gal activity in both dividing and non-dividing epithelial cells after a single dose infection into the trachea of newborn rabbits.[17] No inflammatory reactions were observed. One disadvantage of AAV vectors is that they require co-infection of a producer cell line with adenovirus and therefore viral stocks must be rigorously checked to ensure that they are not contaminated with replication-competent adenovirus. The safety of AAV vectors would be enhanced and viral production greatly simplified by the generation of a good viral producer line.

Non-viral

Cationic liposomes

Liposomes consist of an aqueous suspension of phospholipid. The majority of liposomes used in CF gene therapy studies are cationic and therefore bind to both DNA and the cell surface. Following fusion of the lipid bilayer with the cell surface, DNA is delivered inside the cell. Much of this is degraded through the lysosomal pathways but a proportion is delivered as a transient transformation to the cell nucleus. DNA delivered by this route does not integrate efficiently.

Liposomes can be administered into the lungs as an aerosol[18,19] or by direct lavage.[20] Intravenous injection of liposomes can also be used to deliver DNA to a variety of organs including the lungs but it is not yet clear that this results in delivery to the surface epithelial cells.[21]

Extensive safety trials have been performed with pigs, rabbits and mice to demonstrate that these liposomes are non-toxic, non immunogenic and do not deliver plasmid DNA to the gonads.[22–25]

Liposomes are a relatively inefficient vehicle for gene delivery. Even under optimum conditions only about 5% of primary epithelial cells are transfected. This is probably not a major concern for CF gene therapy as it appears that as few as 6% of cells in an epithelial sheet need express CFTR to generate normal Cl^- currents. Much of the DNA delivered by liposomes is degraded by lysosomal enzymes. Techniques to reduce this, such as encapsulation of certain anti-lysosomal viral proteins, might increase the efficiency of liposome mediated gene delivery.[26]

The feasibility of using liposomes for CF gene therapy has been clearly illustrated independently by 2 groups using CF animal models. Hyde et al[20] delivered a liposome/CFTR expression plasmid complex into the lungs of CF mice by direct tracheal instillation while Alton et al[19] aerosolised the complex. In both cases, a cAMP regulated Cl^- channel was restored to the upper airways. Alton et al[19] also managed to partially correct the Cl^- transport defect in the intestine following rectal delivery. Hyde et al[20] used *in situ* hybridisation to demonstrate that the plasmid was delivered deep into the lungs, both to small airway epithelial cells and type II alveolar cells.

SAFETY CONSIDERATIONS

The safety of any gene therapy procedure is paramount. Phase I clinical trials are designed to test the safety of a treatment and will not necessarily give any indication of a physiological or clinical benefit.

Gene therapy may be approached by the use of viral vectors where the potential for cellular infection and genetic transfection by the virus is subverted to deliver the required gene. In this case it is vital that any pathological effects of the virus *per se* are eliminated. There is also a major question of safety, not only for the patient but also for the human population in general where modified viral pathogens are being used. It is important that reversion or recombination with wild type organisms cannot occur to produce a proliferating modified pathogen. Non-viral vector systems in addition to being incapable of propagation, may also be manufactured to more stringent requirements for purity and are likely to be safer. On the other hand with present technology they are likely to be less efficient at gene transfer.

A large number of studies have been performed by several groups to assess the safety and efficiency of adenovirus vectors for CF gene therapy.[14] One concern is the possible production of a replication competent virus either from a contaminated viral stock or by recombination with an endogenous adenovirus in the host. While *in vitro* infection of cell cultures and *in vivo*administration to animals have both failed to detect any infectious virus production, high multiplicity of infection in HeLa cells gave trace vector DNA synthesis.

Another important consideration in using adenovectors is the generation of any acute cellular response to viral infection and whether these responses will increase upon subsequent applications of virus. Animal studies using rabbits, cotton rats, mice, goats, lambs and baboons have shown that moderate viral titres of adenovectors are not associated with any major clinical side-effects and can efficiently infect epithelial cells.[27] Some of these studies, however, describe more favourable results than the others and this may reflect the different animals used in each safety trial.

No inflammatory responses were noted following either a single or multiple treatment of Rhesus monkey airway epithelium.[28] In contrast, application of high doses of an adenovector to the lungs of baboons produced a dose-dependent inflammation with perivascular lymphocytic and histiocytic infiltrates.[29]

It is not yet clear which of these primates (Rhesus monkey or baboon) will produce responses to adenovectors similar to what might occur in humans but the recent Phase I clinical trial reported by Crystal et al[30] suggests that it may be the response of the baboons.

In view of the possible inflammatory side-effects associated with adenovectors, a number of second generation vectors are currently being developed which will hopefully be safer. Current adenovectors typically delete the E1A and E1B regions (and sometimes the E3 region) of the virus thus rendering it replication defective. However, these adenovectors often allow other viral proteins to be expressed which may contribute to the generation of cellular immune responses.[31,32]

CLINICAL TRIALS

Of all the vector systems proposed for CF gene therapy, adenovectors are the most advanced with the results of two clinical trials already published and several more forthcoming. The first report of using a CF adenovector was by Zabner et al[33] who showed that a single dose of Ad(CFTR) to the nasal epithelium of 3 CF patients corrected the defective Cl^- channel with no serious inflammatory reactions or evidence of viral replication. In contrast, when Crystal et al[30] administered a different CF adenovector into the lungs of 4 CF patients, the patient who received the highest dose (2×10^9 pfu) showed several adverse reactions. These included headache, fatigue, fever, tachycardia, hypertension, dysporea and a decrease in vital and total lung capacity and forced expiratory volume and diffusing capacity in the lung. In addition, an increase in circulating levels of IL-6 were also observed consistent with an inflammatory mediated reaction of the lower respiratory tract. Fortunately this patient recovered to pre-clinical parameters after about one month. Encouragingly, the remaining 3 CF patients who received up to 2×10^7 pfu of Ad(CFTR) did not show any serious adverse effects and the presence of both CFTR mRNA and protein was detected in the nasal epithelia of one of the patients and CFTR protein in the bronchial epithelia of another patient – although mRNA expression was not detected in this individual.

Ongoing clinical trials using adenovectors are aimed at confirming these initial results and extending the number of patients treated to gauge how frequently side-effects might occur.

A phase I clinical trial of liposome mediated CFTR delivery to the nasal epithelium of patients has now been sucessfully completed and although results from this have not yet been fully reported Middleton et al[34] have published a short summary showing that there were no adverse treatment-related side effects. At the highest dose used (600 μg of pSV CFTR plasmid) changes in basal PD, sodium and chloride transport in the direction towards restoration of normality were observed in all patients. These are very encouraging results but lack of toxicity of the liposome route is counterbalanced by its apparent low efficiency of gene transfer.

KEY NOTES FOR CLINICIANS

There are two main approaches being used at present in clinical trials based on adenoviruses and upon cationic liposomes. Most investigators regard both of these as first generation technologies. It is expected that greatly improved viral vectors will become available and that non-viral methods with much greater efficiency of cell targeting and gene transfer will be developed. The adenovector trial reported by Crystal et al,[30] raises several concerns about the safety and usefulness of this route for CF gene therapy and provides lessons in the way such trials should be approached. Whilst pre-clinical studies in animals will not always predict the response in humans, it is important that exhaustive testing is undertaken in animals and the results are interpreted critically before initiating clinical trials. The fact that adenoviruses cause a dose-dependent inflammation in the airways of primates followed by a mononuclear cell infiltrate, although with no clinical manifestations, would suggest a very cautious approach to their use for gene therapy.

REFERENCES

1. Riordan JR. The cystic fibrosis transmembrane conductance regulator. Annu Rev Physiol 1993; 55 (609): 609–630.
2. Welsh MJ, Smith AE. Molecular mechanisms of CFTR chloride channel dysfunction in cystic fibrosis. Cell 1993; 73 (7) :1251–1254.
3. Mearns MB. Cystic Fibrosis; The first 50 years. In: Dodge JA, Brock DJH, Widdicome JH, eds. Cystic Fibrosis: Current Topics. Chichester: John Wiley, 1993: vol 1).
4. Clarke LL, Grubb BR, Gabriel SE, Smithies O, Koller BH, Boucher RC. Defective epithelial chloride transport in a gene-targeted mouse model of cystic fibrosis. Science 1992; 257 (5073): 1125–1128.
5. Colledge WH, Ratcliff R, Foster D, Williamson R, Evans MJ. Cystic fibrosis mouse with intestinal obstruction [letter]. Lancet 1992; 340(8820).
6. Snouwaert JN, Brigman KK, Latour AM et al. An animal model for cystic fibrosis made by gene targeting. Science 1992; 257 (5073): 1083–1088.
7. Ratcliff R, Evans MJ, Cuthbert AW et al. Production of a severe cystic fibrosis mutation in mice by gene targeting. Nature Genet 1993; 4 (1): 35–41.
8. O'Neal WK, Hasty P, P.B. M et al. A severe phenotype in mice with a duplication of Exon 3 in the Cystic Fibrosis locus. Hum Mol Genet 1993; 2: 1561–1569.
9. Dorin JR, Dickinson P, Alton EWFW et al. Cystic fibrosis in the mouse by targeted insertional mutagenesis. Nature 1992; 359: 211–214.
10. Dorin JR, Stevenson BJ, Fleming S, Alton EWFW, Dickinson P, Porteus DJ. Long-term survival of the exon-10 insertional cystic fibrosis mutant mouse is a consequence of low-level residual wild-type gene expression. Mammalian Genome 1994; 5 (8): 465–472.

11 Porteous DJ. Cystic fibrosis in the mouse and progress towards gene therapy. In: Escobar H, Baquero CF, Suarez L, eds. Clinical Ecology of Cystic Fibrosis. Amsterdam: Elsevier, 1993
12 Engelhardt JF, Yankaskas JR, Wilson JM. In vivo retroviral gene transfer into human bronchial epithelia of xenografts. J Clin Invest 1992; 90 (6): 2598–2607.
13 Kozarsky KF, Wilson JM. Gene therapy: adenovirus vectors. Curr Opin Genet Dev 1993; 3(3): 499–503.
14 Mastrangeli A, Danel C, Rosenfeld MA et al. Diversity of airway epithelial cell targets for in vivo recombinant adenovirus-mediated gene transfer. J Clin Invest 1993; 91(1): 225–34.
15 Flotte TR, Solow R, Owens RA, Afione S, Zeitlin PL, Carter BJ. Gene expression from adeno-associated virus vectors in airway epithelial cells. Am J Respir Cell Mol Biol 1992; 7(3): 349–356.
16 Flotte TR, Afione SA, Conrad C et al. Stable in vivo expression of the cystic fibrosis transmembrane conductance regulator with an adeno-associated virus vector. Proc Natl Acad Sci USA 1993; 90(22): 10613–10617.
17 Chu S, Flotte TR, Guggino WB, Zeitlin PL. Single dose AAV gene delivery to the newborn rabbit pulmonary epithelium. Paediatr Pulminol 1994;.
18 Stribling R, Brunette E, Liggitt D, Gaensler K, Debs R. Aerosol gene delivery in vivo. Proc Natl Acad Sci USA 1992; 89(23): 11277–11281.
19 Alton EWFW, Middleton PG, Caplen NJ et al. Non-invasive liposome-mediated gene delivery can correct the ion transport defect in cystic fibrosis mutant mice. Nature Genet 1993; 5: 135–142.
20 Hyde SC, Gill DR, Higgins CF et al. Correction of the ion transport defect in cystic fibrosis transgenic mice by gene therapy. Nature 1993; 362(6417): 250–255.
21 Zhu N, Liggitt D, Liu Y, Debs R. Systemic gene expression after intravenous DNA delivery into adult mice. Science 1993; 261(5118): 209–211.
22 Stewart MJ, Plautz GE, Del BL et al. Gene transfer in vivo with DNA-liposome complexes: safety and acute toxicity in mice. Hum Gene Ther 1992; 3(3): 267–275.
23 Canonico AE, Plitman JD, Conary JT, Meyrick BO, Brigham KL. No lung toxicity after repeated aerosol or intravenous delivery of plasmid-cationic liposome complexes. J Appl Phys 1994; 77(1): 415–419.
24 Nabel EG, Gordon D, Yang ZY et al. Gene transfer in vivo with DNA-liposome complexes: lack of autoimmunity and gonadal localization. Hum Gene Ther 1992; 3(6): 649–656.
25 Middleton PG, Caplen NJ, Gao X et al. Nasal application of the cationic liposome DC-Chol:DOPE does not alter ion transport, lung function or bacterial growth. Eur Respir J 1994; 7(3): 442–445.
26 Gao L, Wagner E, Cotten M et al. Direct in vivo gene transfer to airway epithelium employing adenovirus-polylysine-DNA complexes. Hum Gene Ther 1993; 4(1): 17–24.
27 Siegfried W. Perspectives in gene therapy with recombinant adenoviruses. Exp Clin Endocrinol 1993; 101: 7–11.
28 Zabner J, Petersen DM, Puga AP et al. Safety and efficacy of repetitive adenovirus-mediated transfer of CFTR cDNA to airway epithelia of primates and cotton rats. Nature Genet 1994; 6: 75–83.
29 Engelhardt JF, Simon RH, Yang Y et al. Adenovirus-mediated transfer of the CFTR gene to lung of nonhuman primates: biological efficacy study. Hum Gene Ther 1993; 4(6): 759–769.
30 Crystal RG, McElvaney NG, Rosenfield MA et al. Administration of an adenovirus containing the human CFTR c-DNA to the respiratory tract of individuals with cystic fibrosis. Nature Genet 1944; 8: 42–51.
31 Wold WS, Gooding LR. Region E3 of adenovirus: a cassette of genes involved in host immunosurveillance and virus-cell interactions. Virology 1991; 184: 1–8.
32 Yoshimura K, Rosenfield MA, Seth P, Crystal RG. Adenovirus-mediated augmentation of cell transfection with unmodified plasmid vectors. J Biol Chem 1993; 268: 2300–2303.

33 Zabner J, Couture LA, Gregory RJ, Graham SM, Smith AE, Welsh MJ. Adenovirus-mediated gene transfer transiently corrects the chloride transport defect in nasal epithelia of patients with cystic fibrosis. Cell 1993; 75(2): 207–216.
34 Middleton PG, Caplen NJ, Gao X et al. The electophysiological effects of in vivo liposome mediated cftr delivery to the nasal epithelium. Pediatr Pulminol 1994;(Suppl 10): 229–230.

British Medical Bulletin (1995) Vol.51, No.1, pp.91–105

Prospects for gene therapy of haemophilia A and B

G G Brownlee
Chemical Pathology Unit, Sir William Dunn School of Pathology, University of Oxford, Oxford, UK

Haemophilia A and B are relatively rare, X-linked inherited bleeding disorders which are life-threatening to patients unless treated by regular injections of factors VIII or IX, respectively. Gene therapy offers the prospect of a cure for the disease, thus potentially freeing patients from the existing regimens of regular intravenous injection of proteins and the risks of infection by contaminating viruses. Although, in theory, gene therapy is very attractive to patients and clinicians, in practice, preclinical experiments in animal models suggests that it may be difficult to obtain adequate therapeutic levels of either factors VIII or IX for long periods of time in patients unless improved methods can be devised. Progress in the preclinical studies is more encouraging with haemophilia B than with haemophilia A. Clinical trials for haemophilia B patients have started in China.

INTRODUCTION AND ETHICAL CONSIDERATIONS

Haemophilia has been known since biblical times as an inherited, bleeding condition affecting males but not females. The two forms of haemophilia were not distinguished from one another until 1952, since both are X-linked, recessive, conditions with similar clinical manifestations. The commoner disease, haemophilia A or classical haemophilia, occurs about once in every 6000 male births. The rarer disease, haemophilia B or Christmas disease, occurs about once in every 30,000 male births. In the case of haemophilia A, there is a defect in clotting factor VIII, whereas for haemophilia B it is in clotting factor IX (Table 1). These factors are both essential proteins in the clotting cascade (Fig. 1).

Both forms of haemophilia (*see* references 1 and 2) are life-threatening unless treated by frequent, often weekly, intravenous injec-

Table 1 Vital statistics of the haemophilias and factors VIII and IX

Disease	Frequency (in males)	Gene defect	MW kDa	Plasma protein concentration (μg/ml)	Plasma protein (No. of amino acids)	cDNA coding length (no. of nucleotides)[a]	Half-life of clotting factor (h)
Haemophilia A (classical haemophilia)	1 in 6000	Factor VIII	280	0.1–0.2	2332	7056	~10
Haemophila B (Christmas disease)	1 in 30,000	Factor IX	68	~5	415	1389[b]	~20

[a]Excluding 5′and 3′non-coding regions, but including the signal peptide domain, the translation terminator codons and the propeptide domain in the case of factor IX; [b]Assuming that the most 5′of the 3 possible AUG initiating codons is used.

tions of clotting factors. These factors have traditionally been purified from plasma pooled from blood donors, although recently recombinant factor VIII has become available. The traditional treatment, which was introduced in the mid-1960s, has proved effective in controlling bleeding in patients and the life-expectancy of those haemophiliacs who are not infected with HIV approaches that of the normal population. Nevertheless, patients are still at risk of bleeding into joints, which is painful and may lead to crippling. Before 1985 most large-pool blood product concentrates carried a high risk of transmitting HIV and hepatitis C virus (HCV). Since then, the introduction of blood donor screening for antibodies to HIV and HCV and the use of virocidal steps during manufacture have greatly reduced the risk of viral transmission.

It is well known that patients with >2–3% of normal factor VIII or IX levels rarely suffer from spontaneous muscle or joint bleeding, although they will still bleed excessively following injury or surgery. For this reason most regimens of prophylaxis aim to maintain the clotting factors at about 4–5% of normal.

For gene therapy a gene, or more usually a cDNA, is required and those for factors VIII and IX were cloned in early 1980s. In 1986, in a review of the molecular pathology of haemophilia B, I suggested[3] that the haemophilias would 'provide an excellent if challenging model' to study gene therapy. I doubt that this suggestion was taken seriously then. Even now some clinicians and scientists believe that haemophilia is not a valid target for gene therapy, because the present treatment is wholly satisfactory. In fact, the present treatment is inconvenient for patients, does not prevent all bleeding and may still not be completely safe. Moreover, only a small percentage of the World's haemophiliacs have access to this expensive life-long therapy. Most clinicians now believe that, if a safe gene therapy procedure were available, it would have many advantages over the existing therapy. It would free patients from their dependence on regular injections of clotting factors and the risk of bleeding not to say the risk, albeit remote, of being infected by blood-borne viruses.

FACTORS VIII & IX – Biosynthesis and protein domains

A brief overview of the biosynthesis and protein domain organization of factors VIII and IX will be presented in order to highlight some features relevant for gene therapy. For further details consult the following paper[4] or reviews.[5–7] Factors VIII and IX are synthesized in the liver and, after processing in the endoplasmic reticulum (ER) and Golgi apparatus, are secreted as glycoproteins into the blood. Messenger RNA for both proteins has been detected in extra-hepatic tissues and it seems probable, at least for factor VIII, that some fraction of the

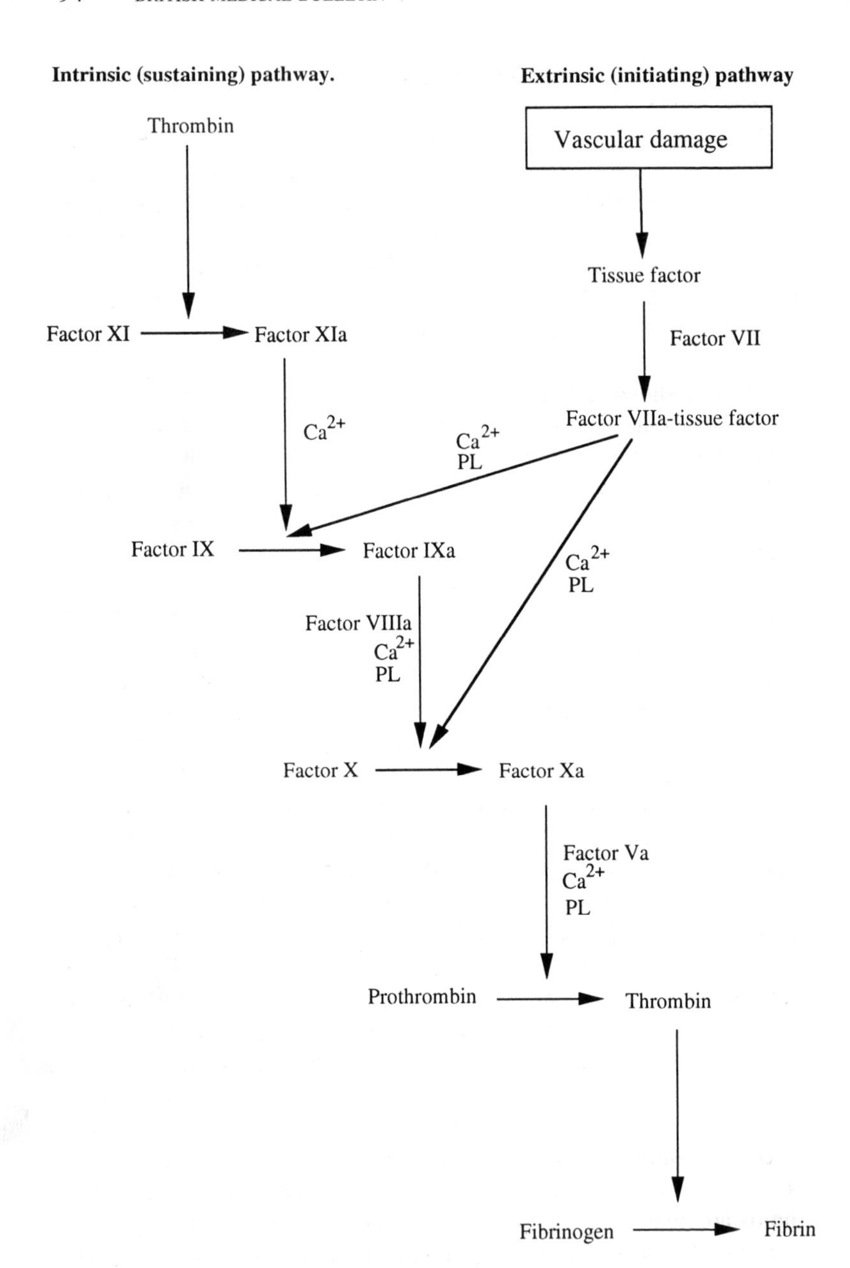

Fig. 1 The clotting cascade. One current model[31] stresses the importance of the extrinsic pathway in initiating clotting and excludes factor XII. Thrombin, formed by the action of factor Xa, activates factor XI thereby sustaining clotting through the intrinsic pathway. PL represent phospholipid. This scheme omits many details for clarity.

circulating protein is synthesized in spleen, lymph nodes, kidney and possibly other tissues.

Factor IX circulates as a monomer. Some factor IX may be complexed to endothelial and possibly other cells by binding to a cellular receptor. Factor VIII, on the other hand, circulates as a complex with von Willebrand factor, which is, itself, multimerized to form a high molecular weight complex. Without complex formation with von Willebrand factor, factor VIII is extremely unstable. Even as a complex, its half-life is only about 10 h, which is much shorter than that of factor IX (Table 1).

Figure 2 shows the domain structures of factors VIII and IX. Both proteins are synthesized as slightly longer precursor molecules containing a classic N-terminal **signal peptide**, which is cleaved during vectorial transport into the ER. In addition, factor IX contains a **propeptide** sequence of 18 amino-acids, which is cleaved intracellularly by a furin-type protease[8] late in the secretory pathway. Without this cleavage, factor IX is known to be inactive.[9] The **propeptide** and **gla** domains are required to target the vitamin K-dependent γ-glutamyl carboxylase[10] present in the ER. This enzyme modifies 12 glutamyl residues of the **gla** and **hydrophobic** domains to give γ-carboxyglutamic acid, which is an essential post-translational modification both to ensure correct protein folding of factor IX in the presence of calcium and to allow binding to phospholipid. The **EGF** (epidermal growth factor-like) domains are of unknown function although the **first EGF** domain binds calcium with high affinity, probably in association with the adjacent **gla** and **hydrophobic** domains. The **activation** domain is cleaved by factors XIa or VIIa giving rise to factor IXa. The **serine protease** domain is homologous to serine proteases and is the catalytic domain responsible for factor X cleavage.

Factor VIII is processed in the Golgi apparatus, by proteolytic cleavage at the carboxy-terminal side of amino-acid 1648, to generate a heterodimer consisting of a heavy and light chain stabilized by metal ion binding. This heterodimer is highly glycosylated and is secreted into the blood. The **A domains** of factor VIII (Fig. 2) are homologous to ceruloplasmin – a plasma copper-binding oxidase. The **B domain** is carbohydrate-rich and non-essential for function, while the **2 C domains** are homologous to discoidin I – a phospholipid-binding protein of *Dictyostelium*, suggesting they are involved in phospholipid binding.

GENE THERAPY FOR HAEMOPHILIA B

When the first attempts were made to test the feasibility of gene therapy for haemophilia B in 1987[11] defective retroviruses provided the only generally available methodology. An ex vivo approach was envisaged

Table 2 Summary of amounts of factor IX synthesized ex vivo by various cell types[a]

Cell type and species	Primary or transformed	Vector	Promoter/enhancer	Factor IX[b] (μg/10^6cells/24 h)	Biological activity[c] (% of normal)	References
Hepatocytes (human)	Transformed	Retrovirus	Metallothionine	0.01	86	11
Fibroblasts (human)	Transformed	"	Metallothionine	0.01	~100	11
Fibroblasts (rat)	Primary	"	Various	0.1–4.6	NT[f]	12
Fibroblasts (human)	Primary	"	Various	0.08–3.4	72–100[d]	12
Fibroblasts (mouse)	Transformed	"	LTR	0.01–0.04	10–100[d]	33
Hepatocytes (rabbit)	Primary	"	CMV[e]	0.45	90	34
Endothelial cells (rat)	Primary	"	LTR	0.84	~100	35
Fibroblasts (dog)	Primary	"	Various	0.02–1[g]	96	36
Endothelial cells (bovine)	Primary	"	CMV	1	83	36
Myoblasts (mouse)	Transformed	"	LTR	2.6	~85	37
Myoblasts (mouse)	Primary	"	Various	0.1–0.5	NT[h]	17
Keratinocytes (human)	Primary	"	LTR	0.58	42	13
Fibroblasts (rabbit)	Primary	"	Various	0.5–2.5	NT[h]	16
Fibroblasts (human)	Primary	"	Various	0.2–0.3	70	24
Fibroblasts (mouse)[i]	Transformed	Plasmids	Various	0.01	70	14

[a]Not all results from each report are included. [b]Mostly human, but in some reports dog, factor IX. These figures were usually determined by ELISA. [c]Determined by a quantitative one stage clotting assay using factor IX-deficient plasma. Cells were usually cultured in the presence of vitamin K, which is a cofactor for the carboxylase. Strictly, 'biological activity' is 'specific biological activity', since all values were normalised with respect to antigen. 'Normal' refers to normal plasma factor IX. [d]Determined in part, by ELISA with Ca^{2+} specific antifactor IX antibody. [e]Human cytomegalovirus, immediate early enhancer/promoter. [f]NT = not tested. [g]Highest values were observed only if basic fibroblast growth factor was included. [h]Barium citrate adsorption suggested a substantial proportion was active. [i]Microencapsulated.

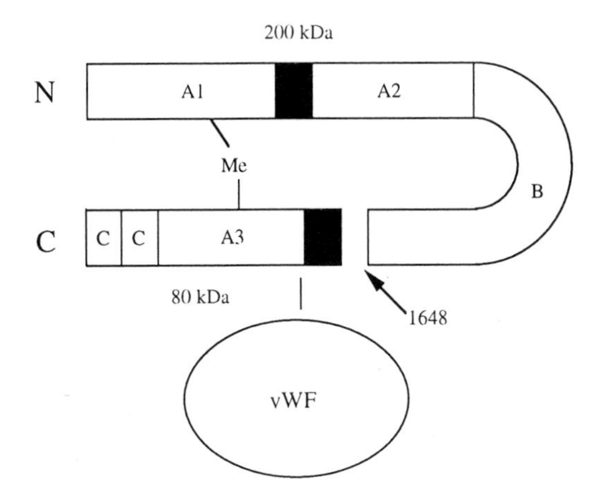

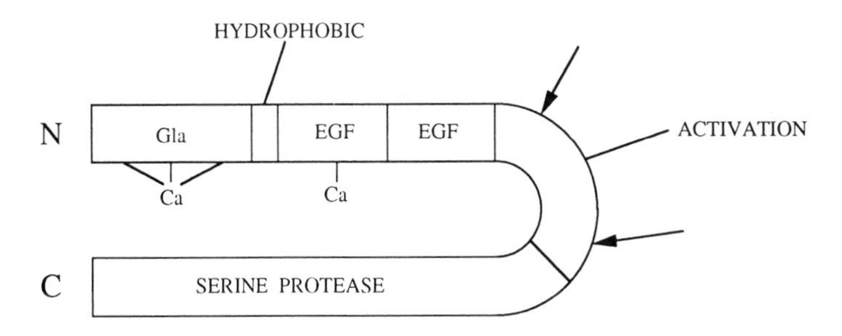

Fig. 2 Factor VIII (above) and IX (below) protein domains. In factor VIII, the N-terminal heavy chain (200 kD) and the C-terminal light chain (80kD) are shown, stabilized as a complex by metal (Me) binding. A proposed site of binding to the multimeric von Willebrand factor is shown (from Hoeben[32] with permission). In factor IX, Ca is calcium and arrows mark the sites of cleavage, in the **activation** domain, by factor XIa or VIIa. For further details, see text.

in which the virus would be used to infect (or transduce) in culture cells that had been derived from a biopsy of some tissue of the patient. After characterization of the transduced cells and safety testing, these transduced cells would then be re-introduced into the patient by transplantation. Since then a number of other methods, using either viral or non-viral vectors, have been developed for use in gene therapy in general and some have now been tested for haemophilia B. Some of these more recent methods envisage the introduction of the factor IX cDNA by in vivo delivery directly into patients, since this is obviously much simpler than the ex vivo approach.

Gene therapy for haemophilia B has become a model for diseases in which an extracellular glycoprotein is required. The idea of using a cell other than the hepatocyte[11] was initially considered to be controversial, because of the requirement for adequate levels of γ-glutamyl carboxylase necessary for factor IX activity. It is clear, however, that this enzyme is widely distributed, since many different cell types have been successfully targeted.

Ex vivo studies

Since the discovery[11] that fibroblasts could produce active factor IX, there have been many other reports (Table 2) of successful expression in cells as diverse as endothelial cells, myoblasts and keratinocytes as well as hepatocytes. Retroviral vectors based on the Moloney murine leukaemia/sarcoma virus were used in most studies and factor IX was secreted ex vivo at between 0.01–4.6 μg/10^6 cells/24 h. Fibroblasts appear to secrete the highest yields of factor IX ex vivo.[12] Undoubtedly, the low yields of secreted factor IX reported in the early studies[11] were caused by the use of weak promoter/enhancer elements to control factor IX expression. Where strong promoter/enhancers such as the immediate-early cytomegalovirus (CMV) promoter-enhancer were used,[12] higher yields were obtained. Although transformed cells have been widely used as models, they are not suitable in general as in vivo models for gene therapy because of the obvious risk of cancer. There remains some doubt as to whether there is sufficient γ-glutamyl carboxylase present in all cell types tested for **full** biological activity of factor IX, since in some cells – e.g. in primary keratinocytes, factor IX was not fully active.[13] In fibroblasts, also, it was suggested that the cells secreting most factor IX may be least active, possibly because the carboxylase was limiting.[12] It may be necessary to co-express the carboxylase cDNA[10] with the factor IX cDNA to obtain maximal activity, although initial attempts at doing this in Chinese hamster ovary cells have failed.[8] However, co-expression of a cDNA which expresses furin (the enzyme required for propeptide cleavage) did improve factor IX activity.[8]

A particularly interesting non-viral approach is being developed by Chang's group who propose enclosing fibroblasts secreting factor IX within immunoprotective membraneous capsules. Such capsules, containing transformed mouse fibroblasts transfected by various factor IX expression plasmids, secrete factor IX ex vivo[14] (Table 2).

Animal model studies

The significant yields of factor IX secreted by cells in tissue culture encouraged early studies in animal models, in particular in rodents (Table 3). Retrovirally-transduced human, rat or mouse primary fibroblasts, after subcutaneous or intraperitoneal transplantation into mice and rats, secreted easily detectable quantities of factor IX into the bloodstream.[12] However, secretion was transient up to a maximum of a month. (The transport and half-life of human factor IX from a subcutaneous site to the bloodstream has been separately studied in nude mice. Transport appears to occur via lymphatic drainage and is surprisingly efficient.[15]) The reason for only transient production of factor IX in vivo in mice and rats was unclear.[12] A possible scenario, however, is that those fibroblasts which survived the transplantation continued to divide and secrete factor IX until they came under the control of the (largely unknown) mechanisms that limit their growth in vivo, when they became quiescent. Under these conditions the fibroblasts presumably fail to synthesize one or more of the large number of transcription factors and enhancer-binding proteins required for the heterologous promoter/enhancer used to express the factor IX mRNA, so that factor IX secretion stops.

A recent report from China, in which human and rabbit fibroblasts secreting human factor IX were grafted subcutaneously into rabbits, showed that factor IX secretion continued at significant levels for up to 10 months.[16] Why fairly long-term expression of factor IX occurred in rabbits, but not in rats and mice, is unclear.

Human primary keratinocytes, transduced with a human factor IX retrovirus ex vivo and grafted into nude mice, secreted very small amounts of factor IX into the bloodstream for only 1 week.[13] In an interesting and well-controlled study using primary mouse myoblasts, Dai et al[17] found that a muscle-specific enhancer, derived from the creatine kinase gene and incorporated into the provirus upstream of a CMV enhancer/promoter, was critical for long term expression in mice of small amounts of canine factor IX. This conclusion has been recently challenged,[18] but the results obtained may depend on the particular combination of tissue-specific enhancer and viral promoter/enhancer used, which differed in these separate studies.

In vivo studies

In vivo studies (Table 3) in which factor IX retroviruses are directly injected into the portal vasculature of haemophilia B dogs, partially hepatectomized so as to stimulate hepatocyte proliferation, have been pioneered by Woo's and Brinkhous' laboratories.[19] Small amounts of recombinant normal canine factor IX were secreted into blood over 5

Table 3 Studies in animal models[a] and in haemophilia B patients

Cell type used (or targeted)	Human or animal model (species)	Vector	Ex vivo or in vivo	Site injected	Plasma[b] Factor IX (% normal)	Duration[c]	References
Fibroblasts (human, mouse, rat)	Mouse & rat	Retrovirus	ex vivo	i.p. & s.c.	<4	1 week– 1 month	12
Fibroblasts (rabbit, human)	Rabbit	”	”	i.p. & s.c.	1–10	4–10 months	16
Fibroblast (human)	Human	”	”	s.c	0-3[f]	6 months	24
Keratinocytes	Mouse	”	”	s.c.	0.1	1 week	13
Myoblasts (mouse)	Mouse	”	”	i.m.	0.1–0.3	>5 months	17,18
Hepatocytes	Dog[d]	”	in vivo	intraportal	0.1	5 months	19
All tissues	Mouse	Adenovirus[e]	”	Various	7	9 weeks	21
All tissues	Dog	Adenovirus[e]	”	intraportal	300	1-2 months	20
Hepatocytes	Mouse	Herpes simplex virus 1	”	liver	10	1 week	22
Hapatocytes	Rat	Galactosylated poly (L-lysine)	”	i.v.	0.1–35	4.5 months	23

[a]Excluding studies with transformed cells. [b]Determined by ELISA and/or clotting activity. [c]Time to baseline factor IX or when experiment ended. [d]Partially hepatectomized. [e]A second injection of recombinant adenovirus failed to boost plasma factor IX levels suggesting that neutralising antibodies were present. [f]One patient showed a 3% increase in clotting activity, the other showed no increase.

months and there was a marginal improvement in a functional assay for clotting, implying that the secreted factor IX was biologically active. The use of factor IX adenoviral vectors, because they can infect non-dividing cells, eliminates the need for hepatectomy. When a defective factor IX adenovirus was directly injected into the portal vasculature of haemophilia B dogs,[20] huge quantities of biologically active factor IX were secreted into the blood but the amounts rapidly decreased to baseline within 1–2 months. The reason for this decline is unknown.[20] It is, however, likely that host-derived cytotoxic T cells, specific for adenoviral antigens, will proliferate and eventually result in the elimination of virally-infected cells. Lower but still very significant amounts of factor IX were present in plasma when a factor IX adenovirus was directly injected into the tail vein of mice.[21] In both the adenoviral vector approaches[20,21] there was evidence that the liver was the major, but not the sole target of the virus. In particular, the ovary of a heterozygous female carrier haemophilia B dog was shown to be infected.[20]

Despite their interest, it is doubtful whether any of the above in vivo approaches would be ethically acceptable for patients, because of the risks associated with hepatectomy in the case of the retroviral approach, and the probability that the retrovirus or adenovirus would be dispersed throughout the body and would infect cells other than hepatocytes, including the germ line cells. The transient nature of the response is clearly a severe limitation to the use of adenoviral vectors. Similar criticisms apply to the in vivo approach with replication-defective factor IX herpes simplex virus vectors,[22] injected directly into the liver of a mouse (Table 3).

Receptor-mediated gene transfer, targeting factor IX cDNA to the asialoglycoprotein receptor of the hepatocyte, seems promising if the variability associated with the initial studies reported in rats can be resolved.[23]

The Chinese clinical trial

In late 1991, Hsueh and colleagues in Shanghai, China, started a clinical trial on 2 brothers, aged 9 and 13 with moderately severe haemophilia B using autologous fibroblasts transduced with factor IX retroviruses. The protocol was based on experience with the rabbit model studies[16] in which an improved transplantation procedure was devised whereby the fibroblasts were simply premixed with rat collagen just before injection. About 10^9 fibroblasts, in 3 or 4 treatments over a period of 3–4 months, were injected subcutaneously in the abdominal area. A brief general anaesthetic was used and the patients tolerated the procedures well. Their report,[24] in English, claimed that both the plasma factor IX antigen and clotting activity gradually rose, in the younger patient, from a base line of about 3% to a value of about 6%, with accompanying clinical improvement in bleeding, and maintained that level 6 months after the start of the gene therapy. No improvement, however, was seen in the older patient. The possible reasons advanced for the failure in the older patient were the fact that his fibroblasts grew less well in culture, that he received only 60% of the number of fibroblasts as his younger brother and that he was about 50% heavier. The presence of the *neo* gene in the vector used by the Chinese group may be a problem, because antigen processing of neomycin phosphotransferase (the product of the *neo* gene) within transduced fibroblasts and their presentation by host-derived Major Histocompatibility Complex (MHC) Class I molecules at the cell surface to specific cytotoxic T cells would be expected in time to result in cell death. Further work is obviously needed to validate this approach.

GENE THERAPY FOR HAEMOPHILIA A

Gene therapy for haemophilia A is theoretically more attractive than for haemophilia B, because of the significantly lower amounts of protein required for haemostasis (Table 1). Unfortunately, the shorter half-life of factor VIII (Table 1), its inefficient secretion due to retention within the endoplasmic reticulum and the presence of a possible transcriptional repressor sequence (see below) within its mRNA coding region all negate this advantage and complicate studies aimed at testing the feasibility of gene therapy.

A further difficulty is the length of the factor VIII mRNA, which is believed to be too long (Table 1) to package into a viable retrovirus. Fortunately, the in-frame removal of an internal region of the mRNA coding for a non-essential B domain (Fig. 2), generates a shorter 4.4 kb mRNA which is packaged and codes for active factor VIII (Fig. 1).

There are few reports[25–29] of successful expression of factor VIII in experiments aiming towards gene therapy, and in all studies defective retroviral vectors were used. Since some factor VIII is probably synthesized outside the liver, many cell types are potential targets. Transformed fibroblasts and primary human fibroblasts, transduced with various factor VIII retroviruses, secrete low amounts of factor VIII (1–40 $\mu g/10^6$ cells/24 h) when grown in tissue culture and, where it was tested, the factor VIII was found to be fully biologically active.

The low amounts of factor VIII secreted in tissue culture were not unexpected because of earlier work from Kaufman's laboratory showing that factor VIII expression derived from transfected plasmids was very inefficient compared with von Willebrand factor expression in cell lines co-expressing these proteins.[30] Following up this theme, the Miller and Kaufman group[29] estimated that the yield of factor VIII was about 100 times less than factor IX produced by similar retroviral vectors in the same cell type. The viral titre of the factor VIII vectors was also 2 orders of magnitude less than the factor IX vectors. It emerged from deletion studies[29] that there are dominant inhibitory sequences within the A2 and A3 coding domains of the factor VIII provirus which allow only roughly 1% of the expected mRNA to accumulate. Recent studies (R C Hoeben, personal communication) suggest that these sequences down-regulate the initiation of transcription by an unknown mechanism. It is clearly vital to define this in detail in the hope that the problem can be overcome in the near future.

Despite the low yields of factor VIII synthesized in the cell culture experiments, transplantation experiment have been attempted in nude mice, but with very limited success.[27] After subcutaneous transplantation of various fibroblasts (human primary and transformed lines), transduced with a factor VIII retrovirus, it proved impossible to detect factor VIII in the blood. Transplanted cells could, however, be rescued and were still capable of synthesizing factor VIII in tissue culture. Factor VIII retrovirus was also used[26] to infect murine haematopoietic progenitor cells in culture followed by selection and transplantation into mice. However, no evidence of transcription of the provirus was found in vivo implying that transcription is repressed in the process of differentiation of the blood cells in vivo.

FUTURE PROSPECTS

Despite the considerable progress made in the last few years, it is obvious that all existing gene therapy protocols for haemophilia B have significant limitations: either too little protein is synthesised in animal models, or expression of clotting factors is maintained for too short a time. Thus there will be great difficulty in obtaining normal factor IX clotting levels in the first human gene therapy trials. This has been borne out by the results of the Chinese clinical protocol where only small increases of clotting activity were reported. This trial, while promising, needs to be confirmed. Nevertheless it should be emphasised that, even if gene therapy were to boost the concentration of factor IX by 2–3%, this could be of great benefit to patients clinically and should prevent bleeding into joints. Improvements in existing methodology or new methods of gene delivery, particularly in vivo methods, are required to obtain better and longer-term expression of factor IX in vivo. Progress with gene therapy for haemophilia A has been disappointing, but further research is vital. Despite these uncertainties, I predict that gene therapy for haemophiliacs will become a reality in the not too distant future, although it may take a considerable time before the present protein therapy is superceded.

ACKNOWLEDGEMENTS

I thank Ann Gerrard, Charles Rizza, Sean Page, and Rob Hoeben for critically reading the manuscript, and Suzanne Motyka for secretarial help. Professor Brownlee's research is supported by the Wellcome Trust.

REFERENCES

1 Brettler DB, Levine PH. Factor concentrates for treatment of hemophilia: which one to choose? Blood 1989; 73: 2067–2073.
2 Hedner U, Davie EW. Introduction to hemostasis and the vitamin K-dependent coagulation factors. In: Scriver CR, Beaudet AL, Sly WS, Vale D, eds. The metabolic basis of inherited disease. 5th edn. New York: McGraw-Hill, 1989: 2107–2134.
3 Brownlee GG. The molecular pathology of haemophilia B. Biochem Soc Trans 1987; 15: 1–8.
4 Pittman DD, Kaufman RJ. Proteolytic requirements for thrombin activation of anti-hemophilic factor (factor VIII). Proc Natl Acad Sci USA 1988; 85: 2429–2433.
5 Giannelli F, Green PM, Sommer SS et al. Haemophilia B: database of point mutations and short additions and deletions – fifth edition. Nucleic Acids Res 1994; 22: 3534–3546.
6 Kurachi K, Kurachi S, Furukawa M, Yao S-N. Biology of factor IX. Blood Coagul Fibrinolysis 1993; 4: 953–974.
7 Tuddenham EGD, Schwaab R, Seehafer J et al. Haemophilia A: database of nucleotide substitutions, deletions, insertions and rearrangements of the factor VIII gene Second Edition. Nucleic Acids Res 1994; 22: 3511–3533.
8 Rehemtulla A, Roth DA, Wasley LC, et al. *In vitro* and *in vivo* functional characterization of bovine vitamin K-dependent γ-carboxylase expressed in Chinese hamster ovary cells. Proc Natl Acad Sci USA 1993; 90: 4611–4615.
9 Bentley AK, Rees DJG, Rizza C, Brownlee GG. Defective propeptide processing of blood clotting factor IX caused by mutation of arginine to glutamine at position -4. Cell 1986; 45: 343–348.
10 Wu S-M, Cheung W-F, Frazier D, Stafford DW. Cloning and expression of the cDNA for human γ-glutamyl carboxylase. Science 1991; 254: 1634–1636.
11 Anson DS, Hock RA, Austen D, et al. Towards gene therapy for Haemophilia B. Mol Biol Med 1987; 4: 11–20.
12 Palmer TD, Thompson AR, Miller AD. Production of human factor IX in animals by genetically modified skin fibroblasts: potential therapy for haemophilia B. Blood 1989; 73: 438–445.
13 Gerrard AJ, Hudson DL, Brownlee GG, Watt FM. Towards gene therapy for haemophilia B using primary human keratinocytes. Nature Genet 1993; 3: 180–183.
14 Liu H-W, Ofosu FA, Chang PL. Expression of human factor IX by microencapsulated recombinant fibroblasts. Hum Gene Ther 1993; 4: 291–301.
15 Gerrard AJ, Austen DEG, Brownlee GG. Subcutaneous injection of factor IX for the treatment of haemophilia B. Br J Haematol 1992; 81: 610–613.
16 Zhou J-M, Qiu X-F, Lu D-R, Lu J-Y, Xue J-L. Long-term expression of human factor IX cDNA in rabbits. Science in China (Series B) 1993; 36: 1333-1341.
17 Dai Y, Roman M, Naviaux RK, Verma IM. Gene therapy via primary myoblasts: long term expression of factor IX protein following transplantation *in vivo*. Proc Natl Acad Sci USA 1992; 89: 10892–10895.
18 Yao S-N, Smith KJ, Kurachi K. Primary myoblast-mediated gene transfer: persistent expression of human factor IX in mice. Gene Ther 1993; 1: 1–9.
19 Kay MA, Rothenberg S. Landon CN, et al. *In vivo* therapy of haemophilia B: sustained partial correction in factor IX-deficient dogs. Science 1993; 262: 117–119.
20 Kay MA, Landon CN, Rothenberg SR, et al. *In vivo* hepatic gene therapy: complete albeit transient correction of factor IX deficiency in hemophilia B dogs. Proc Natl Acad Sci USA 1994; 91: 2353–2357.

21 Smith TAG, Mehaffrey MG, Kayda DB, et al. Adenovirus mediated expression of therapeutic plasma levels of human factor IX in mice. Nature Genet 1993; 5: 397–402.
22 Miyanohara A, Johnson PA, Elam RL, et al. Direct gene transfer to the liver with Herpes simplex virus type 1 vectors: transient production of physiologically relevant levels of circulating factor IX. New Biol 1992; 4: 238–246.
23 Perales JC, Ferkol T, Beegen H, Ratnoff OD, Hanson RW. Gene transfer *in vivo*: sustained expression and regulation of genes introduced into the liver by receptor-targeted uptake. Proc Natl Acad Sci USA 1994; 91: 4086–4090.
24 Lu D-R, Zhou J-M, Zheng B, et al. Stage I clinical trial of gene therapy for hemophilia B. Science in China (Series B) 1993; 36: 1342–1351.
25 Hoeben RC, van der Jagt RCM, Schoute F, et al. Expression of functional factor VIII in primary human skin fibroblasts after retrovirus-mediated gene transfer. J Biol Chem 1990; 265: 7318–7323.
26 Hoeben RC, Einerhand MPW, Briet E, van Ormondt H, Valerio D, van der Eb AJ. Towards gene therapy in hemophilia A: retrovirus-mediated transfer of a factor VIII gene into murine haemotopoietic progenitor cells. Thromb Haemost 1992; 67: 341–345.
27 Hoeben RC, Fallaux FJ, van Tilburg NH, et al. Towards gene therapy for hemophilia A: long-term persistence of factor VIII-secreting fibroblasts after transplantation into immunodeficient mice. Hum Gene Ther 1993; 4: 179–186.
28 Israel DI, Kaufman RJ. Retroviral-mediated transfer and amplification of a functional human factor VIII gene. Blood 1990; 75: 1074–1080.
29 Lynch CM, Israel DI, Kaufman RJ, Miller D. Sequences in the coding region of clotting factor VIII act as dominant inhibitors of RNA accumulation and protein production. Hum Gene Ther 1993; 4: 259–272.
30 Kaufman RJ, Wasley LC, Davies MV, Wise RJ, Israel DI, Dorner AJ. Effect of von Willebrand factor co-expression on the synthesis and secretion of factor VIII in Chinese hamster ovary cells. Mol Cell Biol 1989; 9: 1233–1242.
31 Gailani D, Broze GJ. Factor IX activation in a revised model of blood coagulation. Science 1991; 253: 909–912.
32 Hoeben RC. Towards gene therapy for haemophilia A: vectors for the expression of blood clotting factor VIII *in vivo*. Ph.D. thesis, University of Leiden, The Netherlands 1991.
33 St Louis DL, Verma ID. An alternative approach to somatic cell gene therapy. Proc Natl Acad Sci USA 1988; 85: 3150–3154.
34 Armentano D, Thompson AR, Darlington G, Woo SLC. Expression of human factor IX in rabbit hepatocytes by retrovirus-mediated gene transfer: potential for gene therapy of hemophilia B. Proc Natl Acad Sci USA 1990; 87: 6141–6145.
35 Yao S-N, Wilson JM, Nabel EG, Kurachi S, Hachiya JL, Kurachi K. Expression of human factor IX in rat capillary endothelial cells: towards somatic gene therapy for hemophilia B. Proc Natl Acad Sci USA 1991; 88: 8101–8105.
36 Axelrod JH, Read MS, Brinkhous KM, Verma IM. Phenotypic correction of factor IX deficiency in skin fibroblasts of hemophilia dogs. Proc Natl Acad Sci USA 1990; 87: 5173–5177.
37 Yao S-N, Kurachi K. Expression of human factor IX in mice after injection of genetically modified myoblasts. Proc Natl Acad Sci USA 1992; 89: 3357–3361.

British Medical Bulletin (1995) Vol. 51, No. 1, pp.106–122

Gene therapy of lysosomal storage disorders

A Salvetti, J M Heard and O Danos

Retrovirus et Transfert Genétique, Institut Pasteur, Paris, France

Lysosomal storage disorders (LSD) result from deficiencies in enzymes normally implicated in the catabolism of macromolecules inside the lysosome. Many of these enzymes can reach the lysosome after being secreted in the extracellular medium and recaptured by specific cell surface receptors. This has suggested a rationale for therapeutic approaches in LSD, in which the missing enzyme is provided by an external source. Current therapies based on this concept, including the administration of purified enzyme and bone marrow transplantation, have been shown to result in clinical improvements in both animal models and patients. Although considerable difficulties must be surmounted, LSD present a favourable situation for gene therapy. The gene corresponding to the affected enzyme has been identified in most diseases and cDNAs are available. Low and unregulated levels of enzyme activity should be sufficient for correction. Importantly, a variety of gene transfer strategies can be carefully evaluated in animal models.

Most of the catabolism in the living cell takes place in the lysosome. These organelles are formed in the trans Golgi network, from vesicles in which more than 40 different enzymes, mostly acid hydrolases, are selectively packed. The mature lysosome results from a fusion between these enzyme-containing vesicles and late endosomes where macromolecules awaiting disposal are entrapped. The acid pH maintained within the lysosome activates the enzymes, and proteins, nucleic acids and complex sugars are degraded. A deficiency in one of these digestion processes results in the accumulation of the undegraded substrate within the lysosomes, which increase in number and size and can severely impair the physiology of the cell.

More than 30 lysosomal storage disorders (LSD) have been identified which are usually classified according to the undigested macromolecule which accumulates: glycosaminoglycans in **mucopolysaccharidoses** (MPS), sphingolipids in **lipidoses** and glycoproteins in **glycoproteinoses.**[1] Most LSD are due to a failure to synthesize an active form of the relevant enzyme; in some cases, as in the I-cell disease, the defect lies in the inability to target the enzymes to the lysosome (Table). The tissues most affected by the enzyme deficiency are those in which the accumulation of the undigested substrate is the highest. For example, in Krabbe disease the deficiency in galactosylceramidase affects mainly the cells of the central nervous system where the turnover of galactosylceramide is particularly important. In MPS, the missing enzymes are normally implicated in the degradation of glycosaminoglycans which accumulate in spleen, liver, brain and cartilage resulting in bone and joint abnormalities, hepatosplenomegaly, corneal clouding and mental retardation.[2] Similar symptoms are found in patients with Gaucher disease in whom a defect in glucocerebrosidase results in the accumulation of glycosylceramide in monocytes/macrophages.

Many enzymes implicated in LSD are secreted proteins with the notable exception of glucocerebrosidase and acid phosphatase that behave like membrane-associated proteins. In a classic series of experiments, Neufeld and collaborators showed that fibroblasts from MPS patients could be corrected by factors secreted by normal fibroblasts or present in urine concentrates. These ‘corrective factors’ were identified as the normal enzymes themselves, which were taken up by the mutant cells and targeted to the lysosomes.[1] these enzymes are normally synthesized on membrane-bound polysomes in the rough endoplasmic reticulum and are glycosylated during transit through the endoplasmic reticulum and the Golgi apparatus. There, they are specifically modified by phosphorylation of mannose residues and become ligands for the mannose-6-phosphate receptors (M6PRs). These membrane-anchored receptors cycle between the Golgi compartment, lysosome and the plasma membrane, and direct the phosphorylated enzyme precursors to the organelles, either by selectively packing them into pre-lysosomal vesicles, or by capturing mannose phosphorylated molecules in the extra-cellular environment.[3]

The discovery of this secretion/recapture mechanism has suggested that lysosomal deficiencies could be complemented *in trans* by supplying the missing enzyme either as a purified protein or as a graft of cells secreting the protein. Indeed, in some cases of LSD, treatments involving the infusion of purified enzyme or bone marrow transplantation have demonstrated a therapeutic efficiency in both animal models and patients. The gene corresponding to the affected enzyme has been

Table

Type/syndrome	Enzyme deficiency	Cloned cDNA	Animal models	Affected tissues[a]
MUCOPOLYSACCHARIDOSES				
I/Hurler	α-L-iduronidase	human, canine	dog, cat	CNS, JB, LS
I/Scheie				
II/Hunter	iduronate sulfatase	human	–	CNS, JB, LS
III A/San Filippo A	heparan N-sulfatase	–	–	CNS
III B/San Filippo B	N-acetyl-α-glucosaminidase	–	–	CNS
III C/San Filippo C	acetyl CoA: α-glucosaminide -acetyltransferase	–	–	CNS
III D/San Filippo D	N-acetylglucosamine 6-sulfase	human	goat	CNS
IV A/Morquio A	galactose 6-sulfatase	human	–	JB
IV B/Morquio B	β-galactosidase	human	–	JB
VI/Maroteaux-Lamy	arylsufatase B	human, feline	rat, cat	JB
VII/Sly	β-glucuronidase	human, rat, mouse	mouse, dog	CNS, JB, LS
GLYCORPROTEINOSES				
Fucosidosis	α-L-fucosidase	human	dog	CNS, JB
α-Mannosidosis	α-mannosidase	–	cat, cow	CNS, JB, LS
β-mannosidose	β-mannosidase	–	goat, sheep, cow	CNS
Aspartylglycosaminuria	aspartylglycosaminidase	human	–	CNS, LS
Sialidose	sialidase	–	–	CNS, JB
Galactosialidosis	protective protein	human	dog	CNS, JB, LS

(Table continued on following page)

Table Continued...

Type/syndrome	Enzyme deficiency	Cloned cDNA	Animal models	Affected tissues [a]
LIPIDOSES				
Fabry	α-galactosidase	human	–	kidney
Farber	ceramidase	–	–	JB
Gaucher	glucocerobrosidase	human	mouse	CNS, JB, LS
Krabbe	galactosylceramidase	–	mouse	CNS
GM1 gangliosidosis	β-galactosylceramidase	human	dog, cat	CNS, JB, LS
GM2 gangliosidoses:				
Tay-Sachs	β-hexosaminidase alpha-subunit	human	–	CNS
Sandhoff	β-hexosaminidase, β-subunit	human	cat	CNS
Metachromatic Leukodystrophy	aryl sulfatase A	human	–	CNS
Niemann-Pick A and B	sphingomyelinase	human	–	CNS, LS
Niemann-Pick C	–	–	mouse	CNS, LS
OTHER DISORDERS WITH SINGLE ENZYME DEFECT				
Wolman	acid lipase	–	rat	LS
Pompe	α-glucosidase	?	–	Muscle
I-cell disease and	6-phosopho-N-acetylglucosamine	?	–	CNS, JB

Summary of lysosomal storage disorders [a]Predominantly affected tissues in the most severe forms are indicate (CNS: central nervous system; JB: Joint and bone; LS: liver and spleen) identified for most LSD and cDNAs are available (Table). Gene transfer represents an interesting alternative approach for the therapy of LSD. It could be used to provide the enzyme *in trans* or to restore the production of a normal enzyme directly in the affected cells. This review describes possible approaches for gene therapy of LSD and discusses their potential as compared to currently available treatments.

DESCRIPTION OF LYSOSOMAL STORAGE DISORDERS

Genetics

The estimated incidence of LSD is approximately 1:10 000 live births. The most prevalent lysosomal disorder is Gaucher's disease with a significantly higher frequency in Ashkenazi Jew population (approximately 1:600 to 1:2500).[4] The same biased incidence has been found for Tay-Sachs disease which is more frequent in Ashkenazi Jews and the French-Canadian populations.

Most LSD share common clinical features, such as mental retardation and abnormal skeletal development. Many of these disorders also cause hepatosplenomegaly which may be the dominant symptom in the milder forms. Within each type of LSD, different forms can be distinguished on the basis of the severity of symptoms and age of onset. The most severe forms appear early in infancy and the disease has a chronic and progressive course leading to death before adulthood. Milder forms can lead to late onset symptoms that do not cause premature death. A property shared by these disorders is the accumulation of undegraded molecules, which may be excreted in the urine and result at the histological level, in the appearance of cells containing enlarged lysosomes or inclusions. The diagnosis of LSD is usually made on fibroblast or leucocyte extracts, using enzyme assays to identify the deficiency.

The gene encoding the normal enzyme has been identified and cloned in several cases (Table) and molecular studies can identify the most common mutations. Analysis of the mutations found in Gaucher, metachromatic leukodystrophy, GM2 gangliosidoses, aspartylglycosaminuria and several MPS, indicates that these diseases are very heterogenous.[1] In some cases, these genetic studies have established a correlation between the genetic lesions and the severity of the disease. For example, the analysis of several MPS I patients has led to the identification of at least 3 common mutations associated with the development of severe forms.[5–7] In Gaucher disease, over 35 different mutations have been documented including missense and nonsense point mutations, splicing mutations, deletions, insertions and a fusion gene. For some of these mutations a correlation was made with the severity of the disease dependent on whether they provoke a complete or partial lack of the enzyme.[8] However, a certain degree of variability exists among patients bearing the same genotype, impairing the reliability of predictions bout the clinical outcome.

Animal models

The characterization of animal models of LSD (Table 1) makes it possible to evaluate the efficiency of new therapeutic approaches. Small laboratory animals like mouse and rats, which can be easily bred on an homogenous genetic background have been described in the case of MPS VI, MPS VII and Krabbe disease.[9–11] Larger animals, like MPS I, MPS VII and fucosidosis dogs or MPS I and MPS VI cats are useful in preclinical studies designed to evaluate the feasibility and efficiency of a gene transfer protocol on a larger scale.[12–16] Many other animal models of LSD have been described,[17–26] but in most cases the deficiency was only documented at the biochemical level without definitive identification of the genetic defect.

New animal models can also be created in mice by knocking out the relevant gene. This method has been used to engineer a model of Gaucher disease by disrupting the glucocerebrosidase gene. Mice homozygous for this mutation have a very low enzyme activity and die early after birth.[27] Although animal models for milder forms of Gaucher disease have to be created for therapeutic experiments, this first model is important for the investigation of the pathogenesis of the most severe forms of this disease.

CURRENT TREATMENTS

Preclinical studies on animal models

Studies on animal models of LSD mainly consist in enzyme replacement therapy through bone marrow transplantation. The rationale for this approach is that the lysosomal enzyme secreted by the engrafted hematopoietic cells will be distributed to different tissues and taken up by deficient cells. In addition, non-deficient cells differentiating toward the monocyte/macrophage lineage probably reduce storage in surrounding deficient cells by degrading glycosaminoglycans accumulated in the local environment. Bone marrow transplantation has been shown to have beneficial effects in MPS I dogs, with a decrease in glycosaminoblycans storage in various tissues including the brain, and a much slower progression of the disease. However, only a slight impact on the evolution of the skeletal deformities was observed.[28,29] A clinical amelioration was also demonstrated in MPS VI cats and in fucosidosis dogs.[30,31] In the latter case, a rapid improvement in the peripheral nerve and visceral lesions as well as a more gradual improvement in the central nervous system pathology were documented. Notably, these experiments illustrate that the effectiveness of this treatment depends on the age at the time of transplantation. Engraftment at an early age, before the onset of clinical signs reduced the severity and slowed the progression of neurological lesions. Similarly, and effect on skeletal deformities and on brain lysosomal storage was observed only after treatment of neonatal MPS VII mice[32] and of one month-old MPS VII dogs (M Haskins, personal communication). A neurological improvement was also demonstrated in the Twitcher mouse which has a galactocerebrosidase deficiency analogous to Krabbe disease in humans. The increase in galactosylceramidase activity in the brain correlated with the progressive infiltration of donor-derived macrophages.[33] These cells may progressively reduce storage lesions through local enzyme release, cell-to-cell enzyme exchange and phagocytosis of the undigested products. On the other hand, bone marrow transplantation has no effect on the progression of the neurological disease in dogs with GM1 gangliosidosis.[34] The reduction of the neurological lesions observed in some of these experiments is thought to result mainly from the colonization of brain by donor-derived macrophages. However, injection of purified recombinant β-glucuronidase in newborn MPS VII mice have suggested that enzyme molecules can cross the blood-brain barrier when the treatment is initiated very early in life.[35]

Treatment of patients with LSD

The discovery that lysosomal storage in cell culture can be reduced by providing extracellular enzymes has rapidly led to several clinical trials in patients using plasma or cells as sources of enzymes. However, these experiments always resulted in a minimal transient effect.[36]

Allogenic bone marrow transplantation has now been performed on a large number of LSD patients. HLA matched bone marrow transplantation is available to less than half of the patients. Mortalities are 10% and 25% depending whether an HLA-matched relative or an unrelated HLA-matched donor can be found. Biochemical and clinical benefits have been observed in MPS I, MPS II, MPS VI and Gaucher type I patients. Successful engraftment always results in increased enzyme levels in leucocytes and normalization of the liver and spleen sizes. In MPS I and II, a stabilization of skeletal lesions usually occurs, but little improvement of pre-existing lesions is seen. In these cases, severe neurological symptoms appear to be prevented by early transplantation, but definitive conclusions about intellectual development cannot be drawn in the absence of long-term follow up. Successful engraftment can also be effective in mild forms of Krabbe, Niemann-Pick A and metachromatic leukodystrophy, but not in severe cases.[37,38]

Early trials of enzyme infusion conducted in the 1970s on patients affected with Fabry and Gaucher diseases were encouraging.[1] The procedures for large-scale purification of lysosomal enzymes have now been further developed, especially for the treatment of Gaucher's disease. Glucocerebrosidase can be concentrated from human placenta and processed by modifying the oligosaccharide chains, thus exposing the mannose residues necessary for recognition and uptake by macrophages.[39] More than 200 Gaucher patients with the non-neuronopathic form of the disease (type I), have received regular injections of this preparation (Ceredase®). Hematologic recovery, reduction of hepatosplenomegaly and skeletal improvement have been documented.[40,41]

Enzyme therapy could be applied in many other forms of LSD at least as a transient therapy while awaiting a suitable bone marrow donor. However, because of the high cost of the enzyme purification process, this therapy is subject to serious economical constraints.

STRATEGIES FOR GENE THERAPY

Rationale of the approach

The partial success of BMT, which can only be offered to patients with HLA-matched donors, and the economical obstacles associated with enzyme therapy, have stimulated the search for gene therapy approaches. As in the other therapeutic interventions, the goal is to provide tissues with minimal enzyme levels in order to avoid pathological lysosomal storage. Different strategies must be designed according to the nature of the enzyme. A soluble lysosomal enzyme can be distributed to tissues from autologous cells engineered to secrete it into the blood stream. In the case of membrane-associated or membrane-bound enzymes, gene transfer will have to be targeted to the most affected cells.

The cDNAs for nearly 20 human enzymes involved in LSD have been cloned (Table). Some of them have been transfected into COS or CHO cells to overproduce an active enzyme. Some of these studies also demonstrated that the enzyme was secreted in culture medium and that it could be internalized by deficient cells to restore a normal level of enzyme activity. Normal cDNAs have also been introduced in vitro into deficient cells using retroviral vectors and shown to complement the biochemical and phenotypic defect.[42–49]

Gene transfer into hematopoietic cells

Gene transfer into hematopoietic cells can be performed to complement a deficiency affecting the hematopoietic elements themselves, as in the monocyte/macrophage lineage in Gaucher or Niemann-Pick disease, or to reduce lysosomal storage in non-hematopoietic tissues. In this case the stored substrate can be degraded both by the scavenging activity of infiltrating macrophages derived from corrected stem cells and by other cells that have internalized the enzyme secreted by surrounding genetically modified cells. Recent data also suggest that reduction of storage may also result from cell-to-cell transfer of the lysosomal enzyme.[50,51]

Efficient procedures for retrovirus-mediated gene transfer into hematopoietic stem cells have been developed in the mouse. Donor bone marrow cells are infected in vitro in the presence of fibroblasts producing the retroviral vector and used to reconstitute lethally irradiated syngeneic recipients. If gene transfer occurs into a stem cell with long-term reconstituting capacity, it may be permanently amplified in the peripheral blood differentiated cell population. Hematopoietic chimeras stably expressing a foreign gene in a majority of peripheral cells from all lineages have been obtained.[52]

Several investigators have used retroviral vectors expressing the human glucocerebrosidase cDNA under the control of the viral LTR to demonstrate efficient transduction into murine long-term repopulating marrow cells. Analysis of long-term reconstituted mice (up to 8 months after transplantation) demonstrated the presence of the provirus in bone marrow, spleen and thymus). When bone marrow cells from these animals were transplanted into secondary recipients, the provirus was again detected in various hematopoietic lineages up to 4 months after transplantation. The levels of human glucocerebrosidase activity in bone marrow and spleen macrophages were equal to or greater than the endogenous mouse activity.[53–56] Efficient transduction of the human glucocerebrosidase cDNA was obtained in vitro into a substantial fraction of human hematopoietic progenitor cells from Gaucher patients.[44,57] These studies have encouraged several investigators to plan clinical trials involving gene transfer. However, in the absence of an adequate animal model for Gaucher disease, a therapeutic effect of gene transfer still has to be demonstrated.

A corrective effect of gene transfer into hematopoietic stem cells on lysosomal storage has been shown in 2 studies in MPS VII mice. In the first study, a retroviral vector coding for the rat β-glucuronidase cDNA under the control of a thymidine kinase promoter was used to infect bone marrow cells of two MPS VII mice. The analysis of the treated animals, 6 months after bone marrow transplantation, showed a complete disappearance of lysosomal storage lesions in the liver and spleen.[58] In a second study partial hematopoietic chimeras were obtained using a low irradiation dose conditioning of the recipient animals. Mice with less than 5% hematopoietic cells containing the human β-glucuronidase cDNA under the control of the phosphoglycerate kinase 1 promoter, displayed a complete correction of the liver and spleen, suggesting that small amounts of enzyme delivered locally can be sufficient for correction.[59] This observation is hopeful for clinical application in man, since the current available technology in humans does not provide more than a few percent of genetically-modified cells.

Enzyme delivery into the whole organism by genetically modified cells

In LSD involving a secreted enzyme, any cell type could be chosen as a source, provided that efficient methods for ex vivo gene transfer and stable reimplantation exist. Fibroblasts can be easily obtained from skin biopsies, grown in culture and infected with retroviral vectors. The inclusion of fibroblasts into collagen lattices has been shown to result in the formation of transplantable dermis equivalent.[60] The implantation of these lattices into the peritoneal cavity, mixed with bFGF-coated polytetrafluoroethylene (PTFE) fibers was shown to lead to the rapid formation of individualized neo-organs in which the genetically modified fibroblasts are metabolically active for months. A dense vascularisation of the implants brought the enzyme-secreting fibroblasts in permanent contact with the mesenteric circulation.[61] This procedure has been used to secrete human β-glucuronidase in MPS VII mice after retroviral mediated transfer of the human cDNA into skin primary fibroblasts. The implantation into MPS VII mice of lattices containing fibroblasts secreting the human enzyme was followed by a rapid disappearance of lysosomal storage lesions in the liver and the spleen. Human β-glucuronidase activity was found in the liver, spleen, lung, brain, kidney, heart and bone marrow of the implanted animals.[62] These experiments have shown that engineered fibroblasts, if reimplanted in a suitable environment can provide long-term therapeutic levels of enzyme in an MPS model. The cure was not complete however in the animals which displayed severe skeletal abnormalities when they were treated at the age of 6 to 8 weeks.

Experiments are in progress to test whether implanting enzyme-secreting fibroblasts within the first days of life could facilitate the enzyme access to the developing bones and joints and to the central nervous system.

In the perspective of a clinical trial, the procedure has been scaled up in normal dogs. During follow-up of one year uptake of human β-glucuronidase secreted by neo-organs was demonstrated in liver biopsies, in which the canine enzyme was heat-inactivated (P Moullier, unpublished results).

The skeletal muscle has been proposed as a convenient organ for a systemic delivery of therapeutic proteins.[63] Myoblasts have been isolated from MPS VII dog skeletal muscle, grown in culture and infected with a rat β-glucuronidase cDNA-containing retroviral vector. Enzyme expression was documented in both myoblasts and myotubes.[64]

Myoblasts from adult MPS VII mice were also isolated and infected with a retroviral vector coding for human β-glucuronidase. These cells were then injected in MPS VII mice, following muscle injury. The genetically-modified cells were found to efficiently participate to the constitution of regenerated muscle fiber. However, despite an efficient in vitro secretion of the enzyme, only trace amounts of activity were found in the liver and spleen of the treated animals.[65] This suggested that β-glucuronidase was blocked before it could access the blood stream, possibly at the level the muscle basal membrane or immediately reinternalized through binding to M6PRs which are highly expressed in muscle cells.

The liver occupies a strategic position as a provider of proteins into the blood stream. Retrovirus-mediated gene transfer in situ into the liver has been described in mice, rats and dogs.[66,67]Attempts at transferring the β-glucuronidase cDNA into the liver of MPS VII dogs are currently being made. The first results indicate that the fraction of hepatocyte which can be modified by this procedure may be too small to provide therapeutic enzyme levels.

Enzyme delivery to the central nervous system

It is unlikely that a soluble lysosomal enzyme delivered into the serum will cross the blood-brain barrier under normal conditions.[68] The β-glucuronidase found in the brain of MPS VII mice implanted with fibroblasts secreting the enzyme may correspond to enzyme molecules absorbed by monocytes in the periphery and transported across the barrier.[62] In this case, however, the small amount of enzyme found in this tissue may be too low to obtain a correction of the lysosomal storage lesions.

Crossing of the blood-brain barrier could be achieved by coupling the soluble enzyme to an antibody or a ligand recognized by a receptor present on the surface of endothelial cells. It was shown that when NGF was coupled to an antibody against the transferrin receptor, it could cross the blood-brain barrier after peripheral injection in rats.[69] However, in the case of lysosomal enzymes, fusion molecules may loose their catalytic activity or their ability to be recognized by the M6P receptor. Whether these large molecules can be efficiently transported across the endothelial cells also remains to be demonstrated.

Another possible problem may be that, even if the soluble enzyme can cross the blood-brain barrier, it may not be taken up by the cells that need to be corrected. Indeed, delivery of hexosaminadase A to the brain of GM2 gangliosidosis cats, by reversible blood-brain barrier permeabilization lead to a significative concentration of the enzyme in the brain but no detectable uptake by neurons which are the affected cells. Targeting of neurons was obtained in vitro only after coupling of hexosaminidase A via disulfide linkage to the atoxic fragment C of tetanus toxin.[70]

An alternative solution would be to install intracerebral implants of genetically-modified fibroblasts and myoblasts.[71,72] In the case of LSD however, enzyme delivery throughout the brain is needed and the modified cells should be able to migrate after implantation. Genetically-modified astroglial (O2A) progenitors can be used to assess the capacity of a limited number of cells scattered in the brain to eliminate lysosomal storage. However, the difficulty to access the target cell for ex vivo gene transfer makes this procedure of little therapeutic relevance. Multipotent immortalized neural progenitor cell lines with high migration capacity have been described in the mouse[73] and used to obtain long-term diffuse engraftment in the brain of newborn MPS VII animals after the transfer of the β-glucuronidase cDNA (J Wolfe, personal communication). The availability of such cells in humans could be of genuine interest for the treatment of CNS lesions in LSD.

Direct gene transfer into the CNS is feasible with herpesvirus or adenovirus vectors. A recombinant HSV-1 virus encoding for the rat β-glucuronidase was used to infect MPS VII mice by corneal inoculation. After several weeks, few positive neurons were detected by histochemical staining in the trigeminal ganglia and brain stem of treated mice.[74] The disappearance of lysosomal storage in or around the positive cells was not studied. Although this has not been tested in LSD models yet, a more potent gene transfer can be obtained with adenovirus, by stereotactic injection of vector particles in the brain tissue or in the ventricular space. This second approach leads to the infection of the ependymal cells lining the ventricule and can be used to secrete a protein in the CSF. In LSD, this could directly reduce the levels of undegraded molecules in the CSF and might help enzyme diffusion to large areas of the brain.

Perspectives for clinical trials

Four gene therapy trials have already been approved for the treatment of Gaucher disease by retroviral-mediated transfer of the human glucocerebrosidase cDNA into hematopoietic stem cells.[75] Human $CD34^+$ cells will be purified from G-CSF-mobilized peripheral blood stem cells or from bone marrow and transduced with retrovirus containing media. The retroviral vectors used express the human glucocerebrosidase cDNA under the control of the viral LTR. The transduced cells will then be infused into the patient. If peripheral blood stem cells are used this procedure can be repeated several times while if bone marrow is used, only one treatment will be done. The aims of these trials are: (i) to examine the safety and the efficiency of transducing the human glucocerebrosidase into CD34 cells by retrovirus-mediated gene transfer; (ii) to determine the extent of long-term persistence of transduced cells in patients; (iii) to investigate whether the enzyme is expressed efficiently enough to improve the patient conditions. For safety reasons, early trials do not include myeloablative conditioning treatment. It is not known whether a therapeutic effect can be obtained in such conditions, since low levels of engraftment of genetically-modified cells are expected.

Regarding MPS, in vivo gene transfer data have been obtained with MPS VII animals and it would seem logical to consider patients with Sly syndrome as the first candidates for a gene therapy trial. However, these patients are exceedingly rare, with less than 20 known cases of live birth. Hurler disease is one of the more frequent MPS. A genotype/phenotype correlation has begun to be established and pre or perinatal diagnosis is feasible. The mechanisms of synthesis, processing, secretion and uptake of β-glucuronidase and α-L-iduronidase are similar, and it is likely that most of the gene transfer data obtained in MPS VII animals can be extrapolated to MPS I. Analysis of Nude mice implanted with neo-organs secreting the human α-L-iduronidase indicates that the enzyme is internalized in the liver and the spleen as efficiently as β-glucuronidase (A Salvetti, unpublished results). The therapeutic efficacy of the gene therapy approaches defined in MPS VII models can also be tested in MPS I dogs.[12] Two types of intervention on MPS I patients could be proposed in the near future, involving retrovirus-mediated gene transfer to either hematopoietic ($CD34^+$) cells or to skin fibroblasts reimplanted into the peritoneal cavity. The graft of autologous skin fibroblast secreting α-L-iduronidase from vascularised neo-organs could be performed using a minimally invasive surgical procedure. Initial trials will have to assess the feasibility of the procedure, its tolerance by the patient, the efficiency and duration of enzyme secretion and the effect on the course of the disease.

More clinical trials are likely to be organized within the next few years for the treatment of other LSD, and Niemann-Pick A and B or metachromatic leucodystrophy are likely candidates. However, the multiplication of clinical trials will critically depend on the issue of the early ones, which therefore have to be conducted very rigorously. As clinical applications will progress, it will remain essential to perform careful experiments in animal models. The uncommon wealth of animals affected with these diseases provides a unique opportunity to base gene therapy trials on a solid collection of scientific and preclinical data.

REFERENCES

1 Neufeld EF. Lysosomal storage diseases. Annu Rev Biochem 1991; 60: 257–280.
2 Hopwood JJ, Morris CP. The mucopolysaccharidoses: diagnosis, molecular genetics and treatment. Mol Biol Med 1990; 7: 381–404.
3 Pfeffer SR. Targeting of proteins to the lysosome. Curr Top Microbiol Immunol 1991; 170: 43–63.
4 Barranger JA, Ginns EI. Glucosylceramide lipidoses: Gaucher disease. In: Scriver CJ, Beaudet AL, Sly WS and Valle D eds. The metabolic basis of inherited disease. New York: McGraw-Hill 1989; 1677–1698.
5 Scott HS, Litjens T, Nelson PV et al. Identification of mutations in the α-L-iduronidase gene (IDUA) causing Hurler and Scheie syndromes. Am J Hum Genet 1993; 53: 973–986.
6 Scott HS, Litjens T, Nelson PV, Brooks DA, Hopwood JJ, Morris CP. α-L-iduronidase mutations (Q70X and P533R) associate with a severe Hurler phenotype. Human Mutation 1992;1: 333–339.
7 Scott HS, Litjens T, Hopwood JJ, Morris CP. A common mutation for mucopolysaccharidosis type I associated with a severe Hurler syndrome phenotype. Hum Mutation 1992; 1: 103–108.
8 Beutler E. Gaucher disease as a paradigm of current issues regrading single gene mutations of humans. Proc Natl Acad Sci USA 1993; 90: 5384–5390.
9 Yoshida M, Noguchi J, Ikadai H, Takahashi M, Nagase S. Arylsulfatase B-deficient mucopolysaccharidosis in rats. J Clin Invest 1993; 91: 1099–1104.
10 Birkenmeier EH, Davisson MT, Beamer WG et al. Murine mucopolysaccharidosis type VII. Characterization of a mouse with β-glucuronidase deficiency. J Clin Invest 1989; 83: 1258–1266.
11 Kobayashi T, Yamanaka T, Jacobs JM, Teixera F, Suzuki K. The Twicher mouse: an enzymatically authentic model of human globoid cell leukodystrophy (Krabbe disease). Brain Res 1980; 202: 479–483.
12 Shull RM, Munger RJ, Spellacy E, Hall CW, Constantopoulos G, Neufeld E. Canine α-L-iduronidase deficiency: a model of Mucopolysaccharidosis I. Am J Pathol 1982; 109: 244–248.
13 Haskins ME, Desnick RJ, DiFerrante N, Jezyk P, Patterson DF. Beta-glucuronidase deficiency in a dog: a model of mucopolysaccharidosis VII. Pediatr Res 1984; 18: 980–984.
14 Healy PJ, Farrow BRH, Nicholas FW, Hedberg K, Ratcliffe R. Canine fucosidosis: a biochemical and genetic investigation. Res Vet Sci 1984; 36: 354–359.
15 Haskins ME, Jezyk PF, Desnick RJ, McDonoug SK, Patterson DF. Alpha-l-iduronidase deficiency in a cat: a model for mucopolysaccharidosis I. Pediatr Res 1979; 13: 1294–1297.
16 Jezyk PF, Haskins ME, Patterson DF, Mellman WJ, Greenstein M. Mucopolysaccharidosis in a cat with aryl-sulfatase B deficiency: a model of Maroteaux-Lamy syndrome. Science 1977; 198: 834–836.
17 Thompson JN, Jones MZ, Dawson G, Huffman PS. N-acetylglucosamine 6–sulphatase deficiency in a Nubian goat: a model of Sanfilippo syndrome type D (mucopolysaccharidosis IIID). J Inherit Metab Dis 1992; 15: 760–768.
18 Vandevelde M, Faukhauser R, Bichsel P, Weismann V, Herschkowitz N. Hereditary neurovisceral mannosidosis associated with α-mannosidase deficiency in a family of Persian cats. Acta Neuropathol (Berl) 1982; 58: 64–66.
19 Sasaki M, Lovell KL, Moller JR. Myelin-associated glycoprotein (MAG) in myelin deficiency of caprine beta-mannosidosis. Brain Res 1993; 620: 127–132.
20 Pearce RD, Callahan JW, Little PB, Klunder LR, Clarke JT. Caprine beta-D-mannosidosis: characterization of a model lysosomal storage disorder. Can J Vet Res 1990; 54: 22–29.
21 Bryan L, Schmutz S, Hodges SD, Snyder FF. Bovine beta-mannosidosis: pathologic and genetic findings in Salvers calves. Vet Pathol 1993; 30: 130–139.

22 Kaye EM, Alroy J, Raghavan SS et al. Dysmyelinogenesis in animal models of GM1 gangliosidosis. Pediatr Neurol 1992; 8: 255–261.
23 Cork LC, Munnel JF, Lorenz MD, Murphy JV, Baker JH, Rattazzi MC. GM2 ganglioside lysosomal storage in cats with β-hexosaminadase deficiency. Science 1977; 196: 1014–1017.
24 Weintraub H, Abramovici A, Amichai D et al. Morphometric studies of pancreatic acinar granule formation in NCTR-Balb/c mice. J Cell Sci 1992; 102: 141–147.
25 Honda Y, Kuriyama M, Higuchi I, Fujiama J, Yoshida H, Osame M, Muscular involvement in lysosomal acid lipase deficiency in rats. J Neurol Sci 1992; 108: 189–195.
26 Knowles K, Alroy J, Castagnaro M, Raghavan SS, Jakowski RM, Freden GO. Adult-onset lysosomal storage disease in a Scipperke dog: clinical, morphological and biochemical studies. Acta Neuropathol (Berl) 1993; 86: 306–312.
27 Tybulewicz VL. Tremblay ML, LaMarca ME et al. Animal model of Gaucher's disease from targeted disruption of the mouse glucocerebrosidase gene. Nature 1992; 357: 407–410.
28 Shull RM, Walker MA. Radiographic findings in a canine model of Mucopolysaccharidosis I. Invest Radiol 1988; 23: 124130.
29 Shull RM, Hastings NE, Selcer RR et al. Bone marrow transplantation in canine mucopolysaccharidosis I. J Clin Invest 1987; 79: 435–443.
30 Gasper PW, Thrall MA, Wenger DA et al. Correction of feline arylsulfatase B deficiency (mucopolysaccharidosis VI) by bone marrow transplantation. Nature 1984; 312: 467–469.
31 Taylor RM, Farrow BR, Stewart GJ. Amelioration of the clinical disease following bone marrow transplantation in fucosidase-deficient dogs. Am J Med Genet 1992; 53: 628–632.
32 Sands MS, Barker JE, Vogler C et al. Treatment of murine mucopolysaccharidosis type VII by syngeneic bone marrow transplantation in neonates. Lab Invest 1993; 68: 676–686.
33 Hoogerbrugge PM, Suzuki K, Suzuki K et al. Donor-derived cells in the central nervous system of Twitcher mice after bone marrow transplantation. Science 1988; 239: 1035–1038.
34 O'Brien JS, Storb R, Raff et al. Bone marrow transplantation in canine GM1 gangliosidosis. Clin Genet 1990; 38: 274–280.
35 Vogler C, Sands M, Higgins A et al. Enzyme replacement with recombinant β-glucuronidase in the newborn mucopolysaccharidosis type VII mouse. Pediatr Res 1993; 34: 837–840.
36 Neufeld EF, Lim TW, Shapiro LJ, Inherited disorders of lysosomal metabolism. Annu Rev Biochem 1977; 44: 357–376.
37 Krivit W, Shapiro E, Hoogerbrugge PM, Moser HW. State of the art review: bone marrow transplantation treatment for storage disease. Bone Marrow Transplant 1992; 10: 87–97.
38 Hoogerbrugge PM, Brouwer OF, Aubourg P et al. Limited role for allogenic bone marrow transplantation in metabolic diseases. (Submitted 1994)
39 Furbish FS, Steer CJ, Krett NL, Barranger JA. Uptake and distribution of placental glucocerebrosidase in rat hepatic cells and effects of sequential deglycosylation. Biochim Biophys Acta 1981; 673: 425–434.
40 Barton NW, Brady PR, Dambrosia JM et al. Replacement therapy for inherited enzyme deficiency – macrophage-targeted glucocerebrosidase for Gaucher's disease. N Engl J Med 1991; 23: 1464–1470.
41 Pastores GM, Sibille AR, Grabowski GA. Enzyme therapy in Gaucher Disease type I: dosage efficacy and adverse effects in 33 patients treated for 6 to 24 months. Blood 1993; 82: 408–416.
42 Anson DS, Bielicki J, Hopwood JJ. Correction of mucopolysaccharidosis type I fibroblasts by retroviral-mediated transfer of the human a-L-iduronidase gene. Hum Gene Ther 1992; 3: 371–379.

43 Anson DS, Taylor JA, Bielicki J et al. Correction of human mucopolysaccharidosis type-VI fibroblasts with recombinant N-acetylgalactosamine-4-sulphatase. Biochem J 1992; 284: 789–794.
44 Fink JK, Correl PH, Perry LK, Brady RO, Karlsson S. Correction of glucocerbrosidase deficiency after retroviral-mediated gene transfer into hematopoietic progenitor cells from patients with Gaucher disease. Proc Natl Acad Sci USA 1990; 8 7: 2334–2338.
45 Occhiodoro T, Hopwood JJ, Morris CP, Anson DS. Correction of alpha-L-fucosidase deficiency in fucosidosis fibroblasts by retroviral vector-mediated gene transfer. Hum Gene Ther 1993; 3: 365–369.
46 Peters C, Rommerskirch W, Modaressi S, von Figura K. Restoration of arylsulphatase B activity in human mucopolysaccharidosis-type-VI fibroblasts by retroviral-vector-mediated gene transfer. Biochem J 1991; 276; 499–504.
47 Suchi M, Dinur T, Desnick RJ et al. Retroviral-mediated transfer of the human acid phingomyelinase cDNA: correction of the metabolic defect in cultured Niemann-Pick disease cells. Proc Natl Acad Sci USA 1992; 89: 3227–3231.
48 Rommerskirch W, Fluharty AL, Peters C, von Figura K, Gieselman V. Restoration of arylsulfatase A activity in human-metachromatic-leucodystrophy fibroblasts via retroviral-vector mediated gene transfer. Biochem J 1991; 280: 459–461.
49 Wolfe JH, Schuchman EH, Stramm LE et al. Restoration of normal lysosomal function in mucopolysaccharidosis type VII cells by retroviral vector-mediated gene transfer. Proc Natl Acad Sci USA 1990; 87: 2877–2881.
50 Olsen I, Bou-Gharios G, Abraham D, Chain B. Lysosomal enzyme transfer from different types of lymphoid cell. Exp Cell Res 1993; 209: 133–139.
51 Bou-Gharios G, Adams G, Pace P, Warden P, Olsen I. Correction of a lysosomal deficiency by contact-mediated enzyme transfer after bone marrow transplantation. Transplantation 1993; 56: 991–996.
52 Karlsson S. Treatment of genetic defects in hematopoietic cell function by gene transfer. Blood 1991; 78: 2481–2492.
53 Correl PM, Kew Y, Perry LK, Brady RO, Fink JK, Karlsson S. Expression of human glucocerebrosidase in long-term reconstituted mice following retroviral-mediated gene transfer into hematopoietic stem cells. Hum Gene Ther 1990; 1: 227–287.
54 Weinthal J, Nolta JA, Yu XJ, Lilley J, Uribe L, Kohn DB. Expression of human glucocerebrosidase following retroviral-mediated transduction of murine hematopoietic stem cells. Bone Marrow Transplant 1991; 8: 403–412.
55 Correl PM, Colilla S, Dave HPG, Karlsson S. High levels of human glucocerebrosidase activity in macrophages of long-term reconstituted mice after retroviral infection of hematopoietic stem cells. Blood 1992; 80: 311–336.
56 Ohashi T, Boggs S, Robbins P et al. Efficient transfer and sustained high expression of the human glucocerebrosidase gene in mice and their functional macrophages following transplantation of bone marrow transduced by a retroviral vector. Proc Natl Acad Sci USA 1992; 89: 11332–11336.
57 Nolta JA, Yu XJ, Bahner I, Kohn DB. Retroviral mediated transfer of the human glucocerebrosidase gene into cultured Gaucher bone marrow. J Clin Invest 1992; 90: 342–348.
58 Wolfe JH, Sands MS, Barker JE et al. Reversal of pathology in murine mucopolysaccharidosis type VII by somatic cell gene transfer. Nature 1992; 360: 749–753.
59 Marećhal V, Naffakh N, Danos O, Heard JM. Disappearance of lysosomal storage in spleen and liver of mucopolysaccharidosis VII mice after transplantation of genetically-modified bone marrow cells. Blood 1993; 82: 1358–1365.
60 Bell E, Ivarsson B, Merrill C. Production of a tissue-like structure by contraction of collagen lattices by human fibroblasts of different proliferative potential in vitro. Proc Natl Acad Sci USA 1979; 76: 1274–1278.
61 Moullier P, Maréchal V, Danos O, Heard JM. Continuous systemic secretion of a lysosomal enzyme by genetically-modified mouse skin fibroblasts. Transplantation 1993; 56: 427–432.

62 Moullier P, Bohl D, Heard JM, Danos O. Correction of lysosomal storage in the liver and spleen of MPS VII mice by implantation of genetically-modified skin fibroblasts. Nature Genet 1993; 4: 154–159.
63 Dhawan J, Pan LC, Pavlath GK, Travis MA, Lanctot AM, Blau HM. Systemic delivery of human growth hormone by injection of genetically-modified myoblasts. Science 1991; 254: 1509–1512.
64 Smith BF, Hoffman RK, Giger U, Wolfe JH. Genes transferred by retroviral vectors into normal and mutant myoblasts in primary cultures are expressed in myotubes. Mol Cell Biol 1990; 10: 3268–3271.
65 Naffakh N, Pinset C, Montarras D, Pastoret C, Danos O, Heard JM. Transplantation of adult-derived myoblasts in mice following gene transfer. Neuromusc Disord 1994; 3: 413–417.
66 Ferry N, Duplessis O, Houssin D, Danos O, Heard JM. Retroviral-mediated gene transfer into hepatocytes in vivo. Proc Natl Acad Sci USA 1991; 88: 8377–8381.
67 Cardoso JE, Branchereau S, Prema Roy J, Houssin D, Danos O, Heard JM. In situ retrovirus-mediated gene transfer into dog liver. Hum Gene Ther 1993; 4: 411–418.
68 Pardridge WM. Recent advances in blood-brain barrier transport. Ann Rev Pharmacol Toxicol 1988; 28: 25–39.
69 Friden PM, Walus LR, Watson P et al. Blood-brain barrier penetration and in vivo activity of an NGF conjugate. Science 1993; 259: 373–377.
70 Dobrenis K, Joseph A, Rattazzi MC, Neuronal lysosomal enzyme replacement using fragment C of tetanus toxin. Proc Natl Acad Sci USA 1992; 89: 2297–2301.
71 Gage FH, Kawaja MD, Fisher LJ. Genetically modified cells; applications for intracerebral grafting. Trends Neurosci 1991; 14: 328–333.
72 Jiao S, Gurevich V, Wolff JA. Long-term correction of rat model of Parkinson's disease by gene therapy. Nature 1993; 363: 450–453.
73 Snyder EY, Deitcher DL, Walsh C, Arnold-Aldea S, Hartweig EA, Cepko CL. Multipotent neural cell lines can engraft and participate in development of mouse cerebellum. Cell 1992; 68: 33–51.
74 Wolfe JH, Deshmane SL, Fraser NW. Herpesvirus vector gene transfer and expression of β-glucuronidase in the central nervous system of MPS VII mice. Nature Genet. 1992; 1: 379–384.
75 Anderson WF. Gene therapy for genetic disease. Hum Gene Ther 1994; 5: 281–282.

British Medical Bulletin (1995) Vol. 51, No. 1, pp.123–137

Myoblast-based gene therapies

T A Partridge[1] and K E Davies[2]

[1]MRC Clinical Sciences Centre, Royal Postgraduate Medical School, Hammersmith Hospital, London, UK and [2] Institute of Molecular Medicine, John Radcliffe Hospital, Headington, Oxford, UK

Recent identification of the genetic causes of several neuromuscular disorders has aroused interest in gene therapy in skeletal muscle. The genetic constitution of skeletal muscle can be altered by a number of means. Myoblasts can be used to introduce new genes, endogenous or exogenous, into muscle fibres during growth and repair. DNA expression-plasmids can be directly transfected into a small proportion of muscle fibres, showing persistent expression despite their lack of genomic integration. Recombinant replication deficient adenoviruses are efficient vectors into myoblasts and developing muscle fibres; again, the introduced constructs show long-term episomal persistence and expression. By contrast, recombinant replication deficient retroviruses efficiently introduce constructs into the genomes of dividing myoblasts which subsequently fuse into muscle fibres. None of the available methods provides a practical solution for therapy of genetic muscle diseases but might be useful for inducing synthesis of therapeutic non-muscle proteins by skeletal muscle

SPECIAL INTEREST OF SKELETAL MUSCLE AS A TARGET FOR GENE THERAPY

To one unfamiliar with the field, general interest in skeletal muscle as a target for gene therapy might come as a surprise since it has no obvious single quality, apart from its abundance, to commend it. For explanation, one must look to a conjunction of individual factors, including properties of the mature tissue, its developmental biology, its ease of tissue culture and perhaps especially to historical events – such as the elucidation, over the past few years, of the genetic basis of primary muscle diseases such as Duchenne muscular dystrophy[1,2] and myotonic dystrophy.[3]

It is a matter of convenience for experiment, and perhaps eventually for therapy, that skeletal muscle exhibits distinct proliferative and differentiated stages; the proliferative cells, or myoblasts fuse with one another to form new muscle fibres or with existing muscle fibres during the processes of repair or regeneration after injury. In the process they exit permanently from the cell cycle and begin to synthesize the major structural proteins of skeletal muscle, modulating the spectrum of isoforms in accordance with their workload. By analogy with the transplantation of bone marrow to alter the genetic constitution of blood cells[4] it has been proposed that myoblasts could serve as carriers of genes into myofibres, the main difference being, that the skeletal muscle fibre so formed has a life-span of the same order of magnitude as the recipient individual. A recent variant of this idea is that of making genetic modifications to the myoblast before transplanting it, preferably using the patient's own myoblasts. Yet more recently, it has been found that gene constructs may be introduced directly into muscle fibres where, although they do not become incorporated into the genome of the G_0 myonuclei, they do persist and are expressed quite stably for periods of months or years.

Taken overall, skeletal muscle must be the best described of all tissues; providing the archetype in many areas of biochemistry, biophysics, physiology, molecular biology, cell biology and developmental biology. Such a level of understanding is a valuable aid to the design of experimental strategies for introducing genes into skeletal muscle and for controlling their expression within this tissue. This, together with the revelation that skeletal muscle is susceptible to stable genetic modification by a number of simple techniques, doubtless accounts for the growing interest in skeletal muscle as an in vivo 'factory' for making non-muscle proteins of pharmacological interest.

INHERITED MYOPATHIES

Myoblast transplantation

Without doubt, the driving force for development of methods of genetic modification of skeletal muscle is the existence of a number of crippling primary genetic diseases of this tissue, of which the most notorious is the progressive and fatal X-linked childhood disease, Duchenne muscular dystrophy (DMD). Identification of the genetic basis of this condition did not radically alter prospects for its therapy but did rekindle interest in developing research strategies and at the same time provided the tools required, in the form of animal homologues of the disease and biochemical probes with which to make objective assessments of therapeutic success.

Attempts have been made for some years to explore the notion of myoblast transplantation as a means of genetically modifying skeletal muscle in postnatal animals.

One such series of experiments was conducted on the dy/dy mouse,[5] which suffered, as a model, from the lack of biochemical characterization of the defect and the complexity of its pathology – involving, as it does, amyelination of motor and sensory nerves in addition to degeneration of its muscles – and showing many of the hallmarks of a developmental defect.[6] These features made it difficult to interpret the physiological and histological improvements produced by implantation of normal muscle cells (for discussion *see* ref. 7). But, recent reports of deficiency of laminin-M (merosin) in the basement membranes of muscles and nerves of this animal,[8,9] raises the interesting prospect that it may be the fibroblastic rather than the myogenic cells of the implants which produce the beneficial effects, since these cells are required for the formation of muscle basement membranes.[10]

As to the feasibility of myoblast transplantation, biochemical studies showed that myoblasts carrying an allelic variant of glucose-6-phosphate isomerase (GPI), grafted into growing or regenerating muscle of animals carrying a second variant, were able to alter the GPI phenotype of the recipient muscle.[11] Subsequently, this technique was used to introduce phosphorylase-kinase into the muscles of animals with a genetic deficiency of this enzyme, but with barely detectable levels of conversion.[12]

With the recognition of the mdx mouse as a biochemical homologue of DMD, it became possible to evaluate the effectiveness of myoblast transplantation in terms of its ability to elicit the synthesis of the protein dystrophin, absence of which is the primary biochemical defect in these diseases.[13,14]

These findings, together with those of Law on the dy/dy mouse, precipitated a number of experimental trials of myoblast transplantation on DMD boys, overriding protests from many basic scientists that these were premature (*see* [15]). Now that the results of most of these human myoblast transplantation studies have been published, it is clear that this procedure is not detectably damaging to the recipient but neither, in most cases, has it been found effective in terms either of introducing dystrophin into the recipient muscles or of moderating the decline in muscle function.[16–19] The exception is a series of studies in which claims have been advanced of significant production of dystrophin in injected muscles[20] and of significant improvement or stabilization of strength in these muscles.[21,22] These studies suffer throughout from inadequate control for the ameliorating activity of the immunosuppressant cyclosporin A on strength of DMD muscles[21] and in the more recent series[22] for placebo effects.[23] So great was the unease generated in the scientific community by these experiments that a Gordon Conference presentation of one of the better designed studies evoked a condemnatory letter calling for a moratorium.[24]

Although many doubted that myoblast transplantation would prove an immediately applicable therapy for DMD,[7,14] it has come as a surprise that little or no trace of injected myoblasts has been demonstrated in human myoblast transplantation experiments. In this respect, the work of Tremblay's group, implicating immune reactions to myoblasts, even from donors fully matched at the major histocompatibility locus, may have some bearing.[17,18,25] The contrast with the comparative success in the mouse, suggests that this problem is technical rather than one of basic principle, and is therefore soluble.

An obvious problem of myoblast transplantation, one that is unlikely to be resolved by technical tinkering, is the limited dispersal of injected myoblasts from local graft sites through the substantial and widely distributed mass of skeletal muscles in the body. In the mouse, dispersal from an injection site into surrounding muscle tissue has not been shown to exceed a few millimetres and cells of different species show very similar absolute limits on speed of movement. The compartmental structure of muscles of large mammals is likely to further impede movement. Distribution via the blood vascular system offers a potential solution to this problem, but, at present, there is only a single report of dissemination of myoblasts to skeletal muscle by this route,[26] and this is of a transformed cell line which we find to be malignant in nude mice.

There is also the matter of whether it is possible to generate sufficient myogenic cells to alter a useful amount of muscle in the body. If, as in the current experiments on human myoblast transplantation, living relatives act as donors, then at most a few grams of muscle is available as a source of cells. Even assuming 100% survival of injected myoblasts (*see later*), some 10^{11}–10^{12} cells would be needed to replace the satellite cells of the human body, obtainable from 30–40 cell doublings of cloned myoblasts. This has been shown to be feasible for myoblasts obtained from neonatal donors [27] but barely possible from teenage or adult donors. In practice, one study of human myoblast transplantation has reported a loss of myogenicity in otherwise vigorous myogenic cells after 15–18 doublings.[19] Similar conclusions are implicit in a report by Law's group, who, although claiming retention of myogenicity in culture after very extensive proliferation, have been able to demonstrate only the barest traces of dystrophin in large numbers of these cells grafted into immunosuppressed mdx mice.[28]

By analogy with the haemopoietic and keratinocyte systems, this problem might be approached by isolation of stem cells, i.e. cells with extensive scope for asymmetric division, one of the progeny providing self-replacement, the second being committed to generation of a transit population with limited ability to divide prior to differentiation.[29] Even in the high-turnover tissues where such cells have been demonstrated they are rare, difficult to identify, and yet more difficult to isolate, so it is hardly surprising that no evidence has been found, by conventional tissue culture techniques, for their existence in mature skeletal muscle. Recently, we have examined this question in myogenic cells obtained from a mouse transgenic for a thermolabile mutant of the SV40 large T gene driven by the promoter from a mouse histocompatibility gene.[30] These, although they are not stem cells, do exhibit some of their useful properties. The promoter is activated when the cells are treated with interferon-γ and the large T antigen retains its transforming activity at 33°C, causing the cells to proliferate continuously; removal of interferon-γ and/or elevation of the temperature to >37°C removes the transforming effect of the large T antigen and the cells cease proliferation and differentiate into muscle. This study has also provided evidence of rare myoblasts with properties of stem cells. One myoblast clone, on injection into muscles of mdx mice, gave rise both to normal muscle fibres and to rare undifferentiated cells. These were extracted from the muscle, cloned, and injected into a second cell, and, reiterating the regime, a third passage recipient muscle, forming, at each passage, both muscle fibres and further rare non-differentiated cells. Improved manipulability of myogenic cells or identification and isolation of stem cells within this lineage are probably a prerequisite to successful use in man of techniques involving grafting of myoblasts.

Within the recipient muscle, the extent of colonization by implanted myoblasts can be separated into 3 components, namely, the efficiencies of survival, proliferation, and myogenic differentiation of the implanted cells. Because these variables are difficult to assess in vivo, little is known about this topic, but recent studies of survival of ^{3}H-Tdr-labelled murine myogenic cells injected into muscles of nude mdx mice have produced surprising results; less than 1% of injected cells survive more than a few days, but the small surviving fraction proliferate rapidly to produce the readily detectable donor muscle which forms around the injection site (Beauchamp et al, in preparation). Survival at similar levels in grafts of human or canine myoblasts, would need to be combined with only minor differences in the efficiency of proliferation or differentiation to explain the lack of success in these species. It may be, that the small surviving population represents a special subset of myogenic cells, stem cells for example, which are lacking from human or canine myoblasts after extensive tissue culture.

Features of DMD, which would not be susceptible to myoblast transplantation, are the cardiomyopathy and the intellectual deficit. Recently, demonstrations of successful grafting of C2 myoblasts [31] and of isologous fetal cardiomyocytes [32] into heart muscle are of interest in providing a potential means of replacing lost contractile tissue. However, culture of cardiomyocytes in bulk is not currently possible, so this general strategy cannot be applied to the replacement of cardiac muscle degenerating as a consequence of dystrophin deficiency. Furthermore, because cardiomyocytes do not fuse with one another, their dystrophin remains localized within the individual cells and there is no element of the sharing of gene products which makes this option attractive in skeletal muscle. Given the heroic nature of myoblast transplantation, the use of whole heart transplants, would be a comparatively straightforward solution to the cardiac problems. The intellectual deficit, if it is a reflection of a persistent functional abnormality of dystrophin-deficient neural tissue, may eventually be susceptible to gene therapy, but, if it represents a developmental failure, may be irrecoverable post natally.

Gene therapy in skeletal muscle

Insertion of genetic material into muscle fibres by the various means presently available has become of interest both as a route to therapy for primary genetic disease of muscle and for the conversion of skeletal muscle to the production of systemically active gene products unrelated to muscle function. To a large extent, the methods are common to the two goals, and can be divided into those in which the genetically modified myogenic cells are used to construct new muscle and those aimed at direct insertion of genetic material into mature muscle fibres, which, were it achievable by a systemic route, would be the method of first choice for treatment of DMD.

It came as a surprise that circular DNA plasmids, simply injected intramuscularly were taken up quite effectively by a small number of fibres and that their reporter genes (β-galactosidase, luciferase, chloramphenicol acetyl transferase) were expressed.[33] Still more surprising was the persistence of these plasmids in their circular episomal state combined with stable expression of their genes for periods in excess of one year, despite their lack of integration into the genome of the host muscle fibres. Subsequently, it was shown that the dystrophin gene, similarly introduced by direct transfection into the muscles of the mdx mouse, converted up to 1–2% of muscle fibres to the synthesis of dystrophin.[34]

In the search for ways to augment the numbers of fibres transfected in this way, it has been found that regeneration of the recipient muscle increases the level of expression of the transfected gene to some extent, perhaps by increasing the number of fibres transfected;[35,36] although one report suggests that this effect is due to a transient increase in expression rather than an increase in the number of transfected constructs.[37]

Directed targeting of constructs to muscle by linking them to ligands for cell surface receptors has been demonstrated in vitro[38] but has not been reported to be effective in vivo. As a more efficient means of introducing constructs into skeletal muscle fibres, recombinant replication defective adenoviruses appear particularly effective and, as with transfected constructs, their expression within the muscle fibres is persistent.[39] However, the size of construct is limited and at present only 'mini' versions of the dystrophin gene can be carried by adenoviral vectors.[40,41] In addition, efficient infection appears to be restricted to developing or regenerating muscle fibres[42,43] and myopathic effects of the adenovirus have been reported.[44]

Autologous transplantation of genetically modified myoblasts

A major alternative approach, is to secure stable integration of mini-dystrophin constructs into proliferating myogenic cells in tissue culture by use of a replication-defective retroviral vector.[45] In principle these cells could then be grafted back into muscles of the donor as a genetically corrected autologous transplant. This retroviral vector has also been used to introduce the dystrophin mini-gene into the myoblasts of spontaneously regenerating muscle of the mdx mouse to produce 6–10% dystrophin-positive fibres.[46] Adenoviral and retroviral vectors share the problem of the limited size of construct they can carry, falling well below that of the full-length dystrophin gene. In both cases, in vivo transduction is restricted to growing or regenerating muscle fibres.[43,47] However, retrovirally introduced constructs do have the advantage of becoming integrated into the genome of the host cell, thus potentially conferring lifelong expression.

ALTERNATIVE STRATEGIES FOR TREATMENT OF PRIMARY GENETIC MYOPATHIES

Repair of defective genes

In most cases of DMD, the major part of the Duchenne gene is still present having suffered a minor deletion or duplication or a point mutation such that it would be possible, in theory, to repair the defect by homologous recombination. In practical terms, however, this is not a credible option at present. Not only would it require great improvement in the efficiency of homologous recombination, it would also entail the resolution of all of the problems of distribution, antigenicity etc., which afflict all approaches to genetic modification of skeletal muscle.

Eliciting expression from defective genes

Many DMD patients and all of the animals with dystrophinopathies exhibit a low frequency of small groups of 'revertant' fibres which express protein products of the dystrophin gene.[48] This phenomenon appears to involve loss of exons from the message around the site of the original mutation, possibly by an alternative splicing mechanism, restoring the open reading frame,[49] although further genomic mutations to restore the reading frame have not been formally excluded. It may be possible in some instances to potentiate this process to obtain a useful degree of expression of what, in some cases at least would be a partially active product of the dystrophin gene, as appears to be the case in a small proportion of individuals in which low levels of dystrophin are produced despite frame-shifting deletions within their dystrophin gene.[50,51]

Promoting expression of developmental isoforms

Treatment of human genetic disease by upregulation of other related genes is not a novel idea: there is a current clinical trial, involving β-thalassaemia patients who lack the normal adult β-globin gene.[52] These patients are being treated with butyrate which upregulates the fetal γ-globin gene. This agent has no serious side effects, even though it upregulates other genes in a variety of different tissues, and some patients have shown expression of therapeutic levels of the fetal globin gene.

It has been suggested that over-production of the highly homologous autosomal utrophin (dystrophin related protein) in muscle could theoretically compensate for the lack of dystrophin in DMD patients.[53] There are several observations that suggest that this may be feasible. Utrophin is found at the sarcolemma in early human fetal life but becomes restricted to the neuromuscular junction once dystrophin is expressed.[54] Utrophin expression is high in mdx mouse muscle at birth but declines during the first few weeks of life, during which time the animal begins to develop myonecrotic lesions.[55,56] Formal evidence as to whether utrophin can replace dystrophin awaits the production of an mdx mouse which is transgenic for the utrophin gene under the control of a strong muscle promoter.

In addition it may be possible to make use of some of alternative transcripts of the dystrophin gene itself. Some DMD patients produce small amounts of dystrophin. Since the gene contains promoters for expression in skeletal muscle, brain and Purkinje cells,[57–59] it may be possible to upregulate these alternative promoters if the skeletal muscle promoter is not functioning efficiently enough.

USE OF SKELETAL MUSCLE FOR PRODUCTION OF NON-MUSCLE PROTEINS

In parallel with the developing interest in muscle gene therapy for primary genetic myopathies, there has been some exploration of the use of skeletal muscle as a site for in vivo expression of a variety of non-muscle genes encoding peptide products with systemic activities. For this purpose, there is no need to achieve dispersed genetic conversion of skeletal muscle fibres and the main problem associated with the treatment of genetic primary myopathies is thus avoided. Indeed, the restriction of genetically modified muscle to an identifiable locality within the body would be an important feature of experimental design during the development of any given strategy and only when a completely satisfactory construct has been developed and tested might it be ethical to contemplate diffuse introduction of that construct into the skeletal muscles of the body.

A prerequisite was the demonstration that a marker gene introduced means of a retroviral vector into tissue cultured myoblasts remained stably expressed in muscle fibres formed when these cells were injected into sites of muscle regeneration.[60] It was also shown that this idea could be applied to substances of therapeutic interest such as the multi-drug resistance gene.[61] Similarly, expression of the human growth hormone gene from the retrovirally transduced C2C12 cell line was shown to be sufficient to raise in vivo serum concentrations to levels which would be of therapeutic value in man.[62,63]

Another area of interest is the blood clotting cascade, particularly factor IX which could have therapeutic benefit at very low levels of expression. Here again, stable but low level expression of the factor has been generated by implantation of myogenic cell lines transduced by means of retroviral vectors containing constructs encoding the human factor IX gene.[64,65] Recently, this same strategy has been applied to the genetic modification of primary mouse myoblasts with the resultant production of physiologically relevant concentrations of human factor IX in the serum of mice, and the confirmation that this is properly processed and secreted from the muscle cells as biologically active peptide;[66] this is an important point, bearing in mind the general lack of data on uptake and secretory mechanisms in skeletal muscle.

The obliging versatility on the part of muscle fibres in the production and secretion of substances, which are not part of their normal repertoire, extends to neurotransmitters. Myoblasts transfected in vitro with a plasmid encoding tyrosine hydroxylase and subsequently injected into rat brains, fuse to form muscle fibres which act as a stable source of dopamine production and produce biochemical correction in a rat model of Parkinsonism.[67]

Primary genetic diseases, which would be suitable candidates for a myoblast-based gene therapy, are the mucopolysaccharidoses, where the missing lysosomal enzyme can be passed from competent to non-competent cells. In the canine animal model of β-glucuronidase deficiency it has been shown that the gene can be introduced into proliferating myoblasts by means of a retroviral vector and expressed as active enzyme in the myotubes formed in tissue culture from these cells.[68]

CAVEATS, PROBLEMS, POTENTIAL SOLUTIONS

Uncertainty as to the potential and problems of genetic manipulation of skeletal muscle, particularly those associated with viral vectors, will impose considerable constraints on human experimentation, especially as regards its application to those conditions which are not life-threatening. Much developmental work will therefore necessarily be conducted on animal models in which the balance of relevant variables will be different from those which are important in man. In addition, individual experimental models will differ from one another to the point where comparison of the variant methods will be difficult. At a minimum, it would be useful to devise an agreed set of measures by which the efficacy of any schedule of gene or cell therapy can be compared with other studies.

Some caution should be exercised in interpreting the data derived from myogenic cell lines, which tend to form tumours as well as muscle fibres,[69,70] for undifferentiated muscle cells retain many cellular mechanisms which are lost during myogenesis[71] and it is important to exclude the participation of such undifferentiated cells in the production of the protein of interest. This same criticism is also applicable to experiments in which nominally primary myogenic cells derived from rats or mice are used after extensive proliferation in tissue culture, given the high incidence of spontaneous immortalization in these species.[72]

BASIC RESEARCH INTERESTS

Although the main drive in gene therapy is directed at the treatment of various diseases and medical conditions, this research will entail investigation of matters of basic muscle cell biology. Some of the methods involved in gene therapy will themselves directly aid these basic studies and assist in their advance in their own right. For example, genetic manipulation greatly extends the ability to introduce genes which will act as cell markers in studies of cell fate.[30] A second obvious area for exploration is the introduction or 'knockout' of genes implicated in inter-cellular signalling such as cytokine receptors.[73]

PROSPECTS AND CONCLUSIONS

Much current research into gene therapy is driven by the increasing flow of information as to the genetic causes of disease. In the case of skeletal muscle, primary genetic diseases of this tissue are unlikely to be susceptible to available technology, largely because we can not yet come close to fulfilling the requirement of inserting the gene in question into all of the muscle fibres in the main muscles of the body. Of the methods which have been shown to be capable of significantly modifying the genetic constitution of muscle fibres, none has shown to be effective for more than a few hundred muscle fibres around the site of injection: this may look impressive on the scale of a mouse muscle but, if reproduced in absolute terms in man, would be worthless. All of the methods which have been shown to convert dystrophin-negative to dystrophin-positive fibres are similar, within an order of magnitude, in their effectiveness in adult mdx mouse muscle. But myoblast transplantation and direct transfection have so far proved much less effective in other species for reasons which are not clear.

It is possible that some vector or targeting system will permit the preferential, or at least efficient, introduction of DNA constructs into skeletal muscle via the blood vascular system. In spite of the persistence of episomal constructs within muscle fibres, it seems likely that this would have to be repeated periodically and here most vector systems would run into problems of immunity. There is one report of widespread transfection of most tissues, including skeletal muscle by intravenous injection of constructs in cationic liposomes[74] but evidence as to the cell-types transfected is not histologically precise. However, if such methods could be shown to be effective, then the lack of immunogenicity of the construct and the carrier should make it possible to transfect repeatedly, and the lack of tissue specificity in the transfection could be accommodated by choosing muscle-specific promoters to drive the constructs.

For useful expression of non-muscle genes within skeletal muscle, the constraints are less stringent. Widespread introduction of the gene construct is less important and, in the early experimental stages may be disadvantageous. Tissue-specificity of targeting and expression of the construct too, would be of value only to the extent that it would aid control of the level of production of the protein, taking advantage of the fact that expression seems to be more stable in skeletal muscle than in other tissues. Perhaps the main problem to be overcome will be to choose promoters which will drive expression of constructs at high enough levels to produce the proteins/peptides of interest in sufficient quantity.

The ultimate choice of system will depend on the aim and will probably be modified by experience. In the early stages at least, it would be safest and most informative to stably transfect or transduce myogenic cells in vitro and implant these into sites of experimentally induced muscle regeneration. Ultimately, given a simple non-immunogenic delivery system, it may be preferable to transiently transfect mature muscle fibres via a systemic route. For some purposes, such as vaccination,[75] it may prove adequate from the start to use local transient transfection of skeletal muscle with constructs encoding the microbial antigens of interest and to repeat the vaccination as necessary.

REFERENCES

1 Hoffman EP, Brown RJ, Kunkel LM. Dystrophin: the protein product of the Duchenne muscular dystrophy locus. Cell 1987; 51: 919–928.
2 Koenig M, Hoffman EP, Bertelson CJ, Monaco AP, Feener C, Kunkel LM. Complete cloning of the Duchenne muscular dystrophy (DMD) cDNA and preliminary genomic organization of the DMD gene in normal and affected individuals. Cell 1987; 50: 509–517.
3 Johnson K. Inheritance and pathogenicity of myotonic dystrophy. In: Partridge TA, ed. Molecular and Cell Biology of Muscular Dystrophy. London: Chapman & Hall, 1993: 85–110.
4 O'Reilly RJ. Allogeneic bone marrow transplantation: current status future directions. Blood 1983; 62: 941–964.
5 Law PK, Goodwin TG, Wang MG. Normal myoblast injections provide genetic treatment for murine dystrophy. Muscle Nerve 1988; 11: 525–533.
6 Hermanson JW, Moschella MC, Ontell M. Effect of neonatal denervation/innervation on the functional capacity of a 129/ReJ dy/dy murine dystrophic muscle. Exp Neurol 1988; 102: 210–216.
7 Partridge TA. Myoblast transfer: a possible therapy for inherited myopathies? Muscle Nerve 1991; 14: 197–212.
8 Arahata K, Hayashi YK, Koga R, et al. Laminin in animal models for muscular dystrophy: defect of Laminin M in skeletal and cardiac muscles and peripheral nerve of the homozygous dystrophic dy/dy mouse. Proc Jpn Acad 1993; 69: 259–264.
9 Sunada Y, Bernier SM, Kozak CA, Yamada Y, Campbell KP. Deficiency of merosin in dystrophic dy mice and genetic linkage of laminin M chain gene to dy locus. J Biol Chem 1994; 269: 13729–13732.
10 Sanderson RD, Fitch JM, Linsenmayer TR, Mayne R. Fibroblasts promote the formation of a continuous basal lamina during myogenesis in vitro. J Cell Biol 1986; 102: 740–747.
11 Watt DJ, Morgan JE, Partridge TA. Use of mononuclear precursor cells to insert allogeneic genes into growing mouse muscles. Muscle Nerve 1984; 7: 741–750.
12 Morgan JE, Watt DJ, Sloper JC, Partridge TA. Partial correction of an inherited defect of skeletal muscle by grafts of normal muscle precursor cells. J Neurol Sci 1988; 86: 137–147.
13 Karpati G, Pouliot Y, Zubrzycka GE, et al. Dystrophin is expressed in mdx skeletal muscle fibers after normal myoblast implantation. Am J Pathol 1989; 135: 27–32.
14 Partridge TA, Morgan JE, Coulton GR, Hoffman EP, Kunkel LM. Conversion of mdx myofibres from dystrophin-negative to -positive by injection of normal myoblasts. Nature 1989; 337: 176–179.
15 Griggs RC, Karpati G, eds. Myoblast transfer therapy. New York: Plenum Press, 1990.

16 Gussoni E, Pavlath GK, Lanctot AM, et al. Normal dystrophin transcripts detected in Duchenne muscular dystrophy patients after myoblast transplantation. Nature 1992; 356: 435–438.
17 Huard J, Bouchard JP, Roy R, et al. Human myoblast transplantation: preliminary results of 4 cases. Muscle Nerve 1992; 15: 550–560.
18 Huard J, Roy R, Bouchard JP, Malouin F, Richards CL, Tremblay JP. Human myoblast transplantation between immunohistocompatible donors and recipients produces immune reactions. Transplant Proc 1992; 24: 3049–3051.
19 Karpati G, Ajdukovic D, Arnold D, et al. Myoblast transfer in Duchenne muscular dystrophy. Ann Neurol 1993; 34: 8–17.
20 Law PK, Bertorini TE, Goodwin TG, et al. Dystrophin production induced by myoblast transfer therapy in Duchenne muscular dystrophy. Lancet 1990; 336: 114–115.
21 Law PK, Goodwin TG, Fang QW, et al. Myoblast transfer therapy for Duchenne muscular dystrophy. Acta Paediatr Jpn 1991; 33: 206–215.
22 Law PK, Goodwin TG, Fang Q, et al. Cell Transplantation as an experimental treatment for Duchenne muscular dystrophy. Cell Transplant 1993; 2: 485–505.
23 Thompson L. Cell-transplant results under fire. Science 1992; 257: 472–474.
24 Epstein HF, Fischman DA, Bader D, et al. Myoblast Transplantation. Science 1992; 257: 738.
25 Labrecque C, Roy R, Tremblay JP. Immune reactions after myoblast transplantation in mouse muscles. Transplant Proc 1992; 24: 2889–2892.
26 Neumeyer AM, DiGregorio DM, Brown RHJ. Arterial delivery of myoblasts to skeletal muscle. Neurology 1992; 42: 2258–2262.
27 Webster C, Blau HM. Accelerated age-related decline in replicative life-span of Duchenne muscular dystrophy myoblasts: implications for cell and gene therapy. Somat Cell Mol Genet 1990; 16: 557–565.
28 Chen M, Li HJ, Fang Q, Goodwin TG, Florendo JA, Law PK. Dystrophin cytochemistry in mdx mouse muscles injected with labelled normal myoblasts. Cell Transplant 1992; 1: 17–22.
29 Hall PA, Watt FM. Stem cells: the generation and maintenance of cellular diversity. Development 1989; 106: 619–633.
30 Morgan JE, Beauchamp JR, Peckham M, et al. Myogenic cell lines derived from transgenic mice carrying a thermolabile T antigen: A model system for the derivation of tissue-specific and mutation-specific cell lines. Dev Biol 1994; 162: 486–498.
31 Koh GY, Klug MG, Soonpaa MH, Field LJ. Differentiation and long-term survival of C2C12 myoblast grafts in heart. J Clin Invest 1993; 92: 1548–1554.
32 Soonpaa MH, Koh GY, Klug MG, Field LJ. Formation of nascent intercalated discs between grafted fetal cardiomyocytes and host myocardium. Science 1994; 264: 98–101.
33 Wolff JA, Malone RW, Williams P, et al. Direct gene transfer into mouse skeletal muscle in vivo. Science 1990; 247: 1465–1468.
34 Acsadi G, Dickson G, Love DR, et al. Human dystrophin expression in mdx mice after intramuscular injection of DNA constructs. Nature 1991; 352: 815–818.
35 Davis HL, Whalen RG, Demeneix BA. Direct gene transfer into skeletal muscle in vivo: factors affecting efficiency of transfer and stability of expression. Hum Gene Ther 1993; 4: 151–159.
36 Wells DJ. Improved gene transfer by direct plasmid injection associated with regeneration in mouse skeletal muscle. FEBS Lett 1993; 332: 179–182.
37 Danko I, Fritz JD, Jiao S, Hogan K, Latendresse JS, Wolff JA. Pharmacological enhancement of in vivo foreign gene expression in muscle. Gene Ther 1994; 2: 114–121.
38 Curiel DT, Agarwal S, Wagner E, Cotten M. Adenovirus enhancement of transferrin-polylysine mediated gene delivery. Proc Natl Acad Sci USA 1991; 88: 8850–8854.
39 Stratford-Perricaudet LD, Makeh I, Perricaudet M, Briande P. Widespread long-term gene transfer to mouse skeletal muscles and heart. J Clin Invest 1992; 90: 626–630.

40 Ragot T, Vincent N, Chafey P, et al. Efficient adenovirus-mediated transfer of a human minidystrophin gene to skeletal muscle of mdx mice. Nature 1993; 361: 647–650.
41 Vincent N, Ragot T, Gilgenkrantz H, et al. Long-term correction of mouse dystrophic degeneration by adenovirus-mediated transfer of a minidystrophin gene. Nature Genet 1993; 5: 130–134.
42 Davis HL, Demeneix BA, Quantin B, Coulomb J, Whalen RG. Plasmid DNA is superior to viral vectors for direct gene transfer into adult mouse skeletal muscle. Hum Gene Ther 1993; 4: 733–740.
43 Karpati G, Acsadi G. The potential for gene therapy in Duchenne muscular dystrophy and other genetic muscle diseases. Muscle Nerve 1993; 16: 1141–1153.
44 Alameddine HS, Quantin B, Cartaud A, Dehaupas M, Mandel JL, Fardeau M. Expression of a recombinant dystrophin in mdx mice using adenovirus vector. Neuromusc Disord 1994; 4: 193–203.
45 Dunkley MG, Love DR, Davies KE, Walsh FS, Morris GE, Dickson G. Retroviral-mediated transfer of a dystrophin minigene into mdx mouse myoblasts in vitro. FEBS Lett 1992; 2: 717–723.
46 Dunkley MG, Wells DJ, Walsh FS, Dickson G. Direct retroviral-mediated transfer of a dystrophin minigene into mdx mouse muscle in vivo. Hum Mol Genet 1993; 2: 717–723.
47 Dickson G, Dunckley M. Human dystrophin gene transfer: genetic correction of dystrophin deficiency. In: Partridge TA, ed. Molecular and Cell Biology of Muscular Dystrophy. London: Chapman & Hall, 1993: pp 283–302.
48 Hoffman EP, Morgan JE, Watkins SC, Partridge TA. Somatic reversion/suppression of the mouse mdx phenotype in vivo. J Neurol Sci 1990; 99: 9–25.
49 Sherratt TG, Vulliamy T, Dubowitz V, Sewry CA, Strong PN. Exon skipping and translation in patients with frameshift deletions in the dystrophin gene. Am J Hum Genet 1993; 53: 1007–1015.
50 Winnard AV, Klein CJ, Coovert DD, et al. Characterization of translational frame exception patients in Duchenne/Becker muscular dystrophy. Hum Mol Genet 1993; 2: 737–744.
51 Nicholson LVB. The ‘rescue’ of dystrophin synthesis in boys with Duchenne muscular dystrophy. Neuromusc Disord 1993; 3: 525–531.
52 Perrine SP, Ginder GD, Faller DV, et al. A short-term trial of butyrate to stimulate fetal-globin-gene expression in the β-globin gene disorders. N Engl J Med 1993; 328: 81–86.
53 Tinsley JM, Davies KE. Utrophin: a potential replacement for dystrophin? Neuromusc Disord 1993; 3: 537–539.
54 Clerk A, Morris GE, Dubowitz V, Davies KE, Sewry CA. Dystrophin-related protein, utrophin, in normal and dystrophic human foetal skeletal muscle. Histochem J 1993; 25: 554–561.
55 Barnea E, Zuk D, Simantov R, Nudel U, Yaffe D. Specificity of expression of the muscle and brain dystrophin gene promoters in muscle and brain cells. Neuron 1990; 5: 881–888.
56 Chelly J, Hamard G, Koulakoff A, Kaplan J-C, Kahn A, Berwald-Netter Y. Dystrophin gene transcribed from different promoters in neuronal and glial cells. Nature 1990; 344: 64–65.
57 Gorecki DC, Monaco AP, Derry JMJ, Walker AP, Barnard EA. Expression of four alternative dystrophin transcripts in brain regions regulated by different promoters. Hum Mol Genet 1992; 1: 505–510.
58 Thomason DB, Booth FW. Stable incorporation of a bacterial gene into adult rat muscle in vivo. Am J Physiol 1991; 258: C578–C581.
59 Salminen A, Elson HF, Mickley LA, Fojo AT, Gottesman MM. Implantation of recombinant rat myocytes into adult skeletal muscle: a potential gene therapy. Hum Gene Ther 1991; 2: 15–26.
60 Barr E, Leiden JM. Systemic delivery of recombinant proteins by genetically modified myoblasts. Science 1991; 254: 1507–1509.

61 Dhawan J, Pan LC, Pavlath GK, Travis MA, Lanctot AM, Blau HM. Systemic delivery of human growth hormone by injection of genetically engineered myoblasts. Science 1991; 254: 1509–1512.
62 Dai Y, Roman M, Naviaux RK, Verma IM. Gene therapy via primary myoblasts: long-term expression of factor IX protein following transplantation in vivo. Proc Natl Acad Sci USA 1992; 89: 10892–10895.
63 Yao SN, Kurachi K. Expression of human factor IX in mice after injection of genetically modified myoblasts. Proc Natl Acad Sci USA 1992; 89: 3357-3361.
64 Yao S-N, Smith KJ, Kurachi K. Primary myoblast-mediated gene transfer: persistent expression of human factor IX in mice. Gene Ther 1994; 2: 99–107.
65 Jiao S, Gurevich V, Wolff JA. Long-term correction of rat model of Parkinson's disease by gene therapy. Nature 1993; 362: 450–455.
66 Smith BF, Hoffman RK, Giger U, Wolfe JH. Genes transferred by retroviral vectors into normal and mutant myoblasts in primary cultures are expressed in myotubes. Mol Cell Biol 1990; 10: 3268–3271.
67 Wernig A, Irintchev A, Hartling A, Stephan G, Zimmerman K, Starzinski-Powitz A. Formation of new muscle fibres and tumours after injection of cultured myogenic cells. J Neurocytol 1991; 20: 982–997.
68 Morgan JE, Moore SE, Walsh FS, Partridge TA. Formation of skeletal muscle in vivo from the mouse C2 cell line. J Cell Sci 1992; 102: 779–787.
69 Beauchamp JR, Abraham DJ, Bou-Gharios G, Partridge TA, Olsen I. Expression and function of heterotypic adhesion molecules during differentiation of human skeletal muscle in culture. Am J Pathol 1991; 144: 166–174.
70 Hauschka SD, Linkhart TA, Clegg C, Merrill G. Clonal studies of human and mouse muscle. In: Mauro A, ed. Muscle Regeneration. New York: Raven Press, 1979: pp 311–322.
71 Arbones ML, Austin HA, Capon DJ, Greenburg G. Gene targeting in normal somatic cells: inactivation of the interferon-γ receptor in myoblasts. Nature Genet. 1994; 6: 90–97.
72 Zhu N, Liggit D, Liu Y, Debs R. Systemic gene expression after intravenous DNA delivery into adult mice. Science 1993; 261: 209–211.
73 Davis HL, Michel M-L, Whalen RG. DNA-based immunization induces continuous secretion of hepatitis B surface antigen and high levels of circulating antibody. Hum Mol Genet 1993; 2: 1847–1851.

British Medical Bulletin (1995) Vol. 51, No. 1, pp.138–148

Gene therapy and the brain

H A Jinnah
Department of Neurology, Johns Hopkins University Hospital, Baltimore, MD, USA

T Friedmann
Department of Pediatrics, Center for Molecular Genetics, University of California, San Diego, La Jolla, CA, USA

In this article we describe the application of the emerging concepts of gene therapy to 4 different neurologic disorders. The first of these is Lesch-Nyhan disease, a genetically-determined neurodevelopmental disorder caused by a defect in the gene which encodes the purine salvage enzyme hypoxanthine-guanine phosphoribosyltransferase (HPRT). Two additional disorders, Parkinsonism and Alzheimer's disease, are both neurodegenerative diseases of unknown etiology which affect the elderly. The final disorder involves malignant brain tumors. In each of these disorders, basic research with in vitro systems and animal models has suggested that the tools of gene transfer may provide a novel and potentially effective treatment strategy.

To date, more than 4000 genetic diseases have been identified. In at least 100 of these disorders, the primary manifestations are attributable to dysfunction of the nervous system.[1] Unfortunately, traditional pharmacologic, surgical, or dietary interventions have provided effective treatment for only a very small minority of these diseases. As a result, there has been a great deal of effort devoted to the development of alternative approaches to therapy. Gene therapy is one of these alternative approaches. Conceived more than 20 years ago, the term 'gene therapy' was originally envisioned as a new form of therapy which addressed genetic diseases at the genetic level.[2]

Over the past 5–10 years, rapid technical advances in molecular genetic techniques have brought gene therapy closer to reality. These advances include the ability to clone and manipulate genes responsible for human disease and to re-introduce functional copies of normal genes into living cells and tissues. Along with these technical advances has come the realization that gene therapy will provide a useful therapeutic approach not only for genetic disorders, but non-genetic disorders as well.

In this article, we focus on the application of gene therapy to disorders of the brain. The application of gene therapy to neurologic disease is of particular importance since current treatment is inadequate for so many of these diseases. The lack of effective treatments is undoubtedly related to the complexity of both anatomic and functional organization of the brain, and the fact that the pathophysiology of most neurologic diseases is so poorly understood. The experimental identification of potential gene therapy-based approaches to treatment is further challenged by the relative inaccessibility of nervous system tissues, and the refractoriness of mature neurons and glia to in vitro experimentation and to several of the more common gene transfer methods. Despite these difficulties, significant advances have recently been made. This summary is not meant to be a comprehensive review of the potential for gene therapy in neurologic disease but rather a focus on selected examples which illustrate specific principles. For further details, the reader is referred to several recent reviews.[3,4]

GENERAL PRINCIPLES

General strategies

Two general strategies have been developed for gene therapy: the in vivo approach and the ex vivo approach. These two approaches each have potential advantages and disadvantages which render them appropriate under different conditions. The in vivo approach is conceptually and technically more direct, involving the introduction of a gene directly into the tissues of an affected individual. In principle, it does not depend on the success of cell culture or subsequent survival of transplanted cells. However, it does require a highly efficient method for gene transfer, and until recently such methods have not been available for use in neural tissues.

The ex vivo approach, on the other hand, is technically more demanding. First, a suitable cell type is harvested from a donor and grown in tissue culture. Since mature neurons and glia are notoriously difficult to grow and genetically manipulate in culture, alternative cell types such as fibroblasts and myoblasts have been used. Next, the gene is introduced into the cells in vitro and cells expressing the transgene are amplified. The genetically altered cells are then harvested and reimplanted into an affected host. This approach is labour-intensive and time consuming, and it requires the growth of suitable cells in vitro and their subsequent survival after implantation. However, one advantage of the ex vivo approach is that it does not require a highly efficient method for gene transfer, because genetically altered cells may be amplified in vitro prior to implantation.

Physical methods for gene transfer

Several methods, including calcium phosphate precipitation, lipid carriers, and electroporation have been developed for the transfer of genes into cells. These methods require that the transgene be taken up by cells, bypass normal pathways of lysosomal degradation, and be expressed in the cell. In addition, long-term stable expression requires either that the transgene gain access to the cell nucleus and become incorporated into host genomic DNA or that the transgene remain stable as an independent piece of DNA, an episome. General experience with these methods has demonstrated them to be relatively inefficient.

However, some recent studies have suggested that direct injection of transgenes may be more efficient than previously believed. For example, injection of purified plasmid DNA encoding β-galactosidase into rat muscle in vivo results in expression of β-galactosidase activity for as long as a year.[5,6] The injection of the same DNA into rat muscle or nerve has also been reported to result in expression of β-galactosidase activity in spinal cord motor neurons.[7] The intracellular fate of naked plasmid DNA and the mechanisms by which it is retrogradely transported and expressed in spinal motor neurons remain unclear. Further application of these methods for direct gene transfer awaits confirmation of these reports with more extensive characterization of the efficiency and stability of transgene expression.

Viral vectors for gene transfer

The efficiency and stability of transgene expression has been more thoroughly studied in the case of viral vectors (*see* Vile and Russell, Kremer and Perricandet, Minson and Efstathion, in this issue for full details).

GENE THERAPY MODELS

Lesch-Nyhan disease (LND)

LND is a neurodevelopmental disorder characterized by choreoathetosis, dystonia, self-injurious behaviour, and hyperuricemia. LND was one of the first neurogenetic diseases for which the defective gene was identified and cloned. This gene encodes the purine salvage enzyme hypoxanthine-guanine phosphoribosyltransferase (HPRT), and over the past few years a great deal of effort has been devoted to characterizing the genetic mutations in patients with LND.[13] Despite considerable advance in our understanding of the molecular basis of LND, current treatment remains largely unsatisfactory.

LND was one of the first diseases proposed as a candidate for gene therapy. The earliest work focused on the ex vivo approach to gene therapy, demonstrating that retroviral vectors carrying an HPRT minigene could be expressed in HPRT-deficient cells in tissue culture.[14–16] Expression of HPRT in these cells corrected some of the metabolic abnormalities associated with HPRT deficiency. Subsequent studies demonstrated that human HPRT could be detected in vivo after transplantation of the genetically altered cells into rats or mice.[17,18] More recent work has demonstrated that HPRT can be expressed in the mouse brain using the more direct in vivo approach to gene therapy with herpes virus-based vectors. Unfortunately, the animals used in all of these experiments were not HPRT-deficient, so that the ability of gene transfer to correct the metabolic derangements associated with HPRT deficiency in vivo could not be addressed.

The production of a genetically HPRT-deficient strain of mice as an animal model for LND offers a useful tool to evaluate the effectiveness of gene therapy.[19,20] These mice carry a mutation in the HPRT gene which prevents the expression of HPRT mRNA and protein. They also display some of the metabolic derangements observed in patients with LND, such as a marked increase in de novo purine synthesis[21] and depletion of basal ganglia dopamine.[22–25] They have also been reported to display abnormal behaviours when challenged with amphetamine or 9-ethyladenine.[26–28] Therefore, these mice provide an ideal opportunity to evaluate gene transfer methods, the effect of gene transfer on the metabolic abnormalities associated with HPRT deficiency, and their ultimate effect on the behavioural phenotype. The application of gene therapy to patients affected with LND must await further experiments which demonstrate both feasibility and effectiveness.

Parkinson's disease (PD)

PD is a relatively common neurodegenerative disorder which affects predominantly the elderly. These patients display cogwheel rigidity, resting tremor, and an impairment in the initiation and speed of movements. Although familial PD has been reported, most cases are thought to be acquired. The cause of the disease is unknown, but environmental toxins, metabolic derangements, infectious processes, and normal aging have all been hypothesized to play a role. Pathophysiologically, PD is associated with degeneration of nigrostriatal neurons. These neurons have soma which reside in the substantia nigra, send axonal projections to the basal ganglia, and use dopamine as their neurotransmitter. Features of the disease can be largely controlled by the pharmacologic restoration of dopaminergic transmission. This is typically achieved by the administration of L-DOPA, the metabolic precursor to dopamine which diffuses across the blood-brain barrier more effectively than dopamine itself. Unfortunately as the disease progresses, pharmacologic therapy becomes less and less acceptable as the number and severity of side effects from drug therapy increase.

PD is an ideal candidate for gene therapy for several reasons. The clinical effectiveness of oral L-DOPA indicates that the restoration of lost neuronal circuitry is not essential for controlling the neurologic features of the disease. Therefore, the introduction of genetic material which can drive local synthesis of L-DOPA may prove to be an effective alternative to pharmacologic therapy. Furthermore, the metabolic pathway for the biosynthesis of L-DOPA from the amino acid tyrosine is very simple, requiring only the single enzyme tyrosine hydroxylase. This requirement means that gene therapy might be effective through the expression of only a tyrosine hydroxylase transgene in the areas where neural degeneration is occuring. Finally, several animal models of PD are available in which to test the effectiveness of gene therapy strategies.

An animal model of PD can be produced by the use of a neurotoxin such as 6-hydroxydopamine (6-OHDA) which destroys nigrostriatal dopamine neurons in experimental animals. Rodents and non-human primates treated with this toxin develop motor abnormalities very similar to those observed in PD. One particularly well-characterized model involves the unilateral administration of 6-OHDA to rats.[29] Affected animals display unilateral motor impairment which results in a characteristic circling ambulation. This model is particularly useful because the extent of the disease and the response to therapy can be quantified by measuring the frequency of circling behaviour.

Initial suggestions that a gene therapy approach to PD might be effective came from experiments which showed that rat 208F fibroblasts could produce and release L-DOPA in vitro after being infected with a retroviral vector carrying a rat tyrosine hydroxylase transgene.[30] In essence, these cells could be used as biologic minipumps for continuous and focal delivery of L-DOPA. In fact, the abnormal circling behaviour of rats with unilateral 6-hydroxydopamine lesions of the substantia nigra was significantly reduced by the intrastriatal implantation of these altered fibroblasts.[30] These initial results were subsequently confirmed by introducing human or rat tyrosine hydroxylase transgenes into NIH 3T3 cells, neuroblastoma cells, primary fibroblasts grown from skin biopsies, and even myocytes.[31–37]

The animal experiments clearly support the notion that ex vivo gene therapy might offer an effective therapeutic alternative to traditional pharmacologic therapy in PD. The gene therapy approach offers the theoretical advantage of minimizing side effects of L-DOPA therapy, since the L-DOPA is supplied continuously and locally. However, many questions remain to be answered before these techniques can be applied to affected humans. As mentioned above, the degenerating neurons in PD have soma which reside in the midbrain and extend axons to the forebrain. This fact raises the question of the most appropriate brain region in which to introduce the genetically altered cells. Another question involves the most appropriate surrogate cell type for use in PD. Primary skin fibroblasts offer the advantage of ready accessibility and ease of manipulation in culture, but may have properties which make them undesirable for intracerebral implantation such as the production of a collagen matrix or inappropriate regulation of tyrosine hydroxylase. A further uncertainty is that the intracerebral availability of substrate (tyrosine) or cofactor (tetrahydropterin) may limit the effectiveness of this approach, requiring supplementation with one or both molecules.[36] Finally, it is not yet clear if cells engineered to produce L-DOPA would suffice or if cells engineered to produce dopamine by combined insertion of transgenes encoding both tyrosine hydroxylase and DOPA-decarboxylase would be more effective. Answers to these questions will be forthcoming from further animal experiments.

Alzheimer's dementia (AD)

AD is another relatively common neurodegenerative disorder which affects the elderly. The cause of the disease is unknown, and the majority of cases are acquired. However, familial forms, and a genetic predisposition have been clearly documented.

Pathophysiologically, AD is associated with generalized degeneration of cerebral cortical and hippocampal neurons. Cholinergic neurons in the basal forebrain which project to cortex and hippocampus appear to be particularly vulnerable. Since the progressive dementia results from widespread loss of neuronal connectivity, it seems unlikely that simple replacement of a single neurotransmitter will be effective at reversing the dementia. A more successful approach might be the delivery of neurotrophic factors which prevent the neuronal degeneration. Unfortunately, most known neurotrophic factors are large protein molecules which are likely to be difficult to manufacture and deliver to affected brain areas by traditional parenteral methods. These problems render pharmacologic approach to therapy quite difficult.

Gene therapy may provide an effective alternative to traditional methods for delivery of trophic factors. For example, genes encoding trophic factors can be introduced into cells in tissue culture. Subsequent intracerebral implantation of these cells effectively produces a biologic minipump for constant local delivery of a trophic factor. The effectiveness of this approach has already been demonstrated in several animal models of neurodegeneration. In the first model, surgical lesions of the fimbria-fornix in rodents interrupts cholinergic neurons in the basal forebrain from their normal supply of nerve growth factor (NGF) in the cortex. In the absence of a constant supply of NGF, the cholinergic neurons degenerate. Early studies had documented that the dying neurons could be rescued by the intracerebral delivery of purified NGF via artificial minipumps. Subsequently, it was demonstrated that fibroblasts infected with a retroviral vector carrying a gene encoding NGF could produce and release NGF in vitro.[38,39] Furthermore, grafts of these NGF-producing fibroblasts were shown to rescue dying cholinergic neurons in the fimbria-fornix model.

A second model of neurodegeneration involves the devascularization of the rat cortex. This procedure has a similar effect as fimbria-fornix transection, and results in the degeneration of basal forebrain cholinergic neurons by destroying their source of NGF. Grafts of fibroblasts genetically modified to produce NGF have been shown to prevent death of neurons in this model as well.[40,41] A third model of neurodegeneration takes advantage of the NGF-dependence of neurons in the superior cervical ganglion. These neurons degenerate as a result of axotomy because they are dependent on NGF derived from peripheral target organs. It has been reported that the degenerative changes can be attenuated if the superior cervical ganglion is injected with a herpes-based vector carrying the gene encoding NGF.[42]

The appropriateness of NGF administration as treatment for AD and other neurodegenerative disorders remains a matter of debate. However, the animal experiments demonstrate the principle that gene therapy may be applied to prevent neurodegeneration by directing constant local production of a growth factor either by grafts of growth factor-producing cells, or direct introduction of growth factor genes.

Brain tumors

Neoplastic disease in adults is perhaps best thought of as an acquired genetic disease. Tumors of glial cell origin are clearly the most common brain tumors, and carry a poor prognosis. Even with the most aggressive of interventions including surgical debulking, chemotherapy and radiation treatments, fewer than 5% of patients survive more than 5 years after diagnosis. As a result of the poor success of traditional modalities, treatment strategies based on gene therapy are being developed.

A gene therapy approach to brain tumors exploits differences in the growth characteristics of malignant cells and mature brain cells, and the fact that transgenes introduced into cells by retroviral vectors require cell division for stable expression. Since malignant cells divide rapidly whereas normal brain cells are quiescent, retroviral vectors can be used to deliver genes selectively to the malignant cells. By incorporating a transgene which arrests growth, encodes a toxic product, or confers sensitivity to specific chemotherapeutic agents, tumor growth might be controlled. Most recent studies have focused on the thymidine kinase gene derived from herpes simplex virus (HSV-TK). Although mammalian cells are relatively resistant to the drug ganciclovir, the presence of HSV-TK results in the conversion of the drug to a toxic product which kills cells.

Several studies have demonstrated that normal glioma cells in culture are resistant to the actions of ganciclovir. However, when infected with a retroviral vector encoding HSV-TK, they become sensitive to the drug.[43–45] Initial studies showed that only a small fraction of glial tumors in the rat brain could be infected with a single intracerebral injection of retroviral vector.[46] This poor efficiency is probably related to the fact that the half-life of the retroviral vector in vivo is 2–4 h, and only a small proportion of glial cells are in their growth phase during this period. Subsequent studies demonstrated that a much higher proportion of tumor cells could be infected if they were inoculated with retrovirus producer cells to provide a more continuous supply of retrovirus for several days.[43,44,46]

In principle, a potential limitation of this approach might be that the tumor would continue to grow unless 100% of the tumor cells are infected with the retrovirus and express HSV-TK. Even under the best circumstances, this degree of efficiency is not generally possible with retroviral vectors. In practice however, less than 100% infection efficiency does not appear to impede significant tumor regression. For reasons that have yet to be explained, intracerebral tumors of glioma cells have been shown to regress completely after ganciclovir treatment even when only 10–70% of the cells have been genetically modified to express HSV-TK. This phenomenon, in which non-infected tumor cells die after ganciclovir treatment, has been termed the 'bystander effect' and has been observed by several different investigators.[43,45,47,48] For example, rats with experimentally introduced brain tumors comprised of 9L glioma cells almost always die within one month as a result of the growing tumor mass. However, when inoculated with cells which produce a retroviral vector carrying HSV-TK and treated with ganciclovir, the majority of animals have been reported to survive with apparently complete histologic regression of tumor.[43,48]

The results from experimental work with animals have been sufficiently encouraging that clinical trials have been initiated at several centres.[49] A number of patients with primary or metastatic brain tumors have been treated with the gene therapy approach outlined above. Specifically, mouse fibroblasts producing a retroviral vector carrying HSV-TK have been implanted directly into the tumor bed by stereotactic injection. Several days later, the patients have been treated with ganciclovir. The mouse cells do not survive because they express HSV-TK and are therefore sensitive to ganciclovir. In addition, they would eventually be rejected by the immune system. Firm conclusions from these pilot trials are not yet available, but it is likely that this approach or a modification of this approach will eventually prove useful.

SUMMARY AND CONCLUSIONS

In this brief review we have summarized potential gene therapy-based treatment strategies for 4 neurologic diseases. These are not the only 4 neurologic diseases for which gene therapy might prove effective, and more models are currently being developed. Although the neurologic diseases as a group have traditionally been difficult management problems, it is becoming increasingly clear that newer and more effective genetic treatment modalities are forthcoming.

REFERENCES

1 Martin JB. Molecular genetics in neurology. Ann Neurol 1993; 34: 757–773.
2 Friedmann T, Roblin R. Gene therapy for human genetic disease? Science 1972; 175: 949–955.
3 Jinnah HA, Gage FH, Friedmann T. Gene therapy and neurologic disease. In: Rosenberg RN, Prusiner SB, DiMauro S, Barchi RL, Kunkel LM, eds. The molecular and genetic basis of neurologic disease. Boston: Butterworth-Heinemann, 1993; 969–976.
4 Suhr ST, Gage FH. Gene therapy for neurologic disease. Arch Neurol 1993; 50: 1252–1268.
5 Wolff JA, Malone RW, Williams P et al. Direct gene transfer into mouse muscle in vivo. Science 1990; 247: 1465–1468.
6 Wolff JA, Ludtke JJ, Acsadi G, Williams P, Jani A. Long-term persistence of plasmid DNA and foreign gene expression in mouse muscle. Hum Mol Genet 1992; 1: 363–369.
7 Sahenk Z, Sehareseyon J, Mendell JR, Burghes AHM. Gene delivery to spinal motor neurons. Brain Res 1993; 606: 126–129.
8 Johnson PA, Miyanohara A, Levine F, Cahill T, Friedmann T. Cytotoxicity of a replication-defective mutant of herpes simplex virus type1. J Virol 1992; 66: 2952–2965.
9 Le Gal La Salle G, Berrard JJR, Ridoux V, Stratford-Perricaudet LD, Perricaudet M, Mallet J. An adenovirus vector for gene transfer in neurons and glia in the brain. Science 1993; 259: 988–990.
10 Bajocchi G, Feldman SH, Crystal RG, Mastrangeli A. Direct in vivo gene transfer to ependymanl cells in the central nervous system using recombinant adenovirus vectors. Nature Genet 1993; 3: 229–234.
11 Davidson BL, Allen ED, Kozarsky KF, Wilson JM, Roessler BJ. A model system for in vivo gene transfer into the central nervous system using an adenoviral vector. Nature Genet 1993; 3: 219–223.
12 Akli S, Caillaud C, Vigne E, et al. Transfer of a foreign gene into the brain using adenovirus vectors. Nature Genet 1993; 3: 224–228.

13 Sege-Peterson K, Nyhan WL, Page T. Lesch-Nyhan disease and HPRT deficiency. In: Rosenberg RN, Prusiner SB, DiMauro S, Barchi RL, Kunkel LM, eds. The molecular and genetic basis of neurological disease. Boston: Butterworth-Heinemann, 1992; 241–260.
14 Miller AD, Jolly DJ, Friedmann T, Verma IM. A transmissible retrovirus expressing human hypoxanthine phosphoribosyltransferase (HPRT): gene transfer into cells obtained from humans deficient in HPRT. Proc Natl Acad Sci (USA) 1983; 80: 4709–4713.
15 Willis RC, Jolly DJ, Miller AD, et al. Partial phenotypic correction of human Lesch-Nyhan (hypoxanthine-guanine phosphoribosyltransferase-deficient) lymphoblasts with a transmissible retroviral vector. J Biol Chem 1984; 259: 7842–7849.
16 Chang SMW, Wager-Smith K, Tsao TY, Henkel-Tigges J, Vaishnav S, Caskey CR. Construction of a defective retrovirus containing the human hypoxanthine phosphoribosyltransferase cDNA and its expression in cultured cells and mouse bone marrow. Mol Cell Biol 1991; 7: 854–863.
17 Gage FH, Wolff JA, Rosenberg MB, et al. Grafting genetically modified cells to the brain: possibilities for the future. Neuroscience 1987; 23: 795–807.
18 Miller AD, Eckner RJ, Jolly DJ, Friedmann T, Verma IM. Expression of a retrovirus encoding human HPRT in mice. Science 1984; 225: 630–632.
19 Hooper M, Hardy K, Handyside A, Hunter S, Monk M. HPRT-deficient (Lesch-Nyhan) mouse embryos derived from germline colonization by cultured cells. Nature 1987; 326: 292–295.
20 Kuehn MR, Bradley A, Robertson EJ, Evans MJ. A potential animal model for Lesch-Nyhan syndrome through introduction of HPRT mutations into mice. Nature 1987; 326: 295–298.
21 Jinnah HA, Page T, Friedmann T. Brain purines in a genetic mouse model of Lesch-Nyhan disease. J Neurochem 1993; 60: 2036–2045.
22 Finger S, Heavens RP, Sirinathsinghji DJS, Kuehn MR, Dunnett SB. Behavioral and neurochemical evaluation of a transgenic mouse model of Lesch-Nyhan syndrome. J Neurol Sci 1988; 86: 203–213.
23 Dunnett SB, Sirinathsinghji DJS. Monoamine deficiency in a transgenic (Hprt-) mouse model of Lesch-Nyhan syndrome. Brain Res 1989; 501: 401–406.
24 Williamson DJ, Sharkey J, Clarke AR, et al. Analysis of forebrain dopaminergic pathways in HPRT-mice. Adv Exp Med Biol 1991; 309B: 269–272.
25 Jinnah HA, Wojcik BE, Hunt MA, et al. Dopamine deficiency in a genetic mouse model of Lesch-Nyhan disease. J Neurosci 1994; 14: 1164–1175.
26 Jinnah HA, Gage FH, Friedmann T. Amphetamine-induced behavioural phenotype in a hypoxanthine-guanine phosphoribosyltransferase-deficient mouse model of Lesch-Nyhan syndrome. Behav Neurosci 1991; 105: 1004–1012.
27 Jinnah HA, Langlais PJ, Friedmann T. Functional analysis of brain dopamine systems in a genetic mouse model of Lesch-Nyhan syndrome. J Pharmacol Exp Ther 1992; 263: 596–607.
28 Wu CL, Melton DW. Production of a model for Lesch-Nyhan syndrome in hypoxanthine phosphoribosyltransferase-deficient mice. Nature Genet 1993; 3: 235–239.
29 Miller R, Beninger RJ. On the interpretation of asymmetries of posture and locomotion produced with dopamine agonists in animals with unilateral depletion of striatal dopamine. Prog Neurobiol 1991; 36: 229–256.
30 Wolff JA, Fisher LJ, Xu L, et al. Grafting fibroblasts genetically modified to produce L-dopa in a rat model of Parkinson disease. Proc Natl Acad Sci (USA) 1989; 86: 9011–9014.
31 Uchida K, Takamatsu K, Kaneda N, et al. Transfection of tyrosine hydroxylase cDNA into C6 cells. Proc Jpn Acad 1988; 64: 290–293.
32 Horellou P, Guibert B, Leviel V, Mallet J. Retroviral transfer of a human tyrosine hydroxylase cDNA in various cell lines: regulated release of dopamine in mouse anterior pituitary AtT-20 cells. Proc Natl Acad Sci (USA) 1989; 86: 7233–7237.

33 Horellou P, Brundin P, Kalen P, Mallet J, Bjorklund A. In vivo release of DOPA and dopamine from genetically engineered cells grafted to the denervated rat striatum. Neuron 1990; 5: 393–402.
34 Horellou P, Marlier L, Privat A, Mallet J. Behavioural effect of engineered cells that synthesize L-DOPA or dopamine after grafting into the rat neostriatum. Eur J Neurosci 1990; 2: 116–119.
35 Fisher LJ, Jinnah HA, Kale LC, Higgins GA, Gage FH. Survival and function of intrastriatally grafted primary fibroblasts genetically modified to produce L-DOPA. Neuron 1991; 6: 371–380.
36 Uchida K, Tsuzaki N, Nagatsu T, Kohsaka S. Tetrahydrobiopterin-dependent functional recovery in 6-hydroxydopamine-treated rats by intracerebral grafting of fibroblasts transfected with tyrosine hydroxylase cDNA. Dev Neurosci 1992; 14: 173–180.
37 Jiao S, Gurevich V, Wolff JA. Long-term correction of rat model of Parkinson's disease by gene therapy. Nature 1993; 362: 450–453.
38 Rosenberg MB, Friedmann T, Robertson RC, Tuszynski M, Wolff JA, Breakefield XO, Gage FH. Grafting genetically modified cells to the damaged brain: restorative effects of NGF expression. Science 1988; 242: 1575–1578.
39 Stromberg I, Wetmore CJ, Ebendal T, Ernfors P, Persson H, Olson L. Rescue of basal forebrain cholinergic neurons after implantation of genetically modified cells producing recombinant NGF. J Neurosci Res 1990; 25: 405–411.
40 Piccardo P, Maysinger D, Cuello AC. Recovery of nucleus basalis cholinergic neurons by grafting NGF secretor fibroblasts. NeuroReport 1992; 3: 353–356.
41 Maysinger D, Piccardo P, Goiny M, Cuello AC. Grafting of genetically modified cells: effects of acetylcholine release in vivo. Neurochem Int 1992; 21: 543–548.
42 Federoff HJ, Geschwind MD, Geller AI, Kessler JA. Expression of nerve growth factor in vivo from a defective herpes simplex virus 1 vector prevents effects of axotomy on sympathetic ganglia. Proc Natl Acad Sci (USA) 1992; 89: 1636–1640.
43 Ram Z, Culver KW, Walbridge S, Blaese RM, Oldfield EH. In situ retroviral-mediated gene transfer for the treatment of brain tumors in rats. Cancer Res 1993; 53: 83–88.
44 Takamiya Y, Short MP, Moolten FL, Fleet C, Mineta T, Breakefield XO, Martuza RL. An experimental model of retrovirus gene therapy for malignant brain tumors. J Neurosurg 1993; 79: 104–110.
45 Takamiya Y, Short MP, Ezzeddine ZD, Moolten FL, Breakefield XO, Martuza RL. Gene therapy of malignant brain tumors: a rat glioma line bearing the herpes simplex virus type 1-thymidine kinase gene and wild type retrovirus kills other tumor cells. J Neurosci Res 1992; 33: 493–503.
46 Short MP, Choi BC, Lee JK, Malick A, Breakefield XO, Martuza RL. Gene delivery to glioma cells in rat brain by grafting of a retrovirus packaging cell line. J Neurosci Res 1990; 27: 427–433.
47 Barba D, Hardin J, Ray J, Gage FH. Thymidine kinase-mediated killing of rat brain tumors. J Neurosurg 1993; 79: 729–735.
48 Culver KW, Ram Z, Wallbridge S, Ishii H, Oldfield EH, Blaese RM. In vivo gene transfer with retroviral vector-producer cells for treatment of experimental brain tumors. Science 1992; 256: 1550–1552.
49 Randall T. Gene therapy for brain tumors in trials, correction of inherited disorders a hope. JAMA 1993; 269: 2181–2182.

British Medical Bulletin (1995) Vol. 51, No. 1, pp.149–166

Gene therapy for HIV infection

A M L Lever
University of Cambridge, Department of Medicine, Addenbrooke's Hospital, Cambridge, UK

The genetic approach to HIV infection is still very young and a number of different stages in the viral life cycle are being studied as targets for gene therapy, using a wide variety of modalities for gene delivery. Several gene therapy protocols for AIDS have been approved and when this article is published these may be in progress. In this chapter the scientific background to these in vivo studies is reviewed.

The concept of gene therapy for infectious diseases is relatively novel. Most infections are self limiting or are treatable with the impressive range of anti-bacterial, anti-fungal and, to a lesser extent, anti-viral drugs available today. Using genetically based vaccines as a means of immunisation against infectious disease is, however, perhaps more widely accepted and model systems exist substantiating their efficacy.

Infectious pathogens which integrate their genome into host cell chromosomes, and which can transmit their progeny to daughter cells, may be considered genetic diseases. The fact that the major route of transmission is still cell free rather than 'vertical' does not alter the fact that the deleterious genetic material has become part of the human genome. Thus virus infections such as HIV, and possibly HTLV-1 and hepatitis B, might usefully be tackled by a genetic approach to treatment. This is further supported by the emerging problems of more conventional, pharmaceutical therapies.

Chemotherapeutic agents targeted against a pathogen which can exist as a DNA provirus, which may be latent, are likely to be of limited efficacy. Treatment must be lifelong and, as is already evident in clinical practice, the problems of drug accumulation and toxicity may outweigh the possible benefits of the drug against the limited number of susceptible viral targets. Anti-viral drugs are generally targeted against viral enzymatic processes. The striking ability of HIV to mutate, through the infidelity of its reverse transcriptase (RT), means that the emergence of drug resistant variants can occur extremely rapidly.

This same genetic mutability is particularly a feature of the hypervariable envelope glycoprotein of HIV which has contributed to the difficulties with development of effective vaccines capable of eliciting broad spectrum neutralisation of diverse HIV strains.

AIMS OF GENE THERAPY IN HIV INFECTION

Gene therapy in HIV is designed to fulfil a number of purposes. A genetically based vaccine might be a way to attempt prophylaxis against HIV infection. For the foreseeable future, other active interventional approaches will only be appropriate for individuals who are already HIV infected. There the aims will be to protect residual uninfected cells, to eliminate cells which are already infected or to render the virus within them non-functional. Peripheral to this, but in epidemiological terms of significant importance, is the potential to reduce the infectivity of an infected person and thus check the spread of the virus through the population.

Before discussing the various approaches to HIV gene therapy, it is worth reviewing the retroviral life cycle[1,2] (Fig. 1), and highlighting areas in which a gene therapy approach might be beneficial.

HIV binds to its cell surface receptor, the CD4 molecule, and by interacting with this and at least one other cell surface molecule, a conformational change occurs in the envelope glycoproteins to reveal the hydrophobic sequence of the transmembrane envelope protein. This leads to a fusion of the viral envelope with the cell membrane and delivery of the viral capsid into the cytoplasm of the cell. Within the capsid structure the diploid RNA genome is reverse transcribed by the viral reverse transcriptase (RT) to, first, an RNA/DNA heterodimer containing a complete copy of the viral genes. It is at this point that misincorporation of nucleotides by the RT may generate mutation in the DNA copy. Subsequently, the RNA is degraded and a DNA duplex synthesised. The double-stranded DNA genome is then integrated into the host cell chromosomes where it may become latent or transcriptionally active. Transcriptional activation mediated through promoter sequences in the long terminal repeat (LTR) gives rise initially to RNAs which are spliced and code for the regulatory proteins of HIV *tat* and*rev* (Fig. 2). The *tat* protein is a transcriptional transactivator whose action is dependent on interaction with an LTR encoded RNA stem-loop structure (TAR) in the nascent transcript. In combination with its target sequences it comprises one of the most powerful activator/promoter combinations known in eukaryotic cells. The *tat*/nucleic acid interaction gives rise to large quantities of viral RNA which is initially spliced. The *rev* protein

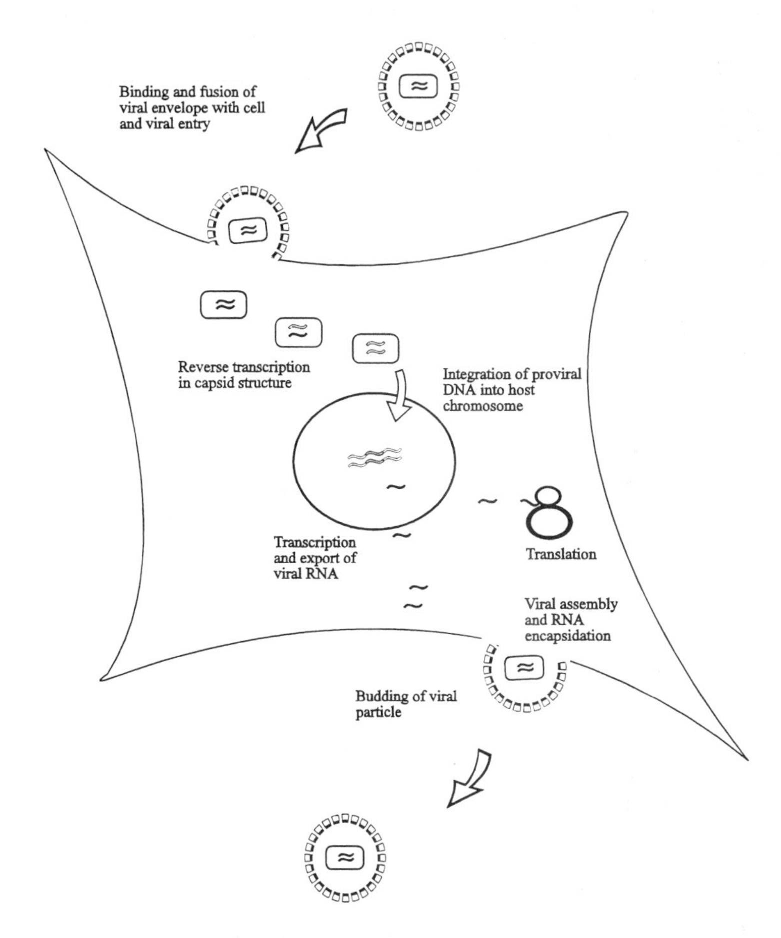

Fig. 1 The retroviral life cycle.

is also encoded on a multiply spliced RNA and this accumulates. Interaction of *rev* protein with a cis-acting stem-loop structure in the 3′end of the full length RNA (the *rev* response element-RRE), inhibits splicing and promotes transport of singly spliced and unspliced RNA to the cytoplasm. *Rev* also facilitates translation of these messages. The singly spliced mRNA codes for the envelope glycoproteins and the unspliced message for the *gag* and *pol* proteins. The former make up the structural proteins of the viral core and the latter code for the viral enzymes. The same full length RNA which codes for *gag* and *pol* can also act as the viral genome. The genome is recognised through a further RNA

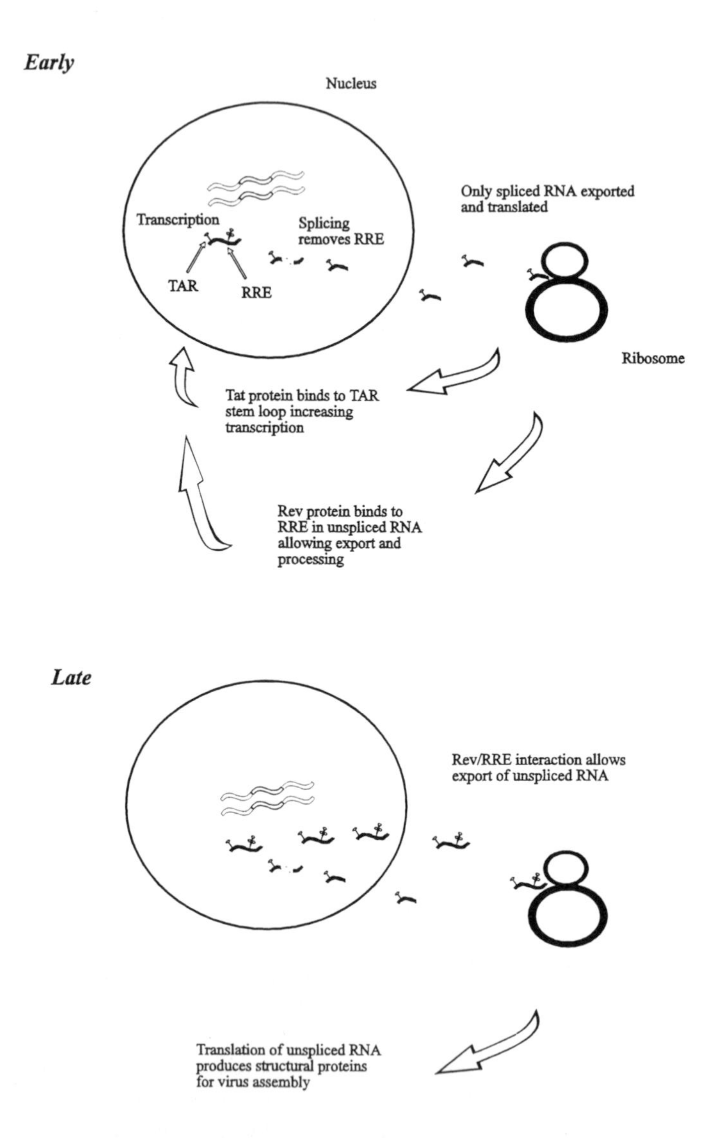

Fig. 2 Simplified diagram of the HIV genes and the messenger RNAs derived from the DNA provirus. A large number of spliced mRNA species have been identified. The proteins encoded by the various RNA species are indicated.

protein interaction involving at least one other structural RNA motif. It is possible that a sub-population of full length RNA molecules is sequestered into a compartment in which such interactions can occur, leading to encapsidation of the RNA genome into the budding virus particle.

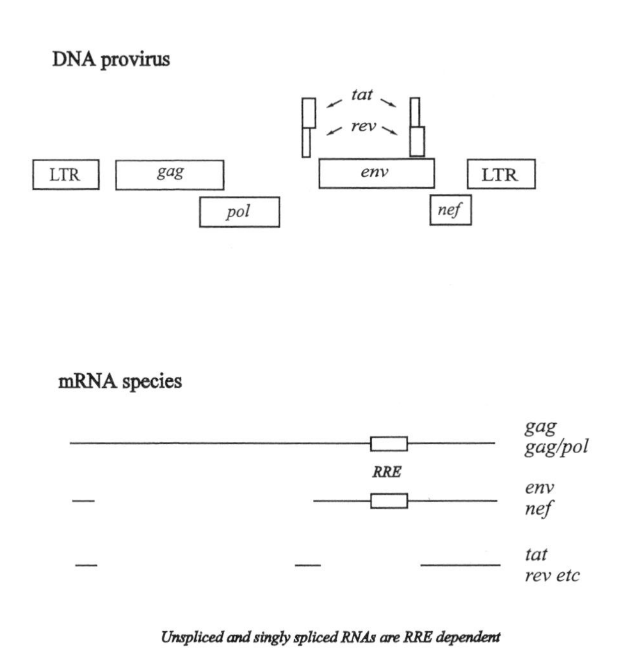

Fig. 3 Regulatory proteins of HIV and the control over early and late stages of the viral life cycle.

Viral assembly[3] in HIV is typical of C-type retroviruses. Envelope glycoproteins have a signal sequence which leads to translocation of the polypeptide into the endoplasmic reticulum lumen where it is processed and glycosylated. Normal cellular exocytic processes then transport the envelope glycoprotein to the cell membrane below which are assembling the unglycosylated *gag* and *gag/pol* polyproteins. The full length RNA which codes for these has a frameshift sequence upstream of *pol*, as *pol* and *gag* are in different open reading frames (Fig. 3) and ribosomal frame shifting leads to an excess of *gag* over *gag/pol* molecules. *Gag* and *gag/pol* assemble at the membrane in association with the envelope glycoproteins and the virus buds from the cell giving rise to a typical C-type virus particle with a doughnut shaped capsid core. Soon after budding auto-catalytic cleavage of the *gag* and *gag/pol*

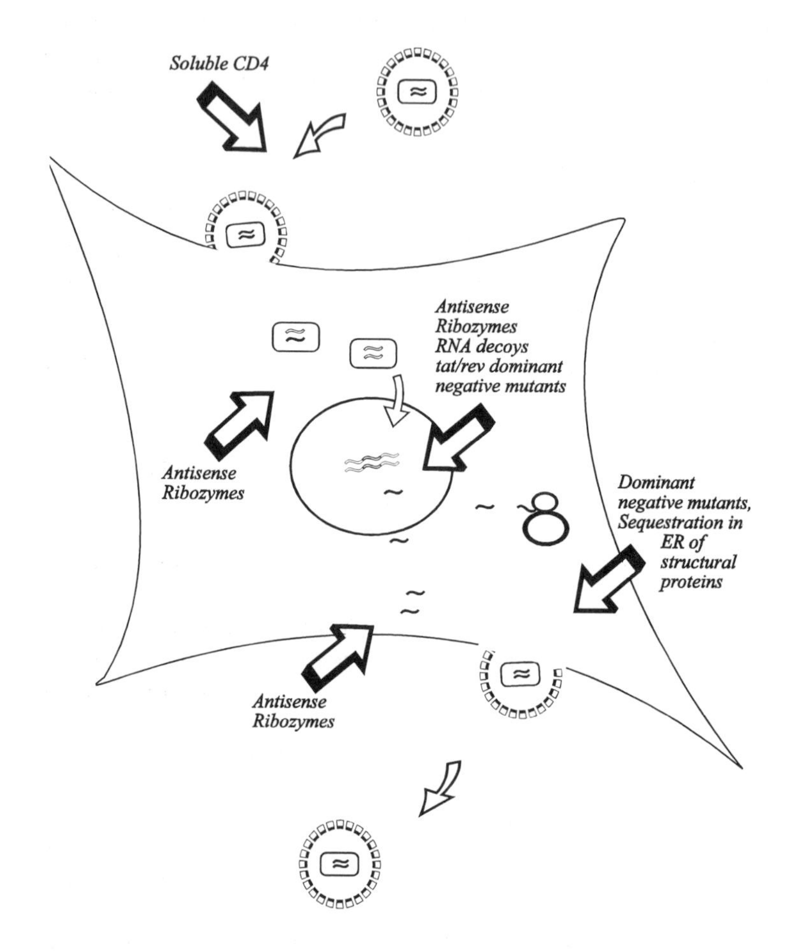

Fig. 4 Potential steps in the life cycle at which genetic based therapies might be targeted.

polyproteins occurs, leading to production of the dense viral core. The viral particle is then infectious for another cell.

POTENTIAL TARGETS FOR GENE THERAPY OF HIV INFECTION

Most processes in the viral life cycle have vulnerable spots which could be disrupted by genetic methods (Fig. 4). Some aspects such as transcription and translation are carried out by the host cell machinery and it is likely that significantly inhibiting these would lead to cell death. However, this may work therapeutically as discussed below. Processes specific to the virus are an obvious choice: entry into the cell, reverse transcription or integration. The *tat* and *rev* RNA/protein interactions are clearly vulnerable and the packaging of the RNA genome is another virus specific function distinct from normal cellular processes.

IMMUNISATION WITH HIV PROTEINS

In vivo expression of viral proteins as a genetic vaccine is one approach to attacking the virus. The advantages of this are that relatively lower level expression of viral protein may be effective in eliciting an immune response than would be required in the case of a direct antiviral protein or RNA molecule.

Animal models using the influenza virus system have shown the efficacy of such a genetic vaccine, in which direct injection of pure plasmid DNA coding for viral proteins has led to persistent viral gene expression[4]. This stimulates development of a cell mediated immune response, which is then protective against lethal challenge with the virus.

In HIV infection it would be important to present highly conserved regions of the virus as immunogens because of the virus' ability to mutate and avoid neutralising responses. In AIDS patients it has already been noted that evasion of immune responses directed against cytotoxic T-cell specific epitopes can occur even in relatively conserved portions of HIV, such as *gag*.[5] Delivery of viral genes together with genes coding for immunostimulatory molecules, such as the B7/BB1 molecule, is another potential development.[6]

gp160, the envelope precursor protein, expressed in syngeneic cells, has been used to induce humoral and cellular immune responses in mice. Homologous gp120 neutralisation has been stimulated.[7,8] Broad spectrum neutralisation has not yet been achieved.

Once immunity develops cells expressing the immunogenic protein are likely to be destroyed along with destruction of any cells containing transcriptionally active virus. The large proportion of the virus infected cells harbouring latent virus will persist and provide a pool from which mutants can arise which may be able to evade the immune response.

INTERFERON MEDIATED INHIBITION

The interferon system is a powerful naturally occurring antiviral mechanism and this has been harnessed in a number of gene therapy approaches to attempt to inhibit HIV replication. Interferon cDNAs have been cloned and inserted into vectors for either constitutive[9] or inducible[10] expression in target cells. Both of these appear to lead to inhibition of replication following a subsequent HIV challenge. Replication escape may occur after a number of weeks. Interferon treatment induces several cellular proteins, one of these (RBP 9–27) apparently interacts with the *rev* responsive element RNA stem-loop structure[11] and may inhibit *rev*-dependent *gag* protein expression.

AUTOLYTIC DESTRUCTION OF INFECTED CELLS

A number of strategies have been developed in which a cell is primed to self destruct on infection with HIV. At first sight this would not appear to be advantageous, as it might lead to serial destruction of large parts of the immune system. On balance, however, the elimination of cells, which act as infectious foci for spread of virus to other cells, might be beneficial. Most in vitro approaches to date have involved the use of potent toxins or conditional lethal genes. The diphtheria toxin A (DT-A) chain gene has been used as an inducible suicide gene.[12] As little as one molecule of DT-A may be enough to kill a cell. Conditional lethal genes used include the herpes simplex virus thymidine kinase (TK),[13] which is innocuous unless the substrate gancyclovir or acyclovir is present. In the presence of the prodrug, which becomes phosphorylated by TK to produce the active moiety, cell death ensues. Studies have shown that either of these genes under the control of the HIV promoter can be induced into transcriptional activity by the entry of replication competent HIV and production of *tat*. Conversely vectors containing *tat* dependent lethal genes which enter *tat* expressing cells can be used to target and destroy infected cells.[14] In the TK system pharmacologically acceptable levels of acyclovir led to virtually complete elimination of HIV replication in vitro.[13] Some promising results have also been noted in vitro using a CD4-pseudomonas toxin chimera[15] which targets cells displaying viral gp120. In most cases, and commonly with most antiviral strategies, the reduction in HIV replication in the gene modified cells is not 100%. It should also be borne in mind that such in vitro experiments usually involve antibiotic selection of cells, so the antiviral gene is expressed in 100% of the cells prior to virus challenge, a situation unlikely to be achieved in vivo unless stem cells are transduced.

This form of inducible therapy has drawbacks if it depends solely on a tat-LTR interaction. The HIV LTR is a very promiscuous promoter which is activated by a large number of proteins other than *tat*[16] including transcription factors such as those of cytomegalovirus. There is limited control over the expression of a *tat* inducible suicide gene, and destruction of cells might occur under circumstances other than HIV infection. Tighter control of induction by HIV can be achieved by making expression of the suicide protein both *tat* and *rev* dependent.[17]

DIRECT INTERFERENCE WITH VIRAL PROCESSES

Interference with viral replication can be achieved by disruption of viral processing either during entry into the cell or, more easily, during exit. The approaches fall into 3 major groups, those concentrating on blocking viral entry and those targeted either to viral protein or to viral RNA intracellularly. The DNA provirus is as yet not a practicable target (Fig. 4).

To enhance the possibility of inhibition occurring prior to integration of HIV, constitutive production of antiviral genes is probably necessary. Activation triggered by viral entry would be ideal. Preintegration events would seem intrinsically difficult to target as most RNA to DNA processing occurs within the structured capsid unit. Intracellular targeting of effector molecules is important as shown by Sullenger, who demonstrated that if there was no other signal motif co-localising effector and target RNAs to the same site,[18] no antisense/ribozyme effect was seen. In this work a retroviral packaging signal sequence on the therapeutic RNA molecule dramatically increased the efficacy of a ribozyme.

Inhibiting virus entry – soluble CD4

Since the CD4 molecule is one of the major receptors for HIV entry into the cell,[19] blocking the gp120 viral envelope with a CD4, truncated beyond the membrane anchoring segment (soluble CD4-sCD4), seemed a hopeful proposition. In vitro studies showed that sCD4 was able to bind to HIV and inhibit infection of CD4+ cells,[20–23] and, when cells producing sCD4 were co-cultivated with HIV susceptible cells, up to a 10-fold decrease in infectivity was noted on challenge with HIV. Early studies showed that the half life in vivo of sCD4 was impractically short for clinical use and a CD4 molecule conjugated to the Fc region of IgG was engineered. This had a longer half life.[24] Early studies in the primate model of HIV showed that soluble CD4 and CD4-IgG chimeric molecules apparently led to some protective effect against subsequent viral challenge.[25–27] The protective effect, however, was far in excess of that which could be accounted for by the levels of sCD4 in the circulation and correlated most closely with production by the animals of an anti-CD4 antibody response. The mode of protection is thus unclear.

One concern about the use of sCD4 is that it might disrupt the normal CD4/MHC Class II contact involved in T-cell/antigen presenting cell interactions.

Expression of mutant CD4 intracellularly designed to complex with the HIV envelope glycoprotein within the cell and prevent viral assembly has also been demonstrated in vitro.[28]

In general, CD4 and its derivatives have not lived up to early promise. Phase I clinical trials of recombinant sCD4 did not demonstrate significant efficacy[29] and virus resistance to neutralisation by sCD4 occurred.[30] The dose of CD4 required to give detectable plasma levels was much higher than expected.[31]One possible use may be as post exposure prophylaxis.

Nucleotide based therapy

There are 3 classes of RNA targeted antivirals: antisense (DNA and RNA), ribozymes (hammerhead and hairpin) and RNA decoys.

Antisense

Antisense oligonucleotides have been widely studied as antiviral agents. Antisense has been targeted to regulatory genes including *tat*, *rev* and *vpu*,[32,33] to *pol*,[34] to structural genes such as *env*[35] and *gag*[17], and cis-acting regulatory sequences including the primer binding site (PBS)[36] and the LTR[37] containing the TAR sequence. Significant inhibition of cell adapted strains of HIV such as HXB2 has been demonstrated. Antisense to the HIV LTR delivered by an adeno-associated virus vector produced a significant (up to 90%) reduction of HIV replication. Rather surprisingly, there was also a reasonably impressive inhibition of SIV, despite the relatively low (< 50%) sequence homology.[37] If this work is reproducible it encourages one to believe that a single antisense sequence might be effective against a large range of HIV variants within an individual. Using antisense to *tat* and *rev* splice acceptors, the optimal length of an antisense molecule against HIV has also been studied.[33] Inhibition of HIV replication was demonstrated in selected cell lines expressing the antisense stably following transduction using a murine retroviral vector. In this study, controls were included and there appeared to be no deleterious effect of antisense expression on the cells. The same group demonstrated inhibition of heterologous HIV strains when longer antisense molecules were used.[38] Further analysis of this and similar antisense RNAs by Homan et al[39] appear to demonstrate the importance of complementarity between the antisense RNA and unpaired (loop) structures in the target RNA as being critical for the efficiency of the antisense effect.

Antisense oligodeoxynucleotides have also been proposed as therapeutic tools against HIV.[40] Phosphorothioate stabilised molecules directed against the TAR, U5 and the PBS[41] and other sites[42] have demonstrated significant antiviral activity. It remains difficult to deliver oligodeoxynucleotides specifically to cells. In a study targeting the *rev* responsive element efficient inhibition of HIV in tissue culture was only seen when the cells were treated every 3 to 4 days with 1μM oligodeoxynucleotide.[43]

RIBOZYMES

Antisense molecules, in general, need to be present in excess of their target sequence. Ribozymes by contrast, in theory, because they are regenerated after each catalytic interaction, should not require such high level expression. The problem of targeting the ribozyme to the same cellular compartment as that of the target RNA still pertains. Anti-HIV ribozymes stably expressed in HeLa- CD4+ cells can inhibit HIV replication as measured by supernatant p24 antigen levels.[44] Targets including the integrase[45] RT[46], *tat*[47], *env*[48] and 5′untranslated region[49–52] have been used, all with some apparent effect on HIV replication. Wong-Staal's group specifically noted that the ribozyme effect was greater than that which could be attributed to the antisense effect of the RNA, by comparing the ribozyme to an identical sequence differing only by mutation of the 'active site' of the ribozyme.[51] The same group has apparently demonstrated that ribozymes may be able to target the incoming genomic RNA prior to reverse transcription,[53] but this has only been shown under conditions where virus and antiviral were co-transfected into cells or where the ribozyme was expressed constitutively.

RNA DECOYS

High level expression of a viral RNA sequence which binds virus specific regulatory proteins such as *tat* and *rev* in a heterologous RNA molecule has been explored to see whether sequestration of the protein could be achieved to a level that would inhibit HIV expression. The *tat* responsive element TAR[54,55] and the *rev* responsive element RRE[56] have both been expressed under the control of an RNA polymerase III specific promoter. Inhibition of viral gene expression was shown using these. Similar results were noted using a sequence containing multiple TAR motifs.[57]

PROTEIN CENTRED STRATEGIES

Mutant forms of protein can sometimes interfere with the function of the wild-type. Interference with protein-protein interaction by a mutant with partial homology to the wild-type protein may be due to its inhibiting normal function or disrupting assembly and/or polymerisation of a viral protein complex. This concept is known as a trans-dominant negative phenomenon in that a relatively small number of mutant proteins can disrupt the effect of a much larger number of wild-type proteins. Both *tat*[58,59] and *rev*[60,61] are favoured targets for this approach. Interaction of *rev* with the RRE is a relatively well characterised process in terms of the important amino acids involved in the various functions. A leucine rich domain near the C-terminus of the protein is conserved and essential for function.[62] Mutants in this region interfere with the activation function of wild-type *rev*,[63] however the ability of *rev* to interact and form polymers is not disrupted. Large mutations in the *tat* protein have also been used[58,59] and both approaches can cause a significant inhibition of HIV replication within cells in which the mutants are expressed. There is some evidence that viral assembly can be disrupted by co-expression of mutant *gag*proteins, although the data is limited.[64] Envelope glycoprotein assembly depends on protein-protein interactions both for the linkage of the SU gp120 glycoprotein to the gp41 transmembrane glycoprotein (TM) and for the ability of this heterodimer to form multimers on the virion surface. Dominant negative mutants of the TM envelope protein can be shown to inhibit HIV production[65]and dominant negatives mutated in the CD4 binding domain will both reduce CD4 gp120 binding and decrease virion production.[66]

Questions remain over the safety of expressing foreign proteins in cells to attempt protection against subsequent HIV infection. Many of these proteins interact strongly with nucleic acid sequences and might disrupt normal cellular function. In addition, expression of peptide derivatives of a foreign protein on the surface of a cell in association with the MHC is very likely to lead to immune-mediated destruction of the cell, hence there will be a slow attrition of the cells expressing the transdominant protein unless this is made inducible by an incoming HIV.

PROTEIN SEQUESTRATION *IN TRANS*

In theory, sequestration of any or all of the structural proteins of the virus could be undertaken.

Sequestration of viral envelope by CD4 containing an endoplasmic reticulum retention signal has already been described.[27,67]Single chain antibodies[68] have also been developed which will bind and sequester the HIV-1 envelope proteins in the endoplasmic reticulum.[69] Co-transfection of single chain antibodies specific for gp120 with proviral DNA led to reduced levels of infectious HIV-1 particles, without affecting the level of *gag* protein produced.

SUMMARY OF GENE THERAPY TECHNIQUES

It is clear from the diversity of approaches that no single methodology has yet proven to be outstandingly effective in inhibiting HIV in vitro. In a majority of cases the inhibition demonstrated by genetic modalities is not permanent.[17] Virus escape commonly occurs within 2–4 weeks in cell culture.[33,42,52] Whether this is by mutational escape or alternative mechanisms is not always clear. Antiviral gene expression is often unchanged. A second problem has been that, in general, the inhibitory effects are only effective at low multiplicities of infection. Challenge with high titre virus, when it has been performed, is generally not inhibited. These two problems do not, however, negate the value of a gene therapy approach in that in vivo a relatively low infectious titre is more likely to be encountered. The fact that there is not complete inhibition of HIV replication is also somewhat artificial, bearing in mind that in vivo there are multiple defences against viral pathogens which are not being assessed in the tissue culture system and that there may be a very significant effect over and above the apparent in vitro phenomenon if it were possible to delay virus infection and decrease cell-cell spread while other immunological defences are recruited. Since it seems unlikely that, once infected, HIV will ever be completely eliminated, genetically produced inhibitory effects should be seen as a therapeutic co-strategy in association with more conventional pharmacological approaches which together may extend the asymptomatic period of HIV infection and prolong disease free life.

MODES OF DELIVERY OF GENE THERAPY MODALITIES

The delivery vehicles for gene therapy are reviewed in other chapters within this volume. It is thus relevant only to mention some of the features which are particularly pertinent to gene delivery in HIV infection. Of the viral vectors available retrovirus, adenovirus, parvovirus and herpesvirus all have been proposed as possible vehicles for delivery of gene therapy in HIV infection. Unless stable episomal gene expression is achieved using, for example, the EBV origin of replication, the greatest efficacy is likely to be obtained from vectors such as retroviruses which are integrated into the cellular genome.

Whilst murine retroviruses have been the preferred vehicle for gene delivery in other diseases, HIV infection is one of the few conditions where an HIV based vector may offer significant advantages. HIV-1, or possibly HIV-2 based vectors would be able to deliver genes highly specifically to cells which are infectable by the wild-type virus and to integrate antiviral genes into susceptible cells. A vector containing an antiviral gene which is packageable inside an HIV virion could also potentially be distributed to other cells by the patient's own virus.

Another major advantage of HIV based vectors is that in common with other lentiviruses they will integrate their genome into non-dividing cells.[70,71] Other gene delivery systems would be unlikely to successfully integrate antiviral constructs into terminally differentiated macrophages or monocytes, or glial cells of the central nervous system, for which HIV itself is tropic.

HIV BASED RETROVIRAL VECTORS

A number of groups have been working on developing HIV as a gene vector system. The initial steps of identifying packaging signals in HIV showed that an important packaging signal exists in the 5′ untranslated region of the virus.[72] This work was confirmed by two other groups[73,74] who demonstrated packaging defects of varying degree when a sequence in the 5′ non-coding region was deleted. Following this a number of reports appeared showing that the same region cloned into a heterologous RNA was sufficient to direct encapsidation of a vector into an HIV particle.[75–77] The situation, however, is not completely clear and evidence for the existence of signals in the 3′ end of the virus enhancing packaging of viral RNA into virus particles in lymphocytes has been published.[78] Delineation of the sequences necessary and sufficient for packaging in HIV is clearly crucial, both for the practicalities of putting vectors into virion particles, but also in terms of co-localisation of antiviral sequences and viral RNA.

NON-VIRAL VECTORS

The chapter by Schofield and Caskey outlines a number of non-viral delivery modalities and the benefits and constraints enumerated there apply no less to HIV gene therapy. Targeting ligands on the outside of non-viral vectors might suitably be targeted towards cells expressing gp120 for modalities which are toxic, or to CD4+ expressing cells (using perhaps gp120 as the targeting ligand) in order to protect uninfected cells. As with much of gene therapy this area is in its infancy.

SUMMARY

From a position five years ago where optimism existed for pharmaceutical methods as being a complete answer to HIV infection, and the development of a vaccine appeared on the face of it to be no more complicated than vaccine development against other similarly sized infectious pathogens, it has now become clear that a new approach is required for the control of HIV infection. Elimination of the virus from an infected person is an unlikely eventuality, therefore the aims must be to maintain the virus in its latent phase for as long as possible and to protect uninfected cells from viral infection and perhaps to enhance the immune response against the virus, (so called post-infectious immunisation). These methodologies are particularly amenable to a gene therapy approach and it seems likely that within the next 5–10 years combination therapy, including both pharmacological agents and gene therapy agents, will be used in concert to minimise the spread of HIV within an infected individual and thus prolong their disease-free life.

A gene therapy based vaccine is also a serious possibility. HIV itself may paradoxically become a valuable therapeutic weapon and the gene therapy of AIDS may become the pioneering ground for development of similar approaches to other infectious agents.

REFERENCES

1 Luciw PA, Leung NJ. Mechanisms of retrovirus replication. In: Levy JA, et. The retroviridae Vol. 1. New York: Plenum Press 1992; pp 159–298.
2 Clements JE, Wong-Staal F. Molecular biology of lentiviruses. Semin Virol 1992; 3: 137–146.
3 Hunter E. Macromolecular interactions in the assembly of HIV and other retroviruses. Semin Virol 1994; 5: 71–83.
4 Ulmer JB, Donnelly JJ, Parker SE et al. Heterologous protection against influenza by injection of DNA encoding a viral protein. Science 1993; 359: 1745–1749.
5 Phillips RE, Rowland-Jones S, Nixon DF, et al. Human immunodeficiency virus genetic variation that can escape cytotoxic T cell recognition. Nature 1992; 354: 433–434.
6 Haffar OK, Smithgall MD, Bradshaw J, Brady B, Damle NK, Linsley PS. Costimulation of T-cell activation and virus production by B7 antigen on activated CD4+ T cells from human immunodeficiency virus type 1- infected donors. Proc Natl Acad Sci USA 1993; 90: 11094–11098.
7 Warner JF, Anderson CG, Laube L et al. Induction of HIV-specific CTL and antibody responses in mice using retroviral vector-transduced cells. Aids Res Hum Retroviruses 1991; 7: 645–655.
8 Jolly D, Chada S, Townsend K et al. CTL cross reactivity between HIV strains. Aids Res Hum Retroviruses 1992; 8: 1369–1371 (1992)
9 Mace K, Seif I, Anjard C, et al. Enhanced resistance to HIV-1 replication in U937 cells stably transfected with the human IFN-β gene behind an MHC promoter fragment. J Immunol 1991; 147: 3553–3559.
10 Bednarik DP, Mosca JD, Raj NBK, Pitha PM. Inhibition of human immunodeficiency virus (HIV) replication by HIV-trans-activated α_2-interferon. Proc Natl Acad Sci USA 1989; 86: 4958.
11 Constantoulakis P, Campbell M, Felber BK, Nasioulas G, Afonina E, Pavlakis GN. Inhibition of Rev-mediated HIV-1 expression by an RNA binding protein encoded by the interferon-inducible 9-27 gene. Science 1993; 259: 1314–1318.
12 Harrison GS, Maxwell F, Long CJ, Rosen CA, Glode LM, Maxwell IH. Activation of a diphtheria toxin A gene by expression of human immunodeficiency virus-1 *Tat* and *Rev* proteins in transfected cells. Hum Gene Ther 1991; 2: 53–60.
13 Caruso M, Klatzmann D. Selective killing of CD4+ cells harboring a human immunodeficiency virus-inducible suicide gene prevents viral spread in an infected cell population. Proc Natl Acad Sci USA 1992; 89: 182–186.
14 Brady HJM, Miles CG, Pennington DJ, Dzierzak EA. Specific ablation of human immunodeficiency virus *Tat*-expressing cells by conditionally toxic retroviruses. Proc Natl Acad Sci USA 1994; 91: 365–369.
15 Winters MA, Merigan TC. Continuous presence of CD4-PE40 is required for antiviral activity against single-passage HIV isolates and infected peripheral blood mononuclear cells. AIDS Res Hum Retrovirus 1993; 9: 1091–1096.
16 Majors J. The structure and function of retroviral long terminal repeats. In: Swanstrom R, Vogt PK, eds. Retroviruses Berlin: Springer-Verlag, 1990: pp 49–92.
17 Sczakiel G, Pawlita M. Inhibition of heterologous immuno-deficiency virus replication in human T cells stably expressing antisense RNA. J Virol 1991; 65: 468–472.
18 Sullenger BA, Cech TR. Tethering ribozymes to a retroviral packaging signal for destruction of viral RNA. Science 1993; 262: 1566–1569.

19 Dalgleish AG, Beverley PC, Clapham PR, Crawford DH, Greaves MF, Weiss RA. The CD4 (T4) antigen is an essential component of the receptor for the AIDS retrovirus. Nature 1984: 312: 763–767.
20 Smith DH, Byrn RA, Marsters SA, Gregory T, Groopman JE, Capon DJ. Blocking of HIV-1 infectivity by a soluble secreted form of the CD4 antigen. Science 1987; 238: 1704–1707.
21 Fisher RA, Bertonis JM, Meier W, et al. HIV infection is blocked in vitro by recombinant soluble CD4. Nature 1988; 331: 76–78.
22 Hussey RE, Richardson NE, Kowalski M et al. Asoluble CD4 protein selectively inhibits HIV replications and syncytium formation. Nature 1988; 331: 78–81.
23 Deen KC, McDougal JS, Inacker R. et al. A soluble form of CD4 (T4) protein inhibits AIDS virus infection. Nature 1988; 331: 82–84.
24 Ward RH, Capon DJ, Jett CM, et al. Prevention of HIV-1 IIIB infection in chimpanzees by CD4 immunoadhesin. Nature 1991; 352: 376–377.
25 Watanabe M, Boyson JE, Lord CI, Letvin NL. Chimpanzees immunized with recombinant soluble CD4 develop anti-self CD4 antibody responses with anti-human immunodeficiency virus activity. Proc Natl Acad Sci USA 1992; 89: 5103–5107.
26 Watanabe M, Levine CG, Shen L, Fisher RA, Letvin NL. Immunization of simian immunodeficiency virus-infected rhesus monkeys with soluble human CD4 elicits an antiviral response. Proc Natl Acad Sci USA 1991; 88: 4616–4620.
27 Watanabe M, Chen ZW, Tsubota H, Lord CI, Levine CG, Letvin NL. Soluble human CD4 elicitis an antibody response in rhesus monkeys that inhibits simian immunodeficiency virus replication. Proc Natl Acad Sci USA 1991; 88: 120–124.
28 Buonocore L, Rose JK. Prevention of HIV-1 glycoprotein transport by soluble CD4 retained in the endoplasmic reticulum. Nature 1990; 345: 625–628.
29 Husson RN, Chung Y, Mordenti J, et al. Phase I study of continuous-infusion soluble CD4 as a single agent and in combination with oral dideoxyinosine therapy inchildren with symptomatic human immunodeficiency virus infection. J Pediatr 1992; 121: 627–633.
30 Daar ES, Ho DD. Relative resistance of primary HIV-1 isolates to neutralization by soluble CD4. Am J Med 1991; 90: 22S–26S.
31 Daar ES, Li XL, Moudgil T, Ho DD. High concentrations of recombinant soluble CD4 are required to neutralize primary human immunodeficiency virus type 1 isolates. Proc Natl Acad Sci USA 1990; 87: 6574–6578.
32 Rhodes A, James W. Inhibition of human immuno-deficiency virus replication in cell culture by endogenously synthesized antisense RNA. J Gen Virol 1990; 71: 1965–1974.
33 Sckakiel G, Oppenlander M, Rittner K, Pawlita M. *Tat* and *Rev* directed antisense RNA expression inhibits and abolishes replication of human immunodeficiency virus type 1: a temporal analysis. J Virol 1992; 66: 5576–5581.
34 Meyer J, Nick S, Stamminger T, Grummt F, Jahn G, Lipps HJ. Inhibition of HIV-1 replication by a high-copy-numner vector expressing antisense RNA for reverse transcriptase. Gene 1993; 129: 263–268.
35 Gyotoku J, el Farrash MA, Fujimoto S, et al. Inhibition of human immunodeficiency virus replication in a human T cellline by antisense RNA expressed in the cell. Virus Genes 1991; 5: 189–202.
36 Joshi S, Van Brunschot A, Asad S, van der Elst I, Read SE, Bernstein A. Inhibition of human immunodeficiency virus type 1 multiplication by antisense and sense RNA expression J Virol 1991; 65: 5524–5530.
37 Chatterjee S, Johnson PR, Wong KK Jr. Dual-target inhibition of HIV-1 in vitro by means of an adeno-associated virus antisense vector. Science 1992; 258: 1485–1488.
38 Rhodes A, James W. Inhibition of heterologous strains of HIV by antisense RNA AIDS 1991; 5: 225–226.
39 Homann M, Rittner K, Sczakiel G. Complementary large loops determine the rate of RNA duplex formation in vitro in the case of an effective antisense RNA directed against the human immunodeficiency virus type 1. J Mol Biol 1993; 233: 000–000.

40 Goodchild J, Agrawal S, Civeira M, Sarin PS, Sun D, Zamecnik PC. Inhibition of human immunodefieciency virus replication by antisense oligodeoxynucleotides. Proc Natl Acad Sci 1988; 85: 5507–5511.
41 Bordier B, Helene C, Barr PJ, Litvak S, Sarih-Cottin L. In vitro effect of antisense oligonucletodies on human immunodeficiency virus type 1 reverse transcription. Nucleic Acids Res 1992; 20: 5999–6006.
42 Lisziewicz J, Sun D, Klotman M, Agrawal S, Zamecnik P, Gallo R. Specific inhibition of human immunodeficiency virus type 1 replication by antisense oligonucleotides: an in vitro model for treatment. Proc Natl Acad Sci USA 1992; 89: 11209–11213.
43 Li G, Lisziewicz J, Sun D, et al. Inhibition of Rev activity and human immunodeficiency virus type 1 replication by antisense oligodeoxynucleotide phosphorothioate analogs directed against the Rev-responsive element. J Virol 1993; 67: 6882–6888.
44 Sarver N, Cantin EM, Chang PS, et al. Ribozymes as potential anti-HIV-1 therapeutic agents. Science 1990; 247: 1222–1225.
45 Sioud M, Drlica K. Prevention of human immuno- deficiency virus type 1 integrase expression in Escherichia coli by a ribozyme. Proc Natl Acad Sci USA 1991; 88: 7303–7307.
46 Joseph S, Burke JM. Optimization of an anti-HIV hairpin ribozyme by in vitro selection. J Biol Chem 1993; 268: 24515–24518.
47 Lo KM, Biasolo MA, Dehni G, Palu G, Haseltine WA. Inhibition of replication of HIV-1 by retroviral vectors expressing *tat*-antisense and anti-rat ribozyme RNA Virology 1992; 190: 176–183.
48 Chen CJ, Banerjea AC, Harmison GG, Haglund K, Schubert M. Multitarget-ribozyme directed to ckeave at up to nine highly conserved HIV-1 env RNA regions inhibits HIV-1 replication - potential effectiveness against most presently sequenced HIV-1 isolates. Nucleic Acids Res 1992; 20: 4581–4589.
49 Ventura M, Wang P, Ragot T, Perricaudet M, Saragosti S. Activation of HIV-specific ribozyme activity by self-cleavage. Nucleic Acids Res 1993; 21: 3249–3255.
50 Ojwang JO, Hampel A, Looney DK, Wong-Staal F, Rappaport J. Inhibition of human immunodeficiency virus type 1 expression by a hairpin ribozyme. Proc Natl Acad Sci USA 1992; 89: 10802–10806.
51 Yu M, Ojwang J, Yamada O, Hampel A, Rappaport J, Looney D, Wong-Staal F. A hairpin ribozyme inhibits expression of diverse strains of human immunodeficiency virus type 1. Proc Natl Acad Sci USA 1993; 90: 6340–6344.
52 Weerasinghe M, Liem SE, Asad S, Read SE, Joshi S. Resistance to human immunodeficiency virus type 1 (HIV-1) infection in human CD4+ lymphocyte-derived cell lines conferred by using retroviral vectors expressing an HIV-1 RNA-specific ribozyme. J Virol 1991; 65: 5531–5534.
53 Yamada O, Yu M, Yee JK, Kraus G, Looney D, Wong-Staal F. Intracellular immunization of human T-cells with a hairpin ribozyme against human immunodeficiency virus type 1. Gene Therapy 1994; 1: 38–45.
54 Sullenger BA, Gallardo HF, Ungers GE, Gilboa E. Overexpression of TAR sequences renders cells resistant to human immunodeficiency virus replication. Cell 1990; 63: 601–608.
55 Sullenger BA, Gallardo HF, Ungers GE, Gilboa E. Analysis of trans-acting response decoy RNA-mediated inhibition of human immunodeficiency virus type 1 transactivation. J Virol 1991; 65: 6811–6816.
56 Lee TC, Sullenger BA, Gallardo HF, Ungers GE, Gilboa E. Overexpression of RRE-derived sequences inhibits HIV-1 replication in CEM cells. New Biol 1992; 4: 66–74.
57 Lisziewicz J, Rappaport J, Dhar R. Tat-regulated production of multimerized TAR RNA inhibits HIV-1 gene expression. New Biol 1991; 3: 82–89.
58 Green M, Ishino M, Loewenstein PM. Mu*tat*ional analysis of HIV-1 Tat minimal domain peptides: identification of trans-dominant mutants that suppress HIV- LTR-driven gene expression. Cell 1989; 58: 215–223.

59 Modesti N, Garcia J, Debouck C, Peterlin M, Gaynor R. Trans-dominant Tat mutants with alterations in the basic domain inhibit Tat mutants with alterations in the basic domain inhibit HIV-1 gene expression. New Biol 1991; 3: 759–768.
60 Mermer B, Felber BK, Campbell M, Pavlakis GN. Identification of trans-dominant HIV-1 *rev* protein mutants by direct transfer of bacterially produced proteins into human cells. Nucl Acids Res 1990; 18: 2037–2044.
61 Malim MH, Bohnlein S, Hauber J, Cullen BR. Functional dissection of the HIV-1 Rev trans-activator-derivation of a trans-dominant repressor of Rev function. Cell 1989; 58: 205–214.
62 Malim MH, McCarn DF, Tiley LS, Cullen BR. Mutational definition of the human immunodeficiency virus type 1 Rev activation domain. J. Virol 1991; 65: 4248–4254.
63 Olsen HS, Cochrane AW, Dillon PJ, Nalin CM, Rosen CA. Interaction of the human immunodeficiency virus type 1 Rev protein with a structured region in env mRNA is dependent on multimer formation mediated through a basic stretch of amino acids. Genes Dev 1990; 4: 1357–1364.
64 Trono D, Feinberg MB, Baltimore D. HIV-1 Gag mutants can dominantly interfere with the replication of the wild-type virus. Cell 1989; 59: 113–120.
65 Buchschacher GL Jr., Freed EO, Panganiban AT. Cells induced to express a human immunodeficiency virus type 1 envelope gene mutant inhibit the spread of wild-type virus. Hum Gene Ther 1992; 3: 391–397.
66 Steffy KR, Wong-Staal F. Transdominant inhibition of wild-type human immunodeficiency virus type 2 replication by an envelope deletion mutant J Virol 1993; 67.
67 Buonocore L, Rose JK. Blockade of human immunodeficiency virus type 1 production in CD4+ T cells by an intracellular CD4 expressed under control of the viral long terminal repeat. Proc Natl Acad Sci USA 1990; 345: 625–628.
68 Winter G, Milstein C. Man-made antibodies. Nature 1992; 349: 293–299.
69 Marasco WA, Haseltine WA, Chen SY. Design, intracellular expression, and activity of a human anti- human immunodeficiency virus type 1 gp120 single-chain antibody. Proc Natl Acad Sci USA 1993; 90: 7889–7893.
70 Lewis P, Hensel M, Emerman M. Human immunodeficiency virus infection of cells arrested in the cell cycle. EMBO Journal 1992; 11: 3053–3058.
71 Conner RI, Ho DD. Pathogenesis of human immunodeficiency virus Seminars in Virology 1992; 3: 213–224.
72 Lever AML, Gottlinger H, Haseltine W, Sodroski J. Identification of a sequence required for efficient packaging of human immunodeficiency virus type 1 RNA into virions. J Virol 1989; 63: 4085–4087.
73 Aldovini A, Young RA. Mutations and protein sequences involved in human immunodeficiency virus type 1 packaging result in production of non-infectious virus. J Virol 1990; 64: 1920–1926.
74 Clavel F, Orenstein JM. A mutant of human immunodeficiency virus with reduced RNA packaging and abnormal particle morphology. J Virol 1990; 64: 5230–5234.
75 Poznansky M, Lever A, Bergeron L, Haseltine W, Sodroski J. Gene transfer into human lymphocytes by a defective human immunodeficiency virus type 1 vector. J Virol 1991; 65: 532–536.
76 Buchschacher GL Jr., Panganiban AT. Human immunodeficiency virus vectors for inducible expression of foresign genes. J Virol 1992; 66: 2731–2739.
77 Shimada R, Fujii H, Mitsuya H, Nienhuis AW. Targeted and highly efficient gene transfer into CD4+ cells by a recombinant human immunodeficiency virus retroviral vector J Clin Invest 1991; 88: 1043–1047.
78 Richardson JH, Child LA, Lever AML. Packaging of human immunodeficiency virus type 1 RNA requires cis-acting sequences outside the 5' leader region. J Virol 1993; 67: 3997–4005.

British Medical Bulletin (1995) Vol. 51, No. 1 pp.167–191

Gene transfer into human hemopoietic progenitor cells

M K Brenner,[2,4] J M Cunningham,[2] B P Sorrentino[2,3] and H E Heslop[1,4]

[1]Division of Bone Marrow Transplantation, [2]Division of Experimental Hematology and [3]Department of Biochemistry, St. Jude Children's Research Hospital, Memphis, Tennessee, USA; and [4]Department of Pediatrics, University of Tennessee, Memphis, Tennessee, USA

Considerable progress is being made in the transfer of genetic material to hematopoietic stem cells. In this chapter we describe how gene transfer is being used to: mark marrow and peripheral blood progenitor cells prior to autologous transplantation, to track their fate on reinfusion and to detect contaminating tumorigenic cells; modulate immunocyte function – important in immunologic disorders and perhaps in cancer therapy; generate tumor vaccines from tumor cells isolated from marrow; correct single gene defects – the 'classical' concept of gene therapy; and finally to modify the drug sensitivity of progenitor cells – enabling them to resist the suppressive effects of cytotoxic drugs during cancer therapy and perhaps providing a mechanism for in vivo selection of gene modified cells.

Hemopoietic progenitor cells are appealing targets for gene transfer, since their genetic modification could be effective in a variety of malignant and non-malignant disorders. These applications are at variable stages of clinical development, but at the moment gene transfer is being used to:

1. Mark marrow and peripheral blood progenitor cells prior to autologous transplantation, to track their fate on reinfusion and to detect contaminating tumorigenic cells.
2. Modulate immunocyte function – important in immunologic disorders and perhaps in cancer therapy.
3. Generate tumor vaccines from tumor cells isolated from marrow.

4. Correct single gene defects – the 'classical' concept of gene therapy. Correction of ADA deficiency and of lysosomal storage disorders are discussed by Hoogerbrugge et al. and Danos respectively elsewhere in this issue. In this article we use sickle cell disease and thalassemia as our illustration.
5. Modify the drug sensitivity of progenitor cells – enabling them to resist the suppressive effects of cytotoxic drugs during cancer therapy and perhaps providing a mechanism for in vivo selection of gene modified cells.

As well as their suitability as targets for a wide range of clinical applications, the use of hemopoietic progenitor cells for gene transfer is attractive because of their logistical characteristics. Both marrow and peripheral blood progenitor cells are readily obtained, manipulated, and returned to the host. Moreover, in principle, successful gene transfer into a single pluripotent stem cell could be sufficient to repopulate each individual with modified cells for their entire life-span. In almost every other type of somatic gene therapy, transfer is required to a vast number of cells which may be spread over a wide anatomical area.

However, to take full advantage of these characteristics, there is a need to use vectors which permanently integrate into hemopoietic stem cell DNA and are therefore present in all the progeny of this cell.[1] At present retroviruses are the only integrating vectors approved for clinical use.[2,3] One of the characteristics of these vectors is that integration occurs almost exclusively in cells which are progressing through cell cycle. Since most mammalian hemopoietic stem cells are in G_0, the efficiency of gene transfer into these cells is generally far below the levels that would be expected to produce benefit in the great majority of gene therapy settings.[2–6] In animal models, a number of techniques have been shown to induce hemopoietic stem cells to cycle and thereby increase the efficiency of retroviral mediated gene transfer.[1,7] These include prior treatment of the animal with cycle specific cytotoxic drugs,[8] or in vivo/ex vivo exposure to hemopoietic growth factors.[9–12] At present, however, the human stem cell has not been precisely identified, and there are no assays which can directly analyze their number or activity. It has therefore been impossible to devize pre-clinical experiments which show how well retroviruses transfer genes to human stem cells and whether manipulation of those stem cells enhanced their susceptibility to retroviral mediated gene transfer. This has been a major constraint on the development of therapeutic protocols. No clinical gene transfer study can be entirely devoid of risk, and when the probability of benefit is unknown and likely to be small, then the risk benefit ratio becomes unacceptably high.[2–4,13] On the other hand, until human studies are performed, it is impossible to make an accurate assessment of the true risks and the true probability of success.

One way of resolving this impasse has been to develop clinical protocols in which even a low efficiency of gene transfer would potentially be of benefit. One example is ADA gene transfer (*see* Hoogerbrugge et al., this issue). In these studies it was anticipated that the ADA gene-corrected population would initially be in an extreme minority, but would ultimately expand because they would have a selective growth advantage over unmodified cells. A more widely applicable example is to use gene transfer simply as a means of marking hemopoietic progenitor cells prior to transplantation, to track their subsequent fate in vivo.[7,14–16] In this instance, the purpose of gene transfer is not to correct a defect in hemopoietic progenitor cells, but rather to improve the **process** of progenitor cell transplantation. As a by product of these studies, information should be obtained to facilitate true gene therapy protocols.

GENE MARKING OF HEMOPOIETIC PROGENITOR CELLS

Gene marking can be used to determine whether harvested progenitor cells in marrow or blood are contaminated with tumorigenic cells and whether attempts to remove such cells are successful.[7,14,15] It may also be used to learn about the contribution of harvested stem cells to long-term engraftment and the impact of ex vivo growth factor treatment on the subsequent behavior of these cells in vivo.[16]

Are harvested hemopoietic progenitor cells contaminated by tumorigenic cells?

While the dose intensification permitted by autologous hemopoietic stem cell (HSC) rescue has shown promise as effective treatment for malignant diseases, including leukemias, lymphomas and breast cancer,[17–21] disease recurrence remains the major cause of treatment failure. When the malignancy originates from or involves the marrow, relapse could originate from malignant cells persisting in the patient, in the rescuing HSC, or in both.[7,14,17–21] The origin of relapse is an important issue to resolve. Concern that the HSC graft may contain residual malignant cells has led to extensive evaluation of techniques for purging these cells, prior to storage and subsequent reinfusion.[22–25] Animal and pre-clinical human studies have shown that these methods do reduce contamination with malignant cells that have been deliberately added to marrow, but no method has been unequivocally shown to reduce the risk of relapse in naturally occurring disease.[26–28]

HSC for autologous transplants are usually harvested at a time when, by definition, no malignant cells are detectable in the marrow.[26,29,30]

It is therefore impossible to undertake any form of quality control after purging to determine whether the putative residual malignant cells have genuinely been eradicated. Unfortunately, these unproven purging techniques almost invariably damage normal progenitor cells, so that engraftment of purged HSC is typically far slower than that of untreated marrow.[28,31,32] Morbidity and mortality from the complications of hemopoietic and immune system failure are correspondingly increased.

If marker genes could be transferred into residual malignant cells in the HSC prior to reinfusion and gene-marked malignant cells subsequently became detectable in the marrow or peripheral blood in patients who relapsed following autologous transplant, this would be powerful evidence that the harvested HSC graft contributes to disease recurrence. Moreover, the finding of marked cells at relapse would permit subsequent evaluation of **ex vivo** purging techniques for their ability to eradicate clonogenic cells. Thus, for the first time it would be possible to directly compare the efficacy of the numerous available techniques for HSC purging.

Method of marking

Marking studies began in September 1991, using 2 closely related retro viral vectors, G1Na and LNL6. Both contain the neomycin phosphotransferase gene (Neo^R) and therefore convey resistance to neomycin and its analogues such as G418. Two-thirds of harvested marrow was frozen directly, and one-third exposed to one or other of the vectors for 6 h at a multiplicity of infection of 10:1. The cells were then recovered, washed and frozen. At the time of transplant, both modified and unmodified cells were thawed and infused.

Marker genes to determine source of relapse in AML and neuroblastoma [15]

12 patients with AML have entered the study and 3 have so far relapsed. In 2 of these patients, the marker gene was present in the malignant population. For example, Patient 2 had blasts in the peripheral blood at 80 days after transplantation which were $CD34^+$ $CD56^+$ dual positive. This is a phenotypic combination not present on normal progenitor cells and allows separation of the leukemic clone by flow cytometry.[15] The clone also contained a genotypic marker, the 1:8:21 complex translocation. The 8:21 portion of this translocation produces a fusion transcript and protein called AML:ETO.[33–35] The leukemic clone contained products of both the malignant gene marker (AML:ETO) and the transferred gene marker (Neo^R).

9 patients with neuroblastoma have also been studied. 3 have relapsed, 2 in the marrow and one in a new site in the right lobe of the liver. In all 3 patients, 0.1–1% of the neuroblasts (phenotypically GD2+ and CD45−) were marker gene positive, as were individual G418 resistant colonies grown from the neuroblast preparation.

Marker genes to determine source of relapse in other malignancies

Related studies are underway to analyze the source of relapse in CML and breast cancer.[36,37]

Conclusions about source of relapse

These data directly demonstrate that autologous marrow, harvested in apparent clinical remission from patients with hematologic and nonhematologic malignancies, may still harbor tumorigenic cells capable of contributing to relapse. Moreover, these cells may contribute to relapse both within the marrow and at extramedullary sites.

Clonality of relapse

Since the provirus may integrate in any of a vast number of possible sites, enumeration of provirus integration sites using inverted PCR[38] has allowed estimation of the clonality of relapse. In one neuroblastoma patient, 4 separate integrants were detected in the malignant population, while in a second patient, 2 such sites were found. Given the efficiency of gene transfer, and that only one-third of the marrow was exposed to the vector, this implies that approximately 100–1000 tumorigenic cells in marrow contribute to disease recurrence.

Use of marking to analyze purging

The implication of these results is that **effective** marrow purging[21,24,25,27,28] will need to be incorporated into protocols of autologous HSC transplantation. It should be possible to use the same sensitive marking technique described here to assess the efficacy of conventional and novel methods of marrow purging. Indeed, as new vectors become available for clinical application, the scope of marker gene investigation should increase greatly. By distinctively marking different aliquots of marrow from the same patient, one could compare several purging technologies simultaneously. Since the end point of such purging studies would be the absence of marked relapse, rather than a prolongation of survival, or a reduction in relapse risk, even small scale clinical trials could be informative. To illustrate this application, our current marker/purging protocol is shown in Figure 1. Marrow is divided into 3 aliquots. One is frozen as a safety back up, one is marked with

G1N, one with LNL6. These vectors can be distinguished because each produces a PCR fragment of different size. The marked portions are then randomized to purging with a pharmaceutical agent, 4HC or an immunological agent IL-2. The purged cells are frozen, and the marrow subsequently reinfused in the standard manner. If patients relapse with marked cells, it will be possible to determine which purging technique failed.

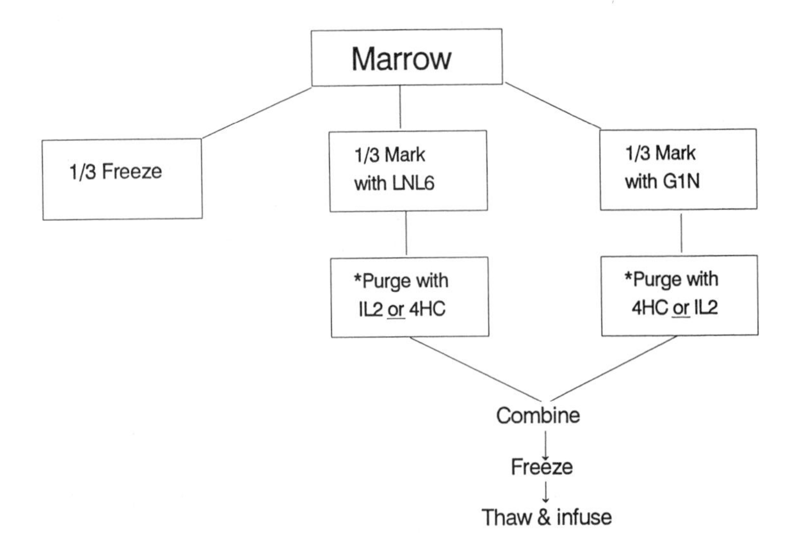

Fig. 1 Outline of AML purging protocol.

Can genes be transferred to normal human stem cells and expressed long-term in their progeny?[16]

During these relapse studies, we also had the opportunity to assess in vivo the ability of retroviral vectors to effect gene transfer to normal hemopoietic stem cells following ex vivo culture. We were also able to determine whether the transferred gene was expressed in the mature progeny of these stem cells.

Studies at one month showed that the infused marrow had contributed to early hemopoietic reconstitution. Semi-quantitative PCR at this time detected the Neo^R gene in the marrow mononuclear cells of 14/18 patients, with gene copy numbers that ranged from approximately 0.005–0.05/cell. The presence of the gene in hemopoietic progenitor cells was confirmed by clonogenic assays which showed gene marked progenitor cells in 15/18 patients. We obtained evidence for the contribution of infused marrow to long-term hemopoietic recovery from the 9 patients who were evaluable 6 months or more after transplantation. We used a clonogenic assay to quantitate the presence of the Neo^R gene in progenitor cells at increasing intervals after transplantation. G418-resistant progenitor cells persisted for 6 months in 9/9 patients and for one year in 5/5; marked progenitor cells remained detectable in marrow from the 2 patients who are more than 2 years post transplant. The gene was also present and expressed long-term in the mature progeny of marrow precursor cells, T and B lymphocytes, monocytes and neutrophils.

These results indicate a major contribution to marrow reconstitution from autologous transplants and strongly suggest that these stem cells can be successfully transduced by retrovirus vectors. Gene-marked marrow progenitor cells were detected for as long as 24 months after autologous bone marrow transplantation; multi-lineage granulocyte-erythroid-monocyte/ macrophage (GEMM) colonies become positive at 6 months, implying transfer into a progenitor at least one stage earlier in differentiation; and detection of the marker gene in both T and B lymphocytes for at least 30 months is consistent with the transfection of a primitive lympho-hemopoietic stem cell. The efficiency of transfer to long-lived progenitor cells was higher than would have been predicted from studies in large animals using similar transduction protocols. This increased transfer rate may be a consequence of harvesting marrow during the hemopoietic recovery phase that follows multiple cycles of intensive (marrow-ablative) chemotherapy. During this recovery period there is substantial proliferation of early marrow progenitor cells that may favor integration of the provirus genome.[8]

Improving stem cell transfer

These marker gene studies[15,16] suggest that modest levels of gene transfer may be effected into normal progenitor cells. They also confirm the need to persist with efforts to increase gene transfer efficiency, if most gene **therapy** applications are to be effective. A number of animal models have suggested that ex vivo treatment with growth factor combinations, with or without the addition of marrow stromal cells or extracellular matrix, can induce stem cells to enter the cell cycle and thereby increase both their number and the efficiency with which they can be transduced.[9–12] In humans, it certainly appears possible to use growth factors such as IL-1, IL-3 and stem cell factor to increase the numbers of hemopoietic progenitor cells by 10-to-50 fold and to increase the efficiency of gene transfer to levels which may exceed 50%.[1] Unfortunately, it is by no means certain that such **ex vivo** data will be reflected by results **in vivo**. In primate studies, transplantation of marrow treated ex vivo with the growth factor combinations have been shown to greatly augment both progenitor numbers and gene transfer rates, but this has been followed by disappointingly low levels of long-term gene expression in vivo (Bodine and Dunbar NIH/NHLBI unpublished). Similarly, in human studies in which SCF, IL-3 and IL-6 were used to stimulate marrow progenitor cells before reinfusion, expansion of CFUs and a high gene-transfer rate ex vivo were associated with in vivo expression that was both scanty and of short duration (Nienhuis, personal communication). The likeliest explanation for this apparent paradox is that many of the growth factors intended only to induce cycling in marrow stem cells also induce their differentiation and the loss of their self renewal capacity.

In the absence of any proven **ex vivo** surrogate method for studying the effects of growth factors on stem cell expansion and transducibility, it is possible to use the marker-gene technique to evaluate whether any increase in progenitor cell numbers and transducibility produced by growth factor combinations and cell culture devices ex vivo has an effect in vivo. By using 2 distinguishable vectors to mark each patient's marrow, we are able to compare treatment regimens **within** a patient. Because each patient acts as their own control, it should be possible to discern the effects of any given growth factor regimen on stem cells, even in a cohort as small as 10 patients (Fig. 2).

By comparing the proportion of clonogenic cells marked long-term with each vector we will have a measure of the impact of ex vivo growth factor treatment on stem cell ***transducibility.***

Is gene transfer to hemopoietic progenitor cells safe?

One of the major concerns about any use of long-lived marrow progenitor cells for retrovirus mediated gene transfer or therapy, is that insertional mutagenesis will occur.[13] This event could occur at the time of initial exposure to the vector, or subsequently – if wild type retrovirus contaminates the vector, or is formed by recombination. This concern has been given extra weight following the discovery of thymomas in monkeys injected with a vector contaminated with wild type virus.[39] In the clinical studies reported here, helper free vector was used, and no evidence has been obtained for any recombinational events with endogenous retroviral sequences that have generated infectious virus. But although no events to date have occurred which are attributable

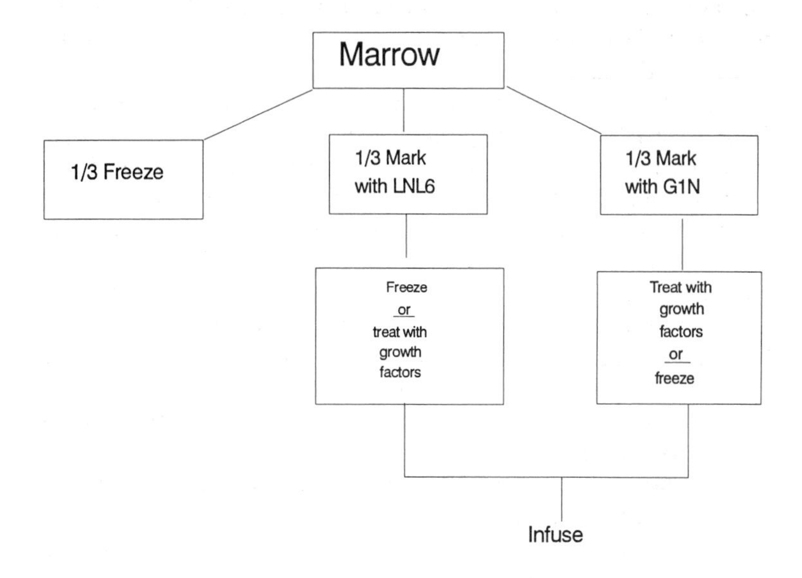

Fig. 2 Outline of growth factor treatment.

to mutagenesis, all patients will have prolonged follow up and genetic analysis of any tumors which do appear within the next 15 years.

GENE TRANSFER TO MODULATE IMMUNOCYTE FUNCTION

Genetic modification of the function of effector cells derived from marrow could have an impact on autoimmune disease, infective illness and malignancy. Initial interest has focussed on the last 2 of these areas because it has been in these conditions that the potential therapeutic role of the immune system[40–42] makes the risk:benefit ratio most attractive. Immunocytes may be altered by changing their effector function or by modifying their receptor specificity.

Therapy of malignant disease

Altered function of effector cells

One way of increasing the anti-tumor activity of immunocytes is to increase the levels of cytotoxic cytokines (such as TNF) which they produce at local tumor sites. This approach is being evaluated in studies with tumor infiltrating lymphocytes (TILs). The problems with this strategy is that it has been difficult to engineer TIL cells to secrete high levels of cytokines and that only scanty data support the belief that reinfused human TIL cells selectively home to tumor sites. In addition, the transduced cytokine gene may act as an autocrine growth factor for the TILs resulting in uncontrolled growth (*See* Friedman, 'Suicide Genes', this issue).

The first patients to receive therapy with cytokine transduced TIL were treated at the NIH in January 1991 in a Phase I dose escalation study. Patients received TNF-transduced TILs either alone or in conjunction with IL-2, in doses from 10^8 to 3×10^{11} cells. The first 6 patients have shown few side effects and one patient has had a sustained response.[43]

Altered specificity of effector cells

A long-term aim of tumor immunology has been to identify tumor specific antigens which might be a target for specific responses. Over the last few years, the molecular basis of antigen recognition by cytotoxic T lymphocytes (CTL) has been elucidated.[44] The demonstration that CTL recognize processed intracellular proteins presented as short peptide fragments in conjunction with MHC molecules on the cell surface, raised the possibility that internal proteins unique to the malignant clone may act as tumor specific antigens for CTL. Several human malignancies indeed contain novel proteins such as mutated oncogenes or fusion proteins generated by chromosomal translocations.[45,46] Other tumors may express immunogenic proteins encoded by Epstein-Barr or papilloma viruses. Finally, even normal proteins can elicit CTL responses if they are expressed in very high quantities, for example the MAGE protein in melanoma cells.[47]

If a tumor is to be recognized by CTL several conditions must be met. First, the tumor must contain a unique antigen that is a target for recognition. Second, the antigen must be processed and expressed in sufficient quantity to induce immune responses to the peptide. Finally, the peptide/MHC complex must be recognizable within the T cell repertoire of the individual and it must be possible to amplify the signal by exogenous help or costimulatory signals. If tumor cells do indeed express weakly immunogenic peptides, it may be possible to enhance the capacity of the immunocyte to recognize the tumor cell target by transfection with appropriate antigen specific T cell receptors. Since a conventional T cell receptor can recognize antigen only in the context of one particular MHC polymorphism, such modified effector T lymphocytes would function only in individuals who shared the relevant MHC restriction element. It would be much simpler practically if a 'universal' T cell could be developed that would recognize a tumor specific antigen regardless of the MHC molecule on which it was present – in other words, if recognition occurred in an analogous way to an antibody molecule.[48,49] One means by which this function could be obtained, would be by transducing a cytotoxic T cell with a construct encoding a hybrid molecule with both a specific antibody-derived binding site and the signal transduction component of the T cell receptor (the zeta chain). When these modified lymphocytes bound to tumor specific antigen on the tumor cell surface, their effector function could be triggered. Many theoretical and many practical concerns remain to be resolved before these techniques will be clinically feasible.

Therapy of viral disease

Lever (this issue) describes the use of genetic modification of lymphocytes for therapy of AIDS: we will take Epstein-Barr virus (EBV) related disease for our illustration of gene therapy of hemopoietic disease.

EBV is a herpes virus that infects the majority of individuals and persists in an asymptomatic state by a combination of chronic replication in the mucosa and latency in peripheral blood B cells.[50] These EBV infected B cells are highly immunogenic and normally susceptible to killing by specific cytotoxic T lymphocytes. However, patients who are severely immunocompromised after organ grafting may develop EBV-driven lymphoproliferation. This event occurs in 1–30% of allograft recipients. The highest incidence is seen in the patients who receive the most immunosuppressive post-transplant regimens, who also have the worst outcome. While it has recently been shown that unmanipulated T cells are effective therapy for this complication,[51] these cells may also induce graft rejection or graft versus host disease. We are evaluating whether adoptive transfer of EBV specific cytotoxic T lymphocytes is effective as prophylaxis and therapy for this complication.[52] To learn more about the survival, distribution and activity of these cells after administration, they are first marked with the neomycin resistance gene. The information gained from this study will allow future gene therapy interventions to be planned. For example, if these CTL cannot persist in vivo in the absence of IL-2, incorporation of the IL-2 gene prior to CTL transfer may provide autocrine growth potential, although the risk of uncontrolled proliferation would need to be considered.

GENETIC MODIFICATION OF TUMOR CELLS ISOLATED FROM MARROW; GENERATION OF TUMOR VACCINES

While conditions have been identified under which the immune system is able to eradicate malignant disease,[40,42,53] it has been suggested that the more general failure of the system to perform this function can be attributed to the poor immunogenicity of most tumors. For example, even if tumors do express immunogenic determinants on their surface (*see above*), there may be insufficient activation of immune system effector cells. In an attempt to enhance immune recognition, investigators have evaluated the effect of transducing tumor cells with cytokine genes or with allogeneic MHC molecules[54] or with B7.1,[55,56] a co-stimulatory molecule which activates cytotoxic T cells after engaging their surface CD28 or CTLA4 ligands.

In a number of different murine model systems, transfection of tumor cell lines with these molecules has augmented immunogenicity. Injection of neoplastic cells in doses that would normally establish a tumor results instead in the recruitment of immune system effector cells and the eradication of injected tumor cells.[57–63] In many cases the animal is then resistant to challenges by further local injections of non-transduced parental tumor. The transduced tumor has therefore acted like a vaccine. In some models, established, non-transduced, parental tumors at distant sites are also eradicated.[59,60]

There are several potential problems in translating this approach to human marrow derived tumors. First, one recent study has suggested that the same effect is attained if tumor cells are admixed with non-specific adjuvants such as *Cryptosporidium parvum*.[64] Since adjuvant dependent cancer immunotherapy has had limited success in treating human cancer, there is a concern that the cytokine gene transfer model in animals will translate no better than any other rodent tumor immunotherapy model. Another risk is that the transferred growth factor may act as an autocrine growth factor for marrow derived tumor. For example, expression of the IL2 gene in a murine T cell line results in autocrine growth **in vitro** and tumorigenicity **in vivo** in immunodeficient mice.[65] Finally, it may only be possible to grow, transduce and select cytokine secreting tumor cells from the marrow of a small minority of patients with malignant disease. In all other patients the approach would have to be modified, using, for example, cytokine transduced patient fibroblasts co-injected with autologous tumor, or cytokine transduced allogeneic but partially HLA-matched tumor cells. While all these alternatives are effective in mice, their relevance to human disease again remains questionable. As of March 1994, the available approaches are being evaluated in 14 different clinical trials.

CORRECTION OF SINGLE GENE DEFECTS: HEMOGLOBINOPATHIES

It has been the goal of several major laboratories to introduce a β-globin gene into the hemopoietic stem cells (HSC) of patients with β-thalassemia syndromes and sickle cell disease (SCD) and obtain correctly regulated and efficient expression in erythroid progenitors. Presently, therapeutic options for these diseases are limited and, with the exception of allogeneic bone marrow transplantation (BMT), non-curative.[66–69] Even allogeneic BMT has limited applicability; it is only available to a minority of patients who have an HLA-matched donor, and even then the procedure is associated with significant morbidity and mortality.[68,69]

Gene therapy for thalassemia requires replacement with a normal functional β-globin gene. While the same approach may be valid for SCD, transfer of a functional γ globin gene may be preferable instead, in view of the ability of γ globin to prevent sickle hemoglobin polymerization.[67] With current methods of gene transfer, however, achieving any clinically significant level of expression of either globin gene is a formidable task. Patient data and animal models indicate that significant amelioration of disease phenotype would require at least 20–30% expression of a transduced gene with respect to endogenous levels.[67,70] To be able to achieve these therapeutic levels requires development of vector systems able to efficiently deliver the gene to stem cells and sufficient understanding of tissue specific expression and regulation of the human β-globin locus to obtain high level expression of the transduced gene in erythroid progenitor cells. Recent advances in these areas are beginning to make these ambitious aims more feasible.

Structure of the β-globin locus

The β-globin locus is located on chromosome 11 and is at least 230 kb in size. The individual globin genes of the locus include the embryonic ϵ-gene, the 2 fetal gamma genes $^{G}\gamma$ and $^{A}\gamma$, and the adult β and δ-genes.[71] These structural elements are arranged in a linear array over a 70 kb interval and regulated at the level of gene transcription. Studies in transgenic mice have demonstrated that cis acting regulating sequences directly adjacent to these genes, the ϵ, $^{G}\gamma$, $^{A}\gamma$, and β promoters and the β enhancer contain all the necessary elements to allow correct developmental and tissue specific expression of the globin genes.[71–73] However, these sequences alone are insufficient for high level expression. Deletions upstream of the globin genes in certain $(\gamma\delta\beta)^0$-thalassemias completely ablates expression although the individual genes remain structurally unaffected. Characterization of these deletions resulted in the identification of a powerful tissue-specific enhancer region, the locus control region or LCR (approximately 15 kb in length) which is required for high level expression in transgenic models.[72,74] There are 4 active sites in the LCR, identified by their sensitivity to the nuclease DNaseI and termed hypersensitivity sites (HSs) 1–4. The core (300–400 bp) of HS 2,3,4 site contains the powerful erythroid specific enhancer element, NF-E2 which is essential for the increase in expression. Individual sites linked to the β-globin gene have been shown to induce levels of expression almost equivalent to that of the endogenous murine gene in transgenic mice.[75]

Transfer of globin sequences to hemopoietic stem cells (HSC)

Gene transfer of globin sequences to HSC has predominantly been explored using retroviral vectors. The ability of retroviruses to transduce HSC[76] and the availability of improved packaging cell lines[77] that produce replication defective retroviruses has stimulated the evaluation of vectors containing either the β- or γ- globin gene. Initially an ecotropic retrovirus, containing a neomycin resistance gene (Neo^R) as a selectable marker and a 3 kb genomic fragment containing the β-gene and its adjacent cis acting regulatory sequences, was used to infect murine erythroleukemia (MEL) cells.[78] Only retroviral constructs containing the globin gene in the reverse orientation were functional and allowed normal viral production. Single copy proviral integration and expression levels of less than 0.1% of endogenous β-globin was demonstrated. Similar results were obtained with an amphotropic vector with a γβ-hybrid and Neo^R construct in MEL cells,[79] although 10% expression of the transgene was obtained. Viral titer was low and the producer lines were prone to rearrangement. Experiments evaluating the efficiency of infection and expression of a β-globin construct in erythroid progenitors, the ultimate target of all gene therapy strategies, showed low levels of infectivity (<0.1%) and 5% expression of the transgene with respect to endogenous levels,[80] although all transduced animals showed trilineage long-term engraftment.[81] Subsequent experiments obtained greatly enhanced transduction efficiency by using improved stem cell isolation and higher viral titer.[82–84] However, globin transgene expression remained unchanged.

Transfer of globin sequences and locus control regions (LCR)

The identification of the LCR[72,73] and its role in high level globin gene expression has prompted subsequent experiments with varying size fragments of the individual or linked hypersensitivity sites to the β- or γ-globin gene. Although relatively high level expression has been demonstrated in MEL cells with HS2β constructs also containing Neo^R,[85] it has not been possible to manufacture high titer unrearranged producer cell lines. Recently a retrovirus containing HS1–4 and a human β-globin gene has been reported to give 70% expression in MEL cells and relatively high expression transplant recipients of infected murine bone marrow.[86] Reproduction of these results in human bone marrow experiments is awaited.

Other vectors

In view of the difficulties with the retroviral approach, other viral vectors have been investigated. There is particular interest in the defective adeno-associated virus (AAV). The structure and biology of this DNA parvovirus is reviewed by Kremer and Perricaudet, this issue. For therapy of the hemoglobinopathies, the major potential advantage of AAV is its ability to stably integrate in a relatively site specific manner, on chromosome 19. Recombinant AAV(rAAV) integrates as 1–3 unrearranged tandem copies and has a packaging limit of 5 kb.[87] Although more complex to assemble than retroviral virions, manipulation of AAV has recently become more accessible with the development of techniques for high titer helper-free stocks.[88] Initial experiments utilizing a HS2$^{A}\gamma$Neo^{R} gene construct demonstrated expression levels 40–110% of the endogenous gene in K562 erythroleukemia cells.[89] Genomic analysis demonstrated a single copy of a unrearranged provirus per cell, albeit with random integration. These encouraging results have led several laboratories to investigate the expression of similar constructs in erythroid progenitors.[90-92] A construct containing core fragments of HS2,3 and 4 and the $^{A}\gamma$gene (v432$^{A}\gamma$) without a selectable marker gives high level expression in human BFU-E (JL Miller and AW Nienhuis, personal communication). Similar results evaluating erythroid specific expression of marker genes linked to HS2 have also been reported. The ability of rAAV containing a lacZ gene to infect CD34^{+} selected cells (S Goodman et al. submitted) suggests that this virus will be valuable in infecting stem cells with therapeutic genes.

Clearly, further advances in gene transfer for correction of hemoglobinopathies will require improved vector technology, a broader understanding of the role of the cis and trans acting elements in globin gene regulation and improved stem cell transduction. Nonetheless, we predict that continued progress in all these areas will allow the first clinical studies to begin in less than a decade.

MODIFY THE DRUG SENSITIVITY OF THE PROGENITOR CELLS

The study of cytotoxic drug resistance in cancer cells has revealed the operation of diverse genetic mechanisms. This increased understanding of drug resistance has not only suggested strategies to circumvent acquired resistance in tumor cells,[93,94] it has also suggested gene therapy approaches to protect normal host tissues from the toxicity of chemotherapy. If hemopoietic stem cells could be rendered re sistant to one or more cytotoxic drugs, this would have two potential advantages for patients. First, it might enable them to resist the myelosuppressive effects of cytotoxic drugs during cancer therapy, allowing longer or more intensive therapy that might cure a higher proportion of patients.[95–97] Secondly, of more standard importance for the field of gene therapy, drug resistance could behave as a dominant selectable marker, allowing in vivo selection of gene modified cells over their unmodified companions.[16,98,99] If the drug resistance gene were linked with a therapeutic gene, this could provide a mechanism of positively selecting gene modified hemopoietic stem cells to a level where therapeutic benefit would be obtained even if the initial gene transfer process were of low efficiency.[99]

Molecular mechanisms of drug resistance include increased expression of normal cellular genes, decreased expression of cellular gene products that are essential for drug induced cytotoxicity, and acquired mutations leading to structurally altered gene products. Table 1 catalogs several examples for each of these mechanisms.

Table

Mechanism of drug resistance	Gene	Drugs	References
Increased expression of structurally normal gene products	human multidrug resistance 1	wide variety of natuarally occurring cytotoxic compounds	100–102
	dihydrofolate reductase	methotrexate	103, 104
	cytosolic aldehyde dehydrogenase	cyclophosphamide	105, 106
Decreased expression of gene products essential for cytotoxicity	topoisomerase II	epipodophyllotoxins, anthracyclines	107, 108
	topoisomerase I	camptothecin, CPT-11	109, 110
	deoxycytidine kinase	arabinosylcytosine	111–113
Acquired **mutations** resulting in structurally altered gene products	dihydrofolate reductase	methotrexate	114–116
	topoisomerase II	epipodophyllotoxins anthracyclines	117
	topoisomerase I	camptothecin, CPT-11	118–120

Pre-clinical studies

The first eukaryotic drug resistance gene to be transferred to reconstituting bone marrow cells was a methotrexate resistant rodent dihydrofolate reductase (mDHFR) gene. These studies showed that mice transplanted with cells transduced with a mDHFR containing retroviral vector were protected from methotrexate induced myelosuppression and had increased survival following methotrexate administration.[121,122] Later experiments have suggested that methotrexate can be used to select for murine hemopoietic cells expressing transferred mDHFR genes.[123] A recent report showed that retroviral vectors containing mutant human DHFR genes can also be used to confer methotrexate resistance **in vitro** to murine hemopoietic cells.[124]

Transfer of the human MDR1 gene to hemopoietic cells has also been described. P- glycoprotein, the product of the MDR1 gene, functions as a drug efflux pump and confers resistance to a wide variety of naturally occurring chemotherapeutics.[100] The feasibility of using the MDR1 gene to protect hemopoietic cells has been demonstrated by transgenic mouse experiments.[125,126] In addition, retroviral transfer of MDR1 to murine clonogenic progenitors resulted in drug resistance **in vitro**.[127] In murine transplant experiments, mice transplanted with MDR1 transduced cells showed attenuation of taxol induced myelosuppression.[99,128] In taxol treated animals, the proportion of circulating leukocytes transduced with the MDR1 virus increased with drug treatment, suggesting that cells expressing the transferred MDR1 gene can be dominantly selected **in vivo** with taxol.[99,129] Recent work has suggested that the MDR1 gene can be used to select for other therapeutic genes when the second gene is linked to the MDR1 cDNA in bicistronic retroviral vectors[130](and M. Gottesman, personal communication).

The experiments with MDR1 and mutant DHFR containing vectors demonstrate the principal that drug resistance genes can be used to attenuate drug induced myelosuppression and can act as dominant selectable markers for genetically altered hemopoietic cells. It is probable that other drug resistance genes may function in an analogous fashion. DNA- methylguanine methyltransferases (MGMT) are enzymes that repair DNA damage done by the nitrosoureas, a class of cancer chemotherapeutic alkylating agents. Preliminary data suggests that retroviral mediated gene transfer of the human MGMT gene to mouse bone marrow cells results in protection of murine progenitors from BCNU toxicity.[131] Some of the other drug resistance genes listed in Table 1 are currently being tested to determine their utility in generating drug resistant hemopoietic cells.

Clinical trials

Based on the preclinical studies described above, 3 trials proposing transfer of the MDR1 gene transfer to bone marrow or peripheral blood stem cells from adult cancer patients have been approved by the National Institutes of Health Recombinant DNA Advisory Committee. The MDR1 vector will be transferred to hemopoietic cells in the setting of autologous bone marrow transplantation. Patients will be treated with taxol after transplantation as clinically indicated. The endpoints of these trials are: (1) to test if MDR1 gene transfer results in toxicity specific to gene transfer, (2) to test if the MDR1 vector can be transferred to human hemopoietic stem cells, (3) to test if MDR1 can be used as a dominant selectable marker **in vivo**, (4) and to test if MDR1 gene transfer will result in amelioration of taxol induced myelosuppression.

Clinical application of drug resistance gene transfer has several potential pitfalls. The low stem cell transduction efficiencies observed with current clinical protocols predict that amelioration of drug induced myelosuppression will not occur unless dramatic **in vivo** selection can be enacted. Other methods to increase the transduction efficiency of pluripotent repopulating stem cells will likely be required for successful application of this approach. A second potential limitation is the risk of transferring drug resistance genes to tumor cells that contaminate the marrow graft. This possibility could theoretically result in a drug resistant relapse. The current protocols exclude patients with documented bone marrow metastases as determined by marrow biopsy and bone scan, however, these conventional methods cannot detect low levels of tumor cells in bone marrow.[132] Despite these considerations, it is not known if clinical vectors would transduce tumor cells, or if transduction of tumor cells would have significant clinical consequences. For example, breast cancer relapse after standard autologous transplant is associated with a uniformly poor prognosis. Furthermore, drugs not affected by P-glycoprotein expression can be used as palliative therapy when relapse occurs in this setting.

CONCLUSION

While hemopoietic progenitor cells are tempting targets for gene transfer, the limited efficiency with which these cells can be transduced currently limits the implementation of clinical protocols. However, by combining some of the strategies outlined in this chapter, it may be possible to make the most of the imperfect systems available. For example, gene marking studies are helping to reveal how best to prepare and manipulate marrow progenitor cells for gene transfer, while co-transfection of drug resistance genes has the potential to provide a dominant selectable marker in vivo. Similarly, co-transfection of cytokine genes may provide a subsequent selective advantage for transduced cells in vivo. However, there remains little doubt that the full potential of hemopoietic stem cell therapy will be realized only after the development of improved gene transfer systems and with an improved understanding of gene regulation in hemopoietic stem cells and their mature progeny.[1]

ACKNOWLEDGEMENTS

We would like to thank all our clinical and laboratory co-workers who made these studies possible. We would also like to thank Nancy Parnell for word processing.
Some of the work presented was supported by ALSAC (American Lebanese Syrian Associated charities).

REFERENCES

1 Hughes PFD, Thacker JD, Hogge D, et al. Retroviral gene transfer to primitive normal and leukemic hematopoietic cells using clinically applicable procedures. J Clin Invest 1992; 89: 1817–1824.
2 Anderson WF. The ADA human gene therapy clinical protocol. Hum Gene Ther 1990; 1: 327–362.
3 Miller AD. Human gene therapy comes of age. Nature 1992; 357: 455–460.
4 Smith C. Retroviral vector-mediated gene transfer into hematopoietic cells: Prospects and issues. J Hematother 1992; 1: 155–166.
5 Schuening FG, Kawahara K, Miller AD, et al. Retrovirus-mediated gene transduction into long-term repopulating marrow cells of dogs. Blood 1991; 78: 2568–2576.
6 Van Beusechem VW, Kukler A, Heidt PJ, Valerio D. Long-term expression of human adenosine deaminase in rhesus monkeys transplanted with retrovirus-infected bone-marrow cells. Proc Natl Acad Sci USA 1992; 89: 7640–7644.
7 Rill DR, Moen RC, Buschle M, et al. An approach for the analysis of relapse and marrow reconstitution after autologous marrow transplantation using retrovirus-mediated gene transfer. Blood 1992; 79: 2694–2700.
8 Wieder R, Cornetta K, Kessler SW, Anderson WF. Increased efficiency of retrovirus-mediated gene transfer and expression in primate bone marrow progenitors after 5-fluorouracil-induced hematopoietic suppression and recovery. Blood 1991; 77: 448–455.
9 Otsuka T, Thacker JD, Eaves CJ, Hogge DE. Differential effects of microenvironmentally presented interleukin 3 versus soluble growth factor on primitive human hematopoietic cells. J Clin Invest 1991; 88: 417–422.
10 Otsuka T, Thacker JD, Hogge DE. The effects of interleukin 6 and interleukin 3 on early hematopoietic events in long-term cultures of human marrow. Exp Hematol 1991; 19: 1042–1048.
11 Stoeckert CJ, Jr, Nicolaides NC, Haines KM, Surrey S, Bayever E. Retroviral transfer of genes into erythroid progenitors derived from human peripheral blood. Exp Hematol 1990; 18: 1164–1170.
12 Dick JE, Kamel-Reid S, Murdoch B, Doedens M. Gene transfer into normal human hematopoietic cells using in vitro and in vivo assays. Blood 1991; 78: 624–634.
13 Cornetta K, Morgan RA, Anderson WF. Safety issues related to retrovirus-mediated gene transfer in humans. Hum Gene Ther 1991; 2: 5–14.
14 Rill DR, Buschle M, Foreman NK, et al. Retrovirus mediated gene transfer as an approach to analyze neuroblastoma relapse after autologous bone marrow transplantation. Hum Gene Ther 1992; 3: 129–136.

15 Brenner MK, Rill DR, Moen RC, et al. Gene-marking to trace origin of relapse after autologous bone marrow transplantation. Lancet 1993; 341: 85–86.
16 Brenner MK, Rill DR, Holladay MS, et al. Gene marking to determine whether autologous marrow infusion restores long-term haemopoiesis in cancer patients. Lancet 1993; 342:1134-1137.
17 Appelbaum FR, Buckner CD. Overview of the clinical relevance of autologous bone marrow transplantation. Clin Haematol 1986; 15: 1–18.
18 Burnett AK, Tansey P, Watkins R, et al. Transplantation of unpurged autologous bone-marrow in acute myeloid leukaemia in first remission. Lancet 1984; 2: 1068–1070.
19 Goldstone AH, Anderson CC, Linch DC, et al. Autologous bone marrow transplantation following high dose chemotherapy for the treatment of adult patients with acute myeloid leukaemia. Br J Haematol 1986; 64: 529–537.
20 Brugger W, Bross KJ, Glatt M, Weber F, Mertelsmann R, Kanz L. Mobilization of tumor cells and hematopoietic progenitor cells into peripheral blood of patients with solid tumors. Blood 1994; 83: 636–640.
21 Shpall EJ, Jones RB. Release of tumor cells from bone marrow. Blood 1994; 83: 623–625.
22 De Fabritiis P, Ferrero D, Sandrelli A, et al. Monoclonal antibody purging and autologous bone marrow transplantation in acute myelogenous leukemia in complete remission. Bone Marrow Transplant 1989; 4: 669–674.
23 Gambacorti-Passerini C, Rivoltini L, Fizzotti M, et al. Selective purging by human interleukin-2 activated lymphocytes of bone marrows contaminated with a lymphoma line or autologous leukaemic cells. Br J Haematol 1991; 78: 197–205.
24 Gorin NC, Aegerter P, Auvert B, et al. Autologous bone marrow transplantation for acute myelocytic leukemia in first remission: A European survey of the role of marrow purging. Blood 1990; 75: 1606–1614.
25 Santos GW, Yeager AM, Jones RJ. Autologous bone marrow transplantation. Annu Rev Med 1989; 40: 99–112.
26 Gribben JG, Freedman AS, Neuberg D, et al. Immunologic purging of marrow assessed by PCR before autologous bone marrow transplantation for B-cell lymphoma. N Engl J Med 1991; 325: 1525–1533.
27 Petersen FB, Buckner CD. Allogeneic and autologous bone marrow transplantation for acute leukemia and malignant lymphoma: current status. Hematol Oncol 1987; 5: 233–243.
28 Yeager AM, Kaizer H, Santos GW, et al. Autologous bone marrow transplantation in patients with acute nonlymphocytic leukemia, using ex vivo marrow treatment with 4-hydroperoxycyclophosphamide. N Engl J Med 1986; 315: 141–147.
29 Campana D, Coustan-Smith E, Behm FG. The definition of remission in acute leukemia with immunologic techniques. Bone Marrow Transplant 1991; 8: 429–437.
30 Uckun FM, Kersey JH, Haake R, Weisdorf D, Nesbit ME, Ramsay NKC. Pretransplantation burden of leukemic progenitor cells as a predictor of relapse after bone marrow transplantation for acute lymphoblastic leukemia. N Engl J Med 1993; 329: 1296–1301.
31 Kaizer H, Stuart RK, Brookmeyer R, et al. Autologous bone marrow transplantation in acute leukemia: a phase I study of in vitro treatment of marrow with 4-hydroperoxycyclophosphamide to purge tumor cells. Blood 1985; 65: 1504–1510.
32 Gorin NC, Douay L, Laporte JP, et al. Autologous bone marrow transplantation using marrow incubated with Asta Z 7557 in adult acute leukemia. Blood 1986; 67: 1367–1376.
33 Miyoshi H, Shimizu K, Kozu T, et al. t(8;21) breakpoints on chromosome 21 in acute myeloid leukemia are clustered within a limited region of a single gene, AML1. Proc Natl Acad Sci USA 1991; 88: 10431–10435.
34 Erickson P, Gao J, Chang K-S, et al . Identification of breakpoints in t(8;21) AML and isolation of a fusion transcript with similarity to Drosophila segmentation gene runt. Blood 1992; (In press)

35 Nucifora G, Birn DJ, Erickson P, et al. Detection of DNA rearrangements in the AML1 loci and of an AML1/ETO fusion mRNA in patients with t(8;21) AML. Blood 1992; (In press).
36 O'Shaughnessy JA, Cowan KH, Wilson W, et al. Pilot study of high dose ICE (ifosfamide, carboplatin, etoposide) chemotherapy and autologous bone marrow transplant (ABMT) with neo-R-transduced bone marrow and peripheral blood stem cells in patients with metastatic breast cancer. Hum Gene Ther 1993; 4: 331–354.
37 Deisseroth AB, Kantarjian H, Talpaz M, et al. Autologous bone marrow transplantation for CML in which retroviral markers are used to discriminate between relapse which arises from systemic disease remaining after preparative therapy versus relapse due to residual leukemia cells in autologous marrow: A pilot trial. Hum Gene Ther 1991; 2: 359–376.
38 Ochman HA, Gerber S, Hart DL. Genetic application of an inverse polymerase chain reaction. Genetics 1988; 120: 621–623.
39 Donahue RE, Kessler SW, Bodine D, et al. Helper virus induced T cell lymphoma in nonhuman primates after retroviral mediated gene transfer. J Exp Med 1992; 176: 1125–1135.
40 Kolb HJ, Mittrmuller J, Clemm Ch, et al. Donor leukocyte transfusions for treatment of recurrent chronic myelogenous leukemia in marrow transplant patients. Blood 1990; 76: 2462–2465.
41 Riddell SR, Watanabe KS, Goodrich JM, Li CR, Agha ME, Greenberg PD. Restoration of viral immunity in immunodeficient humans by the adoptive transfer of T cell clones. Science 1992; 257: 238–241.
42 Rosenberg SA, Spiess P, Lafreniere R. A New Approach to the Adoptive Immunotherapy of Cancer with Tumor-Infiltrating Lymphocytes. Science 1986; 233: 1318–1321.
43 Rosenberg SA. Gene therapy for cancer. JAMA 1992; 268: 2416–2419.
44 Townsend A, Bodmer H. Antigen recognition by class I-restricted T lymphocytes. Annu Rev Immunol 1989; 7: 601–624.
45 Brenner MK, Heslop HE. Graft-versus-host reactions and bone marrow transplantation. Curr Opin Immunol 1991; 3: 752–757.
46 Melief CJ, Kast WM. Potential immunogenicity of oncogene and tumor supressor gene products. Curr Opin Immunol 1993; 5: 709–713.
47 van Der Bruggen P, Traversari C, Chomez P, et al. A gene encoding an antigen recognized by cytolytic T lymphocytes on a human melanoma. Science 1991; 254: 1643–1647.
48 Doherty PC. Cell-Mediated Cytotoxiicty. Cell 1993; 75: 607–612.
49 Lanzavecchia A. Identifying strategies for immune intervention. Science 1993; 260: 937–944.
50 Straus SE, Cohen JI, Tosato G, Meier J. Epstein-Barr virus infections: Biology, pathogenesis and management. Ann Intern Med 1992; 118: 45–48.
51 Papadopoulos EB, Ladanyi M, The Allogeneic Bone Marrow Transplantation Service. Donor leukocyte infusions as treatment of Epstein-Barr virus lymhoproliferative disorders (EBV-LPD) in recipients of unrelated and related allogeneic transplants. Blood 1993; 10 (Suppl 1): 214a.
52 Heslop HE, Brenner MK, Rooney CM, et al. Administration of neomycin resistance gene marked EBV specific cytotoxic T lymphocytes to recipients of mismatched-related or phenotypically similar unrelated donor marrow grafts. Hum Gene Ther 1994; 5: 381–397.
53 Rosenberg SA. The immunotherapy and gene therapy of cancer. J Clin Oncol 1992; 10: 180–199.
54 Nabel GJ, Nabel EG, Yang ZY, et al. Direct gene transfer with DNA-liposome complexes in melanoma: expression, biologic activity, and lack of toxicity in humans. Proc Natl Acad Sci USA 1993; 90(23): 11307–11311.
55 Chen L, Ashe S, Brady WA, et al. Costimulation of antitumor immunity by the B7 counterreceptor for the T lymphocyte molecules CD28 and CTLA-4. Cell 1992; 71: 1093–1102.

56 Townsend SE, Allison JP. Tumor rejection after direct costimulation of CD8+ T cells by B7-transfected melanoma cells. Science 1993; 259: 368–370.
57 Tepper RI, Pattengale PK, Leder P. Murine interleukin-4 displays potent anti-tumor activity in vivo. Cell 1989; 57: 503–512.
58 Golumbek PT, Lazenby AJ, Levitsky HI, et al. Treatment of established renal cancer by tumor cells engineered to secrete interleukin-4. Science 1991; 254: 713–716.
59 Fearon ER, Pardoe DM, Itaya T, et al. Interleukin-2 production by tumor cells bypasses T helper function in the generation of an anti-tumor response. Cell 1990; 60: 397–403.
60 Gansbacher B, Zier K, Daniels B, Cronin K, Bannerji R, Gilboa E. Interleukin 2 gene transfer into tumor cells abrogates tumorigenicity and induces protective immunity. J Exp Med 1990; 172: 1217–1224.
61 Dranoff G, Jaffee E, Lazenby A, et al. Vaccination with irradiated tumor cells engineered to secrete murine GM-CSF stimulates potent, specific, and long lasting antitumor immunity. Proc Natl Acad Sci USA 1993; (In press).
62 Colombo MP, Ferrari G, Stoppacciaro A, et al. Granulocyte colony-stimulating factoe gene transfer suppresses tumorogenicity of a murine adenocarcinoma in vivo. J Exp Med 1991; 173: 889–897.
63 Colombo MP, Forni G. Cytokine gene transfer in tumor inhibition and tumor therapy: where are we now? Immunol Today 1994; (In press).
64 Hock H, Dorsch M, Kunzendorf U, et al. Vaccinations with tumor cells genetically engineered to produce different cytokines: Effectivity not superior to a classical adjuvant. Cancer Res 1993; 53: 714–716.
65 Yamada G, Kitamura Y, Sonoda H, et al. Retroviral expression of the human IL-2 gen in a murine T cell line results in cell growth autonomy and tumorigenicity. EMBO J 1993; 6: 2705–2709.
66 McDonagh K, Nienhuis AW. The thalassemias. In: Nathan DG, Oski FA, eds. Hematology of infancy and childhood, Philadelphia: Saunders, 1992; pp. 783–897.
67 Bunn HF. Sickle hemoglobin and other hemoglobin mutants. In: Stamatoyannopoulos G, Nienhuis AW, Majerus PJ, Varmus H, eds. The molecular basis of blood diseases. Philadelphia: Saunders 1994; pp. 207–256.
68 Lucarrelli G, Galimberti M, Polchi P et al. Bone marrow transplantation in patients with thalassemia. N Engl J Med 1990; 322: 417–421.
69 Ferster A, deValek C, Azzi N, Fondu P, Toppet M, Sariban E. Bone marrow transplantation in severe sickle cell anemia. Br J Haematol 1992; 80: 102–105.
70 Rodgers GP, Dover GJ, Noguchi CT, Schechter AN, Nienhuis AW. Hematologic responses of patients with sickle cell disease to treatment with hydroxyurea. N Engl J Med 1990; 322: 1037–1045.
71 Stamatoyannopoulos G, Nienhuis AW. Hemoglobin switching. In: Stamatoyannopoulos G, Nienhuis AW, eds. The molecular basis of blood diseases. Philadelphia: Saunders 1994; pp. 107–156.
72 Orkin SH. Globin gene regulation and switching: circa 1990. Cell 1990; 63: 665–672.
73 Kollias G, Wrighton N, Hurst J, Grosveld F. Regulated expression of human gamma-, beta- and hybrid gamma beta-globin genes in transgenic mice: manipulation of the developmental expression patterns. Cell 1986; 46: 89–94.
74 Grosveld F, vanAssenfeldt B, Greaves DR, Kollias G. Position independant high level expression of the human β-globin gene in transgenic mice. Cell 1987; 51: 975–985.
75 Fraser P, Hurst J, Collis P, Grosveld F. DNaseI hypersensitive sites 1, 2 and 3 of the human β-globin dominant control region direct position-independent expression. Nucl Acids Res 1990; 18: 3503–3508.
76 Williams DA, Orkin SH, Mulligna RC. Retrovirus-mediated transfer of human adenosine deaminase gene sequences into cells in culture and into muring hematopoietic cells in vitro. Proc Natl Acad Sci USA 1986; 83: 2566–2570.
77 Miller AD. Retroviral vectors. Curr Top Microbiol Immunol 1992; 158: 1–24.
78 Cone RD, Weber-Benarous A, Baorto D, Mulligen RC. Regulated expression of a complete human β-globin gene encoded by a transmissible retrovirus vector. Mol Cell Biol 1987; 7: 887–897.

79 Karlsson S, Papayannopoulo T, Schweiger SG, Stamatoyannopoulos G, Nienhuis AW. Retroviral-mediated transfer of genomic globin genes leads to regulated production of RNA and protein. Proc Natl Acad Sci USA 1987; 84: 2411–2415.
80 Bender MA, Miller AD, Gelinas RE. Expression of the human beta-globin gene after retroviral transfer into murine erythroleukemia cells and human BFU-E cells. Mol Cell Biol 1988; 8: 1725–1735.
81 Dzierzak EA, Papayannopoulou T, Mulligan RC. Lineage-specific expression of a human beta-globin gene in murine bone marrow transplant recipients reconstituted with retrovirustransduced stem cells. Nature 1988; 331: 35–41.
82 Bender MA, Gelinas RE, Miller AD. A majority of mice show long-term expression of a human β-globin gene after retrovirus transfer into hematopoietic stem cells. Mol Cell Biol 1989; 9: 1426–1434.
83 Karlsson S, Bodine DM, Perry L, Papayannopoulo T, Nienhuis AW. Expresssion of the human β-globin gene following retroviral-mediated gene transfer into multipotential hematopoietic progenitors of mice. Proc Natl Acad Sci USA 1988; 85: 6062–6068.
84 Bodine DM, Karlsson S, Nienhuis AW. Combination of interleukins 3 and 6 preserves stem cell function in culture and enhances retrovirus-mediated gene transfer into hematopoietic stem cells. Proc Natl Acad Sci USA 1989; 86: 8897–8891.
85 Novak U, Harris EAS, Forrester W, Groudine M, Gelinas R. High-level β-globin expression after retroviral transfer of locus activation region-containing human β-globin gene derivatives into murine erythroleukemia cells. Proc Natl Acad Sci USA 1990; 87: 3386–3390.
86 Plavec I, Papayannopoulou T, Maury C, Meyer F. A human β-globin gene fused to the human β-globin locus control region is expressed at high levels in erythroid cells of mice engrafted with retrovirus-transduced hematopoietic stem cells. Blood 1993; 81: 1384–1392.
87 Muzyczka N. Use of adeno-associated virus as a general transduction vector for mammalian cells. Curr Top Microbiol Immunol 1992; 158: 97–129.
88 Samulski RJ, Chang LS, Shenk T. Helper-free stocks of recombinant adeno-associated viruses: normal integration does not require viral gene expression. J Virol 1989; 63(9): 3822–3828.
89 Walsh CE, Liu JM, Xiao X, Young NS, Nienhuis AW, Samulski RJ. Regulated high level expression of a human gammaglobin gene introduced into erythroid cells by an adeno-associated virus vector. Proc Natl Acad Sci USA 1992; 89: 7257–7261.
90 Miller JL, Walsh CE, Ney PA, Samulski RJ, Nienhuis AW. Single-copy transduction and expression of human gamma-globin in K562 erythroleukemia cells using recombinant adeno-associated virus vectors: the effect of mutations in NF-E2 and GATA-1 binding motifs within the hypersensitivity stite 2 enhancer. Blood 1993; 82: 1900–1906.
91 Zhou SZ, Li O, Stamatoyannopoulos G, Srivastava A. Adeno-associated virus 2-mediated transduction and erythroid cell-specific expression of a normal human beta-globin gene. Blood 1993; 82(Abstract): 346a.
92 Zhou SZ, Li O, Stamatoyannopoulos G, Srivastava A. Adeno-associated virus 2-mediated gene transfer in murine hematopoietic progenitor cells. Exp Hematol 1993; 21: 928–933.
93 Salmon SE, Dalton WS, Grogan TM, et al. Multidrug-resistant myeloma: laboratory and clinical effects of verapamil as a chemosensitizer. Blood 1991; 78:44.
94 Gottesman MM, Pastan I. Clinical trials of agents that reverse multidrug-resistance. J Clin Oncol 1989; 7: 409.
95 Murphy D, Crowther D, Renninson J, et al. A randomised dose intensity study in ovarian carcinoma comparing chemotherapy given at four week intervals for six cycles with half dose chemotherapy given for twelve cycles. Ann Oncol 1993; 4: 377.
96 Levin L, Hryniuk WM. Dose intensity analysis of chemotherapy regimens in ovarian carcinoma. J Clin Oncol 1987; 5: 756.

97 Levin L, Simon R, Hryniuk W. Importance of multiagent chemotherapy regimens in ovarian carcinoma: dose intensity analysis. J Natl Cancer Inst 1993; 85: 1732.
98 Bodine DM, Moritz T, Donahue RE et al. Long-term in vivo expression of a murine adenosine deaminase gene in rhesus monkey hematopoietic cells of multiple lineages after retroviral mediated gene transfer into CD34+ bone marrow cells. Blood 1993; 82: 1975.
99 Sorrentino BP, Brandt SJ, Bodine D et al. Selection of drug-resistant bone marrow cells in vivo after retroviral transfer of human MDR1. Science 1992; 257: 99.
100 Pastan I, Gottesman MM. Multidrug resistance. Annu Rev Med 1991; 42: 277.
101 Chen CJ, Chin JE, Ueda K, et al. Internal duplication and homology with bacterial transport proteins in the mrd1 (Pglycoprotein) gene from multidrug-resistant human cells. Cell 1986; 47: 381.
102 Roninson IB, Chin JE, Choi KG, et al. Isolation of human mdr DNA sequences amplified in multidrug-resistant KB carcinoma cells. Proc Natl Acad Sci USA 1986; 83: 4538.
103 Tyler-Smith C, Alderson T. Gene amplification in methotrexate-resistant mouse cells. I. DNA rearrangement accompanies dihydrofolate reductase gene amplification in a T-cell lymphoma. J Mol Biol 1981; 153: 203.
104 Flintoff WF, Weber MK, Nagainis CR, Essani AK, Robertson D, Salser W. Overproduction of dihydrofolate reductase and gene amplification in methotrexate-resistant Chinese hamster ovary cells. Mol Cell Biol 1982; 2: 275.
105 Yoshida A, Dave V, Han H, Scanlon KJ. Enhanced transcription of the cytosolic ALDH gene in cyclophosphamide resistant human carcinoma cells. Adv Exp Med Biol 1993; 328: 63.
106 Radin AI, Zhoa X, Woo TH, Colvin OM, Hilton J. Structure and expression of the cytosolic aldehyde dehydrogenase gene in cyclophosphamide-resistant murine leukemia L1210 cells. Biochem Pharmacol 1991; 42: 1933.
107 Takano H, Kohno K, Ono M, Uchida Y, Kuwano M. Increased phosphorylation of DNA topoisomerase II in etoposide-resistant mutants of human cancer KB cells. Cancer Res 1991; 51: 3951.
108 Kasahara K, Fujiwara Y, Sugimoto Y, et al. Determinants of response to the DNA topoisomerase II inhibitors doxorubicin and etoposide in human lung cancer cell lines. J Natl Cancer Inst 1992; 84: 113.
109 Sugimoto Y, Tsukahara S, Oh-hara T, Isoe T, Tsuruo T. Decreased expression of DNA topoisomerase I in camptothecinresistant tumor cell lines as determined by a monoclonal antibody. Cancer Res 1990; 50: 6925.
110 Eng WK, McCabe FL, Tan KB, et al. Development of a stable camptothecin-resistant subline of P388 leukemia with reduced topoisomerase I content. Mol Pharmacol 1990; 38: 471.
111 Drahovsky D, Kreis W. Studies on drug resistance. II. Kinase patterns in P815 neoplasms sensitive and resistant to 1-beta-D-arabinofuranosylcytosine. Biochem Pharmacol 1970; 19: 940.
112 Richel DJ, Colly LP, Arkesteijn GJ, et al. Substrate-specific deoxycytidine kinase deficiency in 1-beta-Darabinofuranosylcytosine-resistant leukemic cells. Cancer Res 1990; 50:6515.
113 Stegmann AP, Honders MW, Kester MG, Landegent JE, Willemze R. Role of deoxycytidine kinase in an in vitro model for Ara-C and DAC-resistance: substrate-enzyme interactions with deoxycytidine, 1-beta-D-arabinofuranosylcytosine and 5-aza-2′-deoxycytidine. Leukemia 1993; 7: 1005.
114 McIvor RS, Simonsen CC. Isolation and characterization of a variant dihydrofolate reductase cDNA from methotrexate-resistant murine L5178Y cells. Nucleic Acids Research 1990; 18: 7025.
115 Simonsen CC, Levinson AD. Isolation and expression of an altered mouse dihydrofolate reductase cDNA. Proc Natl Acad Sci USA 1983; 80: 2495.
116 Blakley RL, Appleman JR, Chunduru SK, Nakano T, Lewis WS and Harris SE. Mutations of human dihydrofolate reductase causing decreased inhibition by

methotrexate. In: Ayling JE, Nair MJ, Baugh CM eds. Chemistry and biology of pteridines and folates. New York: Plenum Press, 1993, p. 473.

117 Bugg BY, Danks MK, Beck WT, Suttle DP. Expression of a mutant DNA topoisomerase II in CCRF-CCEM human leukemic cells selected for resistance to teniposide. Proc Natl Acad Sci USA 1991; 88: 7654.

118 Andoh T, Ishii K, Suzuki Y, et al. Characterization of a mammalian mutant with a camptothecin-resistant DNA topoisomerase I. Proc Natl Acad Sci USA 1987; 84: 5565.

119 Benedetti P, Fiorani P, Capuani L, Wang JC. Camptothecin resistance from a single mutation changing glycine 363 of human DNA topoisomerase I to cysteine. Cancer Res 1993; 53: 4343.

120 Gromova II, Kjeldsen E, Svejstrup JQ, Alsner J, Christiansen K, Westergaard O. Characterization of an altered DNA catalysis of a camptothecin-resistant eukaryotic topoisomerase I. Nucleic Acids Res 1993; 21: 593.

121 Corey CA, DeSilva AD, Holland CA, Williams DA. Serial transplantation of methotrexate-resistant bone marrow: protection of murine recipients from drug toxicity by progeny of transduced stem cells. Blood 1990; 75: 337.

122 Williams DA, Hsieh K, DeSilva A, Mulligan RC. Protection of bone marrow transplant recipients from lethal doses of methotrexate by the generation of methotrexate-resistant bone marrow. J Exp Med 1987; 166: 210.

123 Vinh DB, McIvor RS. Selective expression of methotrexate-resistant dihydrofolate reductase (DHFR) activity in mice transduced with DHFR retrovirus and administered methotrexate. J Pharmacol Exp Ther 1993; 267: 989.

124 Banerjee D, Schweitzer BI, Volkenandt M, et al. Transfection with a cDNA encoding a Ser31 or Ser34 mutant human dihydrofolate reductase into Chinese hamster ovary and mouse marrow progenitor cells confers methotrexate resistance. Gene 1994; 139: 269.

125 Mickisch GH, Licht T, Merlino GT, Gottesman MM, Pastan I. Chemotherapy and chemosensitization of transgenic mice which express the human multidrug resistance gene in bone marrow: efficacy, potency, and toxicity. Cancer Res 1991; 51: 5417.

126 Mickisch GH, Merlino GT, Galski H, Gottesman MM, Pastan I. Transgenic mice that express the human multidrug-resistance gene in bone marrow enable a rapid identification of agents that reverse drug resistance. Proc Natl Acad Sci USA 1991; 88: 547.

127 McLachlin JR, Eglitis MA, Ueda K, et al. Expression of a human complementary DNA for the multidrug resistance gene in murine hematopoietic precursor cells with the use of retroviral gene transfer. J Natl Cancer Inst 1990; 82: 1260.

128 Hanania E, Fu S, Roninson I, et al. cDNA for the multidrug resistance (MDR-1) gene in a transcription unit of a safety modified retrovirus confers in vivo resistance to taxol on early precursor cells in a mouse transplant model and on long-term culture initiating cells in long-term human marrow culture. Blood 1993; 82 (Suppl 1):216a.

129 Podda S, Ward M, Himelstein A, et al. Transfer and expression of the human multiple drug resistance gene into live mice. Proc Natl Acad Sci USA 1992; 89: 9676.

130 Germann UA, Chin KV, Pastan I, Gottesman MM. Retroviral transfer of a chimeric multidrug resistance-adenosine deaminase gene. FASEB J 1990; 4: 1501.

131 Moritz T, Mackay W, Feng LJ, Samson L, Williams DA. Gene transfer of O6-methylguanine methyltransferase (MGMT) protects hematopoietic cells (HC) from nitrosourea (NU) induced toxicity in vitro and in vivo. Blood 1993; 82 (Suppl 1):118a.

132 Leslie DS, Johnston WW, Daly L, et al. Detection of breast carcinoma cells in human bone marrow using fluorescence-activated cell sorting and conventional cytology. Am J Clin Pathol 1990; 94: 8.

British Medical Bulletin (1995) Vol. 51, No. 1, pp.192–204

Gene therapy for solid tumors

K W Culver, T M Vickers, J L Lamsam, H W Walling and T Seregina

Molecular Immunology Laboratory, Human Gene Therapy Research Institute, Des Moines, Iowa, USA.

Advances in molecular biology have proven that there is a genetic basis to the process of carcinogenesis that allows for the consideration of entirely new approaches to the treatment of cancer. The development of an ability to selectively destroy cancer cells through the manipulation of DNA may provide the opportunity to dramatically improve the quality of care and treatment of cancer patients by decreasing systemic toxicities and enhancing efficacy. These new therapies may occur through the restoration of genetic health, such as the insertion of normal tumor suppressor genes or via down-regulation of oncogene or growth factor receptor expression. Other possibilities include the targeting of genetic alterations in tumor cells that will enhance tumor immunogenicity or induce a specific sensitivity to a prodrug. In this chapter, we have reviewed the current status of gene therapy for solid tumors in the United States and evolving new approaches for this emerging clinical discipline.

Further advances in conventional approaches to the treatment of solid tumors by surgery, radiation and chemotherapy is limited by both a lack of sufficient specificity and excessive toxicity to normal tissues. In contrast, targeting the genetic basis of carcinogenesis may allow for the selective destruction of tumor cells improving the specificity of the therapy while reducing systemic toxicity. While there are a number of gene therapy clinical trials in progress, improvements in the methods of gene delivery and expression in tumor cells and other immunologic effector cells are required for the successful application of gene therapies to cancer.

There are a variety of gene delivery systems under development.[1] Murine retroviral vectors, the most commonly used system in clinical trials, require a proliferating target cell to stably integrate and express the vector genes (*see* Russell, this issue). The requirement for proliferation allows the potential for targeting tumor cells in organs where the resident tissues are generally non-proliferative. Use of retroviral vectors is limited by the inability to produce them in high titers.[2] Adenoviral vectors are gaining popularity due to their high titer and efficient gene transfer into target cells regardless of the state of cellular proliferation (*see* Kremer, this issue), however, these vectors do not stably insert their genes into the genome of the target cell.[3] Finally, non-viral gene transfer systems include unconjugated DNA (naked DNA), DNA conjugates (e.g. DNA complexed to antibody or ligands specific to cell surface receptors) and liposomes (DNA encapsulated in a lipid bilayer) – *see* Schofield and Laskey, this issue.[4] These non-viral methods appear to be non-toxic, non-integrating vector delivery systems.

The use of non-integrating in vivo delivery systems may prove useful in the treatment of cancer because the genetic modification is no longer required once the tumor has been destroyed. However, the insertion of genes to prevent cancer (in the case of individuals predisposed to certain cancers) through the restoration of genetic health to the cell (e.g. insertion of a tumor suppressor genes) would require stable, long-term integration and expression throughout the affected tissue. In order to successfully destroy all of the cancer cells in the patient with this method, gene delivery will probably be required in all of the tumor cells. None of the gene delivery techniques available today have a 100% gene transfer efficiency in vivo. Therefore, creative strategies for in vivo gene transfer are under evaluation by many investigators in an attempt to improve the possibilities for complete tumor destruction.

A number of ex vivo gene transfer approaches to cancer gene therapy are attempting to directly enhance tumor immunogenicity.[5] In this approach, poor gene delivery efficiencies and low titers are less of a concern since in vitro gene transfer is generally quite efficient in tumor cells. However, the ability to induce systemic immunity against a malignancy has been complicated by the debilitated state of patients and the lack of a full understanding of the optimal gene combinations for initiation of a potent systemic anti-tumor response. Another ex vivo method involves the protection of tissues against the toxic effects of systemic chemotherapy. Insertion of resistance genes into hematopoietic stem cells (HSC) may allow the administration of higher doses of chemotherapy with decreased marrow toxicity, decreased infections and thus an improved anti-tumor effect. Hopefully, the results of the initial human gene therapy trials described below will begin to define the optimal conditions for gene delivery, gene expression, minimal toxicity and the complete elimination of cancer cells.

EX VIVO GENE ALTERATION OF CANCER CELLS

The concept of genetic modification of a patients own tumor cells for use as a cancer therapeutic was received with some scepticism. An initial report published in 1989 documented that the implantation of IL-4 gene-containing plasmacytoma cells into syngeneic mice resulted in transient tumor growth followed by complete tumor rejection.[6] The anti-tumor effect was mediated by a cellular inflammatory infiltrate. This result has been followed by the insertion of a variety of genes (e.g. cytokines, cell surface proteins) into a number of malignancies (Table 1).[7,8] These studies confirm that a protective systemic anti-tumor response can be elicited in immunocompetent mice. Based upon these types of animal studies, a number of human clinical trials have been developed that focus on ex vivo cell manipulation (Table 2).[9–13] Clinical studies have focused primarily upon the treatment of melanoma, colorectal cancer and renal cell carcinoma due to the observation that these tumors may be more amenable to immunologic manipulation than other solid tumors. Human clinical studies are most commonly performed as follows: (1) A portion of the tumor is surgically resected; (2) the excised tumor is digested with enzymes to obtain a single cell suspension; (3) the tumor is grown in tissue culture; (4) immunostimulatory genes (e.g. IL-2, TNF) are inserted usually with retroviral vectors; (5) successful gene transfer and expression is documented, and (6) the altered tumor cells are injected subcutaneously into the patient. Injections of tumor cells are typically repeated every several weeks to months for as long as 1 year in responding patients.

Table 1 Effect of cytokine gene transfer on tumorigenicity and immunity in mice

Cytokine	Cellular infiltrate	Systemic immunity
Human IL-2	T-cells	Yes
Murine IL-4	Eosinophils/macrophages/T-cells	Yes
Human IL-6	Neutrophils/macrophages/T-cells	Yes
Murine IL-7	Eosinophils/macrophages/T-cells	Yes
Human TNFα	T-cells	Variable
Murine IFNγ	T-cells/macrophages	Yes

Modifications of this technique include the irradiation of the genetically-altered cells, the use of HLA-A2 matched allogeneic human tumor cells and the admixture of genetically-altered autologous fibrob-

Table 2 Approved human cytokine gene therapy trials for cancer in the US

Type of Cancer	Tissue	Genes
Brain tumors	Tumor cells	HS-tk*
Brain tumors	Tumor cells	antisense IGF-1
Brain tumors	Hematopoietic stem cells	MDR-1
Breast cancer	Fibroblasts	IL-4
Breast cancer	Hematopoietic stem cells	MDR-1
Colorectal cancer	Tumor cells	IL-2 or TNF
Colorectal cancer	Fibroblasts	IL-2 or IL-4
Colorectal cancer	Tumor cells	HLA-B7 + β2-microglobulin*
Malignant melanoma	T-cells	TNF
Malignant melanoma	Tumor cells	TNF, IL-2 or IL-4
Malignant melanoma	Fibroblasts	IL-4
Malignant melanoma	Tumor cells	γ-Interferon*
Malignant melanoma	Tumor cells	B7 co-stimulatory molecule
Malignant melanoma	Tumor cells	HLA-B7 + β2-microglobulin*
Neuroblastoma	Tumor cells	IL-2 or γ-Interferon
Non-small cell lung cancer	Tumor cells	antisense K-ras or WTp53*
Ovarian cancer	Hematopoietic stem cells	MDR-1
Ovarian cancer	Tumor cells	HS-tk
Renal cell carcinoma	Tumor cells	IL-2, TNF or GM-CSF
Renal cell carcinoma	Tumor cells	HLA-B7 + β2-microglobulin*
Renal cell carcinoma	Fibroblasts	IL-4
Small cell lung cancer	Tumor cells	IL-2
Solid tumors	Tumor cells	HLA-B7 + β2-microglobulin*

*In vivo gene transfer protocols

lasts with non-genetically-altered autologous tumor cells. Fibroblasts have been chosen because they are more easily grown in tissue culture than many tumors offering greater opportunities for patient treatment. However, it is unclear if fibroblasts producing an immune stimulatory gene product will induce as significant of an immunologic response to the adjacent tumor cells as genetically-altered tumor cells would.[14]

Tumor cells are known to evade immune surveillance through the production of immunosuppressive cytokines. As a result, gene therapy could be potentially used to abolish mechanisms by which tumors hide from the immune system. One example is to genetically arrest the production of insulin-like growth factor-1 (IGF-1) by tumor cells.[15] Many tumors are high producers of IGF-1 (e.g. glioblastoma multiforme, breast cancer). Insertion of an antisense IGF-1 gene inhibits tumor cell production of IGF-1. Implantation of these genetically-modified tumor cells into syngeneic animals results in transient tumor cell growth followed by immunologic rejection of the genetically-altered tumor. This tumor destruction is mediated by T-cytotoxic (CD8+) lymphocytes.[16] The implantation of non-genetically manipulated tumor into the brain of rats followed by the injection of antisense IGF-1 gene-modified tumor cells into the leg resulted in elimination of both tumors. These findings suggest that a systemic immune response can be generated on both sides of the blood-brain barrier. The precise mechanism by which IGF-1 mediates protection of tumor cells in vivo remains unclear.

Despite the large number of ex vivo studies that have been approved, there are no published clinical trial results available. Preliminary reports suggest that the injection of genetically-modified tumor cells containing either the human IL-2 or TNF genes into patients with metastatic melanoma resulted in destruction of the genetically-modified tumor cells but had no significant anti-tumor effect on distant tumor cell deposits. There have been no reported problems with persistent growth of the gene-modified tumor cells in the recipients, with or without irradiation of the innoculum. Information gained in these initial experiments will provide the basis for more efficacious combinations of immunostimulatory genes that may provide our first novel new cancer gene therapies.

IN SITU TRANSFER OF HLA-B7 OR SENSITIVITY GENES AND THE BYSTANDER EFFECT

The first attempts to genetically modify tumors in situ were initiated in 1992. The first trial involves the direct injection of liposomes (DNA encapsulated in lipid) containing the human leukocyte antigen (HLA) B7 gene.[17] The second trial transfers the Herpes Simplex-thymidine kinase (HS-tk) gene in vivo using murine retroviral vectors.[18] Animal studies have demonstrated that the transient expression of foreign major histocompatibility complex (MHC) molecules will result in immunologic destruction of the tumor.[19,20] As a result, a clinical trial was devised involving the direct injection of liposomes containing a foreign HLA B7 gene into melanoma tumor deposits. Liposomes fuse to the tumor cell membrane and are taken up by phagocytosis. Subsequently, exogenous DNA expresses HLA-B7 class molecules transiently on the tumor cell surface. Patients were selected to be HLA A2 positive, HLA B7 negative in an effort to increase the immunogenicity of the tumor.

The first human clinical study utilized HLA B7 gene containing liposomes in a dose escalation phase I design in the treatment of patients with metastatic melanoma. Nabel et al.[21] have published data on the first 5 patients. In 1 of the patients, the injected lesion, as well as distant metastases regressed. This response was mediated by a CD8+ cellular infiltrate. Only the injected lesion responded in the other 4 patients. All of the patients demonstrated evidence of gene transfer without evidence of toxicity related to the procedure. Subsequent patients are being treated with combinations of HLA-B7 and β2-microglobulin genes in an effort to further enhance the immunologic response against the tumor. This protocol has also been expanded to include renal cell carcinoma and colorectal adenocarcinoma involving 4 research centers. These early findings suggest that the use of in vivo gene transfer of foreign HLA antigens may have the potential for inducing a systemic anti-tumor immune response in some patients with melanoma.

The in vivo application of murine retroviral vector-mediated gene therapy was applied to the treatment of human brain tumors beginning in December, 1992. In this protocol, murine fibroblasts, producing retroviral vectors (retroviral vector producer cells or VPC), were directly implanted in situ into growing brain tumors. In a series of animal studies, this approach resulted in a gene transfer efficiency as high as 55% of the cells in the tumor mass.[22] The therapeutic gene being delivered into the tumor is the Herpes Simplex-thymidine kinase (HS-tk) gene, which confers a sensitivity to the anti-herpes drug ganciclovir (Cytovene or GCV).[23] This approach was initially applied to brain tumors because the retroviral vector gene transfer system utilized requires a proliferating target cell population for integration and gene expression. In the brain, the tumor is the predominant mitotic cell type, allowing the potential for selective gene transfer into tumor cells.[24] A series of animal experiments have confirmed the selective nature of the in vivo gene transfer into tumor cells without detectable spread of the vector to the surrounding normal brain tissue.[25]

The stereotactic injection of experimental brain tumors in rats with HS-tk VPC demonstrated complete destruction of microscopic tumor in 80% of rats receiving GCV.[26] In a survival experiment, 50–60% of the rats survived long-term suggesting that this procedure may have the potential to be curative. There were no associated systemic toxicities related to the gene transfer with this form of in vivo gene deliver.[27] This complete tumor ablation occurred despite the fact that less than 100% of the tumor cells contained the HS-tk gene. This finding, the destruction of the adjacent HS-tk negative tumor cells is termed the 'bystander' effect. Since the possibility of achieving 100% gene transfer in vivo is not currently possible, the bystander killing effect has the potential for allowing successful elimination of tumors with current delivery methods.

The etiology of the bystander effect is currently under investigation. When GCV enters an HS-tk positive cell, it is converted to GCV-monophosphate. Endogenous cellular phosphorylases convert the monophosphate to GCV-triphosphate (TP). Studies in HSV infected cells suggest that GCV-TP inhibits DNA polymerase and incorporates into the DNA strand resulting in chain termination (Fig.1).[28] The leading hypothesis for the mechanism of the bystander effect relates to the passage of phosphorylated GCV-derivatives via gap junctions into neighboring cells.[29] Other investigators have suggested that fragments of HS-tk destroyed cells, termed 'apoptotic vesicles', are phagocytized by neighboring tumor cells resulting in their destruction.[30] Elucidation of the mechanism(s) involved in the bystander killing effect may provide an opportunity to magnify the effect, converting a local therapy into a regional or systemic therapy. In none of the animal experiments reported has there been any measurable evidence of bystander destruction to surrounding normal tissues.

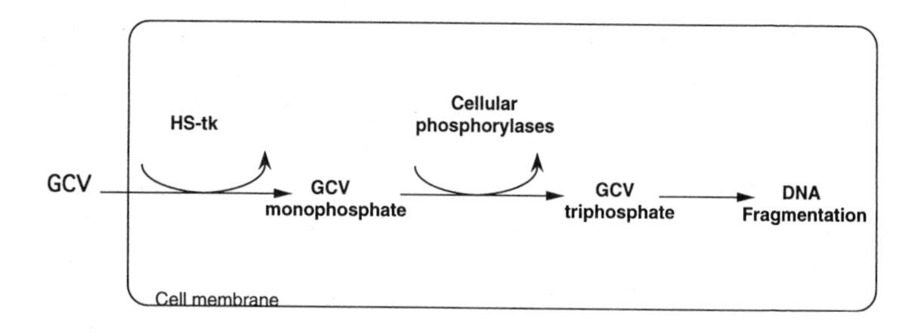

Fig. Tumour cell destruction by HS-tk and GCV. When GCV enters the cell, the HS-tk enzyme converts the drug to GCV-monophosphate. Cellular phosphorylases convert the monophosphate form of GCV to GCV-triphosphate (TP). GCV-TP is thought to destroy tumour cells by incorporating into the elongating DNA chain, inducing chain termination and DNA fragmentation. The current leading hypothesis for the mechanism of the bystander effect is the passage of the GCV-TP through gap junctions into adjacent HS-tk negative cells resulting in their destruction.

As of April, 1994, 14 patients with recurrent glioblastoma multiforme (GBM) or metastatic tumors have been treated with the stereotactic implantation of HS-tk VPC and GCV. There are preliminary data available on the first 8 patients treated (7 with recurrent glioblastoma multiforme and 1 with recurrent metastatic melanoma). HS-tk VPC were stereotactically implanted with MRI guidance only into the portion of the tumor that could be visualized by MRI, so that the effects of the therapy could be monitored. In none of the patients, were all areas of tumor growth directly injected. There has been no evidence of acute toxicity to normal tissues related to the implantation of the murine VPC or treatment with GCV in any of the patients. 3 of the 8 patients (all with GBM) demonstrated no alteration in tumor size following GCV treatment. In 5 of the patients, there was evidence of an anti-tumor effect with a decrease in tumor size and development of cystic changes within the tumor. In 3 of the patients (all GBM), tumor size decreased >50%. These early results suggest that in vivo gene transfer of the HS-tk gene into human brain tumors can be administered safely and may have some biologic activity. The continuing goal of the initial human trial at the National Institutes of Health (NIH) is to determine the toxicities of the treatment, the in vivo gene transfer efficiency and the presence of the bystander effect in human brain tumors.

Additional brain tumor gene therapy clinical trials have been approved by the Recombinant DNA Advisory Committee (RAC) using the HS-tk VPC/GCV technique for the treatment of adults with recurrent glioblastoma multiforme.[31] These trials will test an alternative method for in vivo gene delivery since recurrent tumors are filled with necrosis and gliosis that may interfere with gene transfer and the bystander effect. The new protocols will require patients to undergo a surgical resection to remove as much of the tumor as possible followed by the injection of HS-tk VPC directly into the unresectable margins of the tumor bed at the time of tumor resection. Since most patients die of the local progression of their disease within a 2 cm margin of the resection, the investigators hope that the bystander tumor killing effect will destroy cancer cells within the 2 cm area around the surgical margin. In order to maximize gene delivery, repeated injections of VPC will be administered through an Ommaya reservoir into the tumor bed in responding patients at 5–6 week intervals.

Applications of this form of retroviral-mediated HS-tk in vivo gene transfer are being developed for other solid tumors.[32] Since this method is thought to be a local therapy, the focus has been on the treatment of tumors that do not regularly metastasize, such as hepatocellular carcinoma and stage III ovarian cancer. Investigators have demonstrated that the direct injection of HS-tk VPC into hepatic tumors in rats can produce significant anti-tumor efficacy without toxicity to surrounding normal hepatocytes.[33] Despite the fact that the liver has a higher baseline of proliferation, there was no discernible toxicity either secondarily to gene transfer or the bystander effect. This is consistent with earlier studies that have shown that the transfer of the HS-tk gene into normal cells does not result in toxicity to adjacent normal cells.[34] We have also conducted experiments in the peritoneal cavity that have demonstrated that the direct injection of HS-tk VPC into the abdomen does not result in transduction of the peritoneal lining or evidence of toxicity with GCV injections. Additional clinical trials using this techniqe for the treatment of melanoma, head and neck cancer and liver tumors are expected to be approved in Europe and the USA this year.

Currently, there is one approved clinical trial that attempts to utilize the bystander effect for therapy. Freeman et al. have initiated a gene therapy trial that involves women with stage III ovarian cancer. Their therapeutic agent is a human allogeneic ovarian cancer cell line that has been transduced with an HS-tk retroviral vector. The HS-tk transduced cells are irradiated and injected into the abdomen. The premise of this study is that the HS-tk containing cells will attach adjacent to the patients own tumor cells. Then when GCV is then administered IV, there will hopefully be a bystander tumor killing effect that destroys adjacent tumor cells. Animal studies have demonstrated some evidence of improved survival with this technique. This human trial has only recently begun and there is no preliminary data to report.

There are a number of 'sensitivity' genes in addition to HS-tk that might be useful in the treatment of solid tumors (some of them are listed in Table 3).[35,36] One example is the Cytosine Deaminase (CD) gene, a fungal gene that changes 5-fluorocytidine (5-FC) into 5-fluorouracil (5-FU). When murine retroviral vectors are used to insert the CD gene into tumor cells, the genetically-altered cells can be killed in vitro and in mice.[37] Unfortunately, in vivo studies have shown that the CD bystander effect is much less potent than the one seen with HS-tk.

Table 3 'Sensitivity' enzymes under investigation

Prodrug	Enzyme activator	Toxic byproduct
Doxorubicin phosphate	Alkaline phosphatase	Doxorubicin
Etoposide phosphate	Alkaline phosphatase	Etoposide
5-fluorocytosine (5-FC)	Cytosine deaminase	5-fluorouracil (5-FU)
Ganciclovir (GCV)	HS-tk	GCV-triphosphate
6-methoxypurine arabinucleoside	HS-tk	Ara AMP, ADP and ATP
Mitomycin phosphate	Alkaline phosphatase	Mitomycin C
α-peptidyl methotrexate	Carboxypeptidase	alanyl-methotrexate

IN SITU GENE TRANSFER OF CYTOKINE, ANTISENSE ONCOGENE OR P53 GENES

Approvals have been achieved for in vivo gene transfer by direct injection of retroviral vector supernate into tumor deposits. One group will directly inject retroviral vector supernate containing interferon-γ vectors into melanoma tumor deposits. Animal studies have demonstrated that tumor-associated production of interferon-γ is a potent inducer of anti-tumor immunologic responses.[7]

In a separate experiment, vector supernate will be directly injected into non-small cell endobronchial lung cancers. This gene therapy approach is quite different from other approved trials because the gene insertion targets the genetic mechanisms responsible for the malignancy. If tumor cells are deficient in p53 tumor suppressor gene function, a p53 retroviral vector will be used to transfer a wild-type p53 gene into the tumor mass. In lung cancers that over-express the K-ras oncogene, a vector containing an anti-sense K-ras gene will be transferred. The anti-sense K-ras vector will produce mirror image RNA molecules that will bind and block translation of RNA produced by the oncogene. The RNA:RNA hybrids are then degraded by the cell. Experiments in tissue culture and in animals have demonstrated that either the insertion of the p53 tumor suppressor gene or the anti-sense K-ras oncogene can result in destruction of the genetically-altered tumor.[38,39]

T-LYMPHOCYTE GENE THERAPY PROTOCOLS

A vigorous anti-tumor immune response is critical for the complete elimination of tumor, especially in patients with disseminated malignancy. Since T-lymphocytes are critical for tumor destruction, investi gators have grown T-lymphocytes from tumor biopsies (tumor-infiltrating lymphocytes or TIL) in high dose recombinant IL-2 (rIL-2) in tissue culture, expanded them in number and then reinjected them into patients. These TIL are typically CD8+ T-lymphocytes that will destroy the tumor in vitro in a tumor antigen-specific cytotoxic immune response to high dose rIL-2. Since only about 30% of patients with metastatic melanoma will have a measurable clinical anti-tumor response following the reinfusion of the TIL, investigators wanted to study the trafficking and survival of the TIL in vivo in an effort to learn how to improve the efficacy of the therapy. The initial clinical trial involved the insertion of a marker gene (neomycin phosphotransferase II; NeoR) into a fraction of the TIL to be reinfused.[40] This initial TIL study confirmed the safety of retroviral-mediated gene transfer and the trafficking of TIL to tumor, but did not identify a subset of TIL that contained the anti-tumor activity.

Based on the information that TIL could traffic to tumor, researchers wanted to determine if TIL could be used to deliver cytokine gene products directly to tumor deposits. This approach could theoretically improve both efficacy and the safety of cytokine therapy. The initial experiment proposed the use of human TNF gene-modified TIL to deliver locally high concentrations of TNF directly to the tumor.[41] TNF is a chemical that is normally produced by T-lymphocytes and if infused in sufficient amounts in mice can completely destroy tumors. Unfortunately, the intravenous infusion of TNF in humans has significant adverse side effects, limiting the maximum tolerated dose well below the effective per kilogram dose in mice. This experiment is currently in an early toxicity trial stage. The pace of these human experiments have been slowed due to a poor efficiency of gene transfer into human TIL and a down regulation of cytokine expression by the human

T-lymphocytes.[42] There are no published results available about the human clinical aspects of the trial at this time.

CONCLUSIONS

As investigators focus increasing quantities of resources on the development of gene therapy for cancer, there will undoubtedly be major improvements in current therapies. However, there is no reason to believe that gene therapy will produce a magic bullet for all types of solid tumors as the field evolves. There will likely be problems associated with gene transfer efficiency in humans and unforeseen physiological consequences of the inserted gene. Nonetheless, there appears to be a growing consensus that gene therapy will transform medical practice and the overall health of humankind much as immunization and antibiotics did during the past century. As our knowledge in genetics grows, so does our hope for new opportunities for the prevention and treatment of cancer.

REFERENCES

1 Miller AD. Human gene therapy comes of age. Nature 1992; 357: 455-460.
2 Salmons B, Gunzburg WH. Targeting of retroviral vectors for gene therapy. Hum Gene Ther 1993; 4: 129-141.
3 Rosenfeld MA, Siegfried W, Yoshimura K, et al. Adenovirus-mediated transfer of a recombinant α1-antitrypsin gene to the lung epithelium in vivo. Science 1991; 252: 431-434.
4 Mulligan RC. The basic science of gene therapy. Science 1993; 260: 926-932.
5 Culver KW, Blaese RM. Gene therapy for cancer. Trend Genet 1994; 10: 174-178.
6 Tepper RI, Pattengale PK, Leder P. Murine interleukin-4 displays potent anti-tumor activity in vivo. Cell 1989; 57: 503-512.
7 Colombo MP, Forni G. Cytokine gene transfer in tumor inhibition and tumor therapy: where are we now? Immunol Today 1994; 15: 48-51.
8 Townsend SE, Allison JP. Tumor rejection after direct costimulation of CD8+ T cells by B7-transfected melanoma cells. Science 1993; 259: 368-370.
9 Brenner MK, Furman WL, Santana VM, Bowman L, Meyer W. Phase I study of cytokine-gene modified autologous neuroblastoma cells for treatment of relapsed/refractory neuroblastoma. Hum Gene Ther 1992; 3: 665-676.
10 Gansbacher B, Houghton A, Livingston P. A pilot study of immunization with HLA-A2 matched allogeneic melanoma cells that secrete interleukin-2 in patients with metastatic melanoma. Hum Gene Ther 1992; 3: 677-690.
11 Gansbacher B, Motzer R, Houghton A, Bander N. A pilot study of immunization with interleukin-2 secreting allogeneic HLA-A2 matched renal cell carcinoma cells in patients with advanced renal cell carcinoma. Hum Gene Ther 1992; 3: 691-703.
12 Rosenberg SA, Anderson WF, Blaese RM, et al. Immunization of cancer patients using autologous cancer cells modified by insertion of the gene for interleukin-2. Hum Gene Ther 1992; 3: 75-90.
13 Rosenberg SA, Anderson WF, Asher AL, et al. Immunization of cancer patients using autologous cancer cells modified by insertion of the gene for tumor necrosis factor. Hum Gene Ther 1992; 3: 57-73.
14 Tsai S-CJ, Gansbacher B, Tait L, Miller FR, Heppner GH. Induction of antitumor immunity by interleukin-2 gene-transduced mouse mammary tumor cells versus transduced mammary stromal fibroblasts. J Natl Cancer Inst 1993; 85: 546-553.

15 Trojan J, Blossey BK, Johnson RT, et al. Loss of tumorigenicity of rat glioblastoma directed by episome-based antisense cDNA transcription of the insulin-like growth factor-1. Proc Natl Acad Sci USA 1992; 89: 4874-4878.
16 Trojan J, Johnson TR, Rudin SD, et al. Treatment and prevention of rat glioblastoma by immunogenic C6 cells expressing antisense insulin-like growth factor 1 RNA. Science 1993; 259: 94-97.
17 Nabel GJ, Chang A, Nabel EG, Plautz G. Immunotherapy of malignancy by in vivo gene transfer into tumors. Hum Gene Ther 1992; 3: 399-410.
18 Oldfield EH, Culver KW, Ram Z, Blaese RM. A clinical protocol: Gene therapy for the treatment of brain tumors using intra-tumoral transduction with the thymidine kinase gene and intravenous ganciclovir. Hum Gene Ther 1993; 4: 39-69.
19 Ostrand-Rosenberg S, Thakur A, Clements V. Rejection of mouse sarcoma cells after transfection of MHC class II genes. J Immunol 1990; 144: 4068-4071.
20 Plautz GE, Yang Z-Y, Wu B-Y, et al. Immunotherapy of malignancy by in vivo gene transfer into tumors. Proc Natl Acad Sci USA 1993; 90: 4645-4649.
21 Nabel GJ, Nabel EG, Yang Z, et al. Direct gene transfer with DNA-liposome complexes in melanoma: Expression, biologic activity, and lack of toxicity in humans. Proc Natl Acad Sci USA 1993; 90: 11307-11311.
22 Ram Z, Culver KW, Walbridge S, et al. In situ retroviral-mediated gene transfer for the treatment of brain tumors in rats. Cancer Res 1993; 53: 83-88.
23 Moolten FL. Tumor chemosensitivity conferred by inserted herpes thymidine kinase genes: Paradigm for a prospective cancer control strategy. Cancer Res 1986; 46: 5276-5281.
24 Short MP, Choi JK, Lee A, Malick A, Breakfield XO, Martuza RL. Gene delivery to glioma cells in rat brain by grafting of a retrovirus packaging cell line. J Neurosci Res 1990; 27: 427-433.
25 Ram Z, Culver KW, Walbridge S, Frank JA, Blaese RM, Oldfield EH. Toxicity studies of retroviral-mediated gene transfer for the treatment of brain tumors. J Neurosurg 1993; 79: 400-407.
26 Culver KW, Ram Z, Walbridge S, Ishii H, Oldfield EH, Blaese RM. In vivo gene transfer with retroviral vector producer cells for treatment of experimental brain tumors. Science 1992; 256: 1550-1552.
27 Ram Z, Culver KW, Walbridge S, Frank JA, Blaese RM, Oldfield EH. Toxicity studies of retroviral-mediated gene transfer for the treatment of brain tumors. J Neurosurg 1993; 79: 400-407.
28 Elion GB. The chemotherapeutic exploitation of virus-specified enzymes. Adv Enz Regul 1980; 18: 53-66.
29 Bi WL, Parysek LM, Warnick R, Stambrook PJ. In vitro evidence that metabolic cooperation is responsible for the bystander effect observed with HSV tk retroviral gene therapy. Hum Gene Ther 1993; 4: 725-732.
30 Freeman SM, Abboud CN, Whartenby KA, et al. The 'bystander effect': Tumor regression when a fraction of the tumor mass is genetically modified. Cancer Res 1993; 53: 5274-5283.
31 Culver KW, Van Gilder J, Link CJ, et al. Gene therapy for the treatment of malignant brain tumors with in vivo tumor transduction with the herpes simplex thymidine kinase gene/ganciclovir system. Hum Gene Ther 1994; 5: 343-377.
32 Culver KW, Blaese RM. Gene therapy for adenosine deaminase deficiency and malignant solid tumors. In: Wolff JA, ed. Gene Therapeutics. Boston: Birkhauser, 1994.
33 Caruso M, Panis Y, Gagandeep S, et al. Regression of established macroscopic liver metastases after in situ transduction of a suicide gene. Proc Natl Acad Sci USA 1993; 90: 7024-7028.
34 Plautz G, Nabel EG, Nabel GJ. Selective elimination of recombinant genes in vivo with a suicide retroviral vector. New Biol 1991; 7: 709-715.
35 Senter PD. Activation of prodrugs by antibody-enzyme conjugates: a new approach to cancer therapy. FASEB J 1990; 4: 188-193.

36 Gutierre AA, Lemoine NR, Sikora K. Gene therapy for cancer. Lancet 1992; 339: 715-721.
37 Mullen CA, Kilstrup M, Blaese RM. Transfer of the bacterial gene for cytosine deaminase to mammalian cells confers lethal sensitivity to 5-fluorocytosine: A negative selection system. Proc Natl Acad Sci USA 1992; 89: 33-37.
38 Fujiwara T, Grimm EA, Cai DW, Owen-Schaub LB, Roth JA. A retroviral wild-type p53 expression vector penetrates human lung cancer spheroids and inhibits growth by inducing apoptosis. Cancer Res 1993; 53: 4129-4133.
39 Zhang Y, Mukhopadhyay T, Donehower, et al. Retroviral vector-mediated transduction of K-ras antisense RNA into human lung cancer cells inhibits expression of the malignant phenotype. Hum Gene Ther 1993; 4: 451-460.
40 Rosenberg SA, Aebersold P, Cornetta K, et al. Gene transfer into humans-Immunotherapy of patients with advanced melanoma, using tumor-infiltrating lymphocytes modified by retroviral gene transduction. N Engl J Med 1990; 323: 570-578.
41 Rosenberg SA, Kasid A, Anderson WF, et al. TNF/TIL human gene therapy clinical protocol. Hum Gene Ther 1991; 1: 443-462.
42 Hwu P, Yannelli J, Kriegler M, et al. Functional and molecular characterization of tumor-infiltrating lymphocytes transduced with tumor necrosis factor-α cDNA for the gene therapy of cancer in humans. J Immunol 1993; 150: 4104-4115.

British Medical Bulletin (1995) Vol. 51, No. 1, pp.205–216

Gene therapy and viral vaccination: the interface

G W G Wilkinson and L K Borysiewicz

Department of Medicine, University of Wales College of Medicine, Cardiff, UK

Live viral vaccines have had a major impact on the incidence of acute virus infections world-wide. Virus infections recognised as future vaccine targets will require a modified approach based on a detailed understanding of the immunobiology of specific infections combined with the application of new technologies designed to generate specific and appropriate protective immunity. A similar vector technology directed at in vivo gene delivery is currently being exploited both for gene therapy and vaccination. The induction of an immune response to an expressed transgene represents a potential hazard for a gene therapy protocol but is the object of a vaccine strategy. In vivo gene delivery using replication-competent or replication-deficient viral vector systems and by direct transfer of naked DNA can generate an effective humoral, secretory and cell-mediated immune response to expressed transgenes.

Prevention of acute exanthems of childhood and the eradication of smallpox by vaccination are landmarks in modern medicine. Viral vaccines in clinical use can be classified as: live, inactivated or subunit (Table 1). Most live viral vaccines are attenuated so that they infect but do not produce disease in the vaccinee. Experience has shown that live vaccines have advantages: (i) they can generate a comprehensive immune response (antibody-mediated, cell-mediated and mucosal); (ii) a small inoculum is required making live vaccines relatively inexpensive to produce; (iii) long-lived protection is induced. However, some live vaccines can be either reactogenic or unsuitable for certain popu lations. Future targets for anti-viral vaccination (Table 2) may also not be amenable to this approach. Many of these agents cannot be propagated in vitro, while some can establish persistent infections or are potentially oncogenic; the long-term safety of new live attenuated viruses is of paramount importance. Subunit vaccines are attractive but the advantages associated with using live attenuated viruses in inducing a long lived and wide ranging immune responses may be essential for effective protection. This scenario poses new challenges for vaccine development.

Table 1 Conventional vaccines in common use

Live	Inactivated	Subunit
Polio (OPV)	Polio (IPV)	HBV (recombinant)
Measles	Hepatitis A virus	Influenza A
Mumps	Rabies	
Rubella	Japanese encephalitis	
Yellow fever	Tick-borne encephalitis	
Adenovirus	Influenza A	
Varicella Zoster		
Vaccinia		

Table 2 Virus targets for vaccination

Viruses	Problem for vaccine development
Dengue	Antibody enhancement, variation
EBV	Latency, transforming, immune evasion
HBV	'Latency', age of infection
HCV	'Latency', variability
HIV infection	Variability, immune escape
HSV/CMV	Latency
Influenza	Variability and secondary hosts
Measles	Age of infection (less developed regions)
Papillomavirus	Multiple genotypes, transforming
Rotavirus	Age of infection; immunogen
RSV	Age of infection, vaccine history

Gene therapy can be defined as 'the transfer of new genetic material to the cells of an individual resulting in therapeutic benefit to the individual'.[1] There are therefore parallels with live vaccination in that both involve transfer and expression of new genetic material with potential or actual (in the case of post exposure vaccination) therapeutic benefit. However, there is a conflict of interests since for gene therapy it is essential to limit immune responses to all elements of the vector and the expressed transgene. Expression systems for gene therapy require:

- gene targeting to the appropriate cell.
- appropriate levels, location and duration of expression to correct the disease phenotype.
- delivery should be non-toxic to the target cell.

For vaccination, it is often necessary only to express the transgene long enough to stimulate an effective immune response. Vector technology now being rapidly developed for somatic cell gene therapy, can also be exploited in vaccine design to overcome the constraints of problematical viral targets (Table 2).

At the simplest level, recombinant technology provides for the efficient expression of a gene product in vitro to produce large quantities of antigens for subunit vaccines. This is exemplified by the hepatitis B virus (HBV) surface antigen expressed in yeast. These simple applications have now been extended to human clinical trials with recombinant vectors for both vaccine development and gene therapy. Gene therapy has relied almost exclusively on virus-based systems for gene delivery and has been instrumental in the development of replication-deficient vectors. Direct DNA transfer systems (e.g. DNA inoculation and lipofection) are now also being exploited for in vivo gene delivery. We review the current and potential application of in vivo gene transfer systems in vaccine development.

VACCINIA

The origin of vaccinia virus is uncertain. Although Jenner originally advocated the use of cowpox for smallpox vaccination (vacca *L.* = cow), genetic analysis has shown vaccinia to be distinct from both cowpox virus and variola.[2] Nevertheless vaccinia is an orthopox virus which replicates in the cytoplasm of infected cells, has a large DNA genome of approx 185 kb, can accommodate exceptionally large insertions (in excess of 25 kb) and can promote high level expression of recombinant proteins.[3]It therefore has a number of distinct advantages as a live vector in man for anti-viral immunisation in:

- it is inexpensive
- readily administered by scarification
- induction of superficial lesion is evidence of vaccine take
- long-term protection elicited by single vaccination
- vaccine stable in long-term storage
- incidence of complications well-characterised.

However, potential drawbacks have to be considered especially the safety profile of vaccinia itself. This was well established in the global eradication programme.[2,4] The incidence of complications varies with primary or repeat vaccination, vaccine strain, age of vaccinee, population group (Fig. 1). The generation of the characteristic pustular lesion at the site of scarification, mild fever and lymphadenopathy are accepted consequences of successful vaccination.[2] However, significant complication do arise, which include secondary spread of lesion, rash, progressive vaccinia, eczema vaccinatum and encephalitic disease (Fig. 1). This resulted in restricted vaccination to groups at high risk, including those with immune disorders. Clearly screening for these disorders and avoidance of use in the first year will reduce the overall risk from the vector itself, to levels where the risk:benefit ratio will in many instances make this an acceptable strategy.

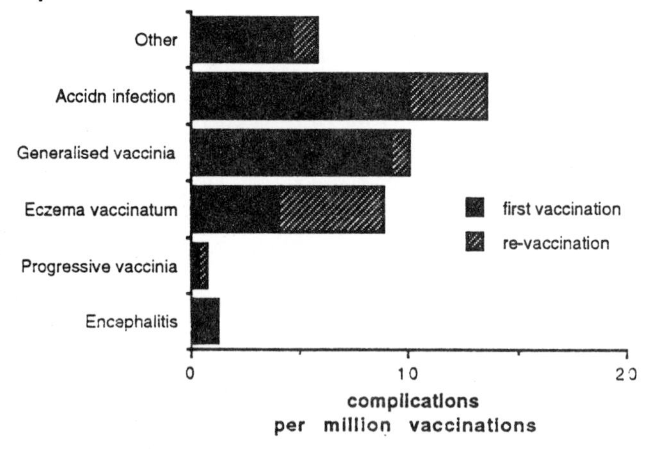

Fig. 1 Complication rates for primary and re-vaccination in the US, 1968. The overall complication rate was 40.4 per million total vaccinations and 72% of complications occured at primary vaccination (complication rate = 74.7/million primary vaccinations). The mortality rate was 0.02% for recorded complications (Lane et al, 1969[4]).

Attempts have been made to produce more disabled orthopox virus vectors.[3] Vaccinia has been further attenuated by introducing defined mutations into genes that are not essential for in vitro replication (e.g. thymidine kinase) and some of these constructs have retained a capacity to generate immune responses to cloned transgenes. An alternative approach has been to insert the gene for IL-2 into vaccinia. IL-2 stimulates the host's response both to vaccinia and the expressed transgenes, such recombinants consequently produce smaller lesions and are less pathogenic. Unfortunately altering the vector may negate the extensive available safety data (Fig. 1). Interest has grown in the application of avipox vectors[4] (e.g. canarypox, fowlpox) which can infect and express recombinant proteins in human cells but are unable to replicate. Although intrinsically safer, the data is much more limited than that for vaccinia. The assessment of risk: benefit will continue to be a problem; it must consider whether an absolute measurement of hazard is essential for vaccination with informed consent for any particular targeted disease.

Immune response to recombinant vaccinia

Vaccinia vectors have played a crucial role in the analysis of the immune response to viruses. Expression of recombinant products using vaccinia, has allowed qualitative and quantitative analysis of the relative importance of immune responses to individual virus gene products, in vivo and in vitro. Such studies have also established the relative contribution of antibody and cell-mediated immunity in combating virus infection.[3]

The ability of live vaccines to induce T cell responses is important if full immunity against a pathogen is to be generated. Although intrinsically safer, non-replicating subunit vaccines are at present inefficient in inducing T cell responses, at least until new adjuvants or delivery methods are developed. Experimentally, vaccinia recombinants can generate a protective CD8 cytotoxic T cell response against lymphocytic choriomeningitis and murine cytomegalovirus, in vivo. This suggests that although vaccinia infection of a cell is associated with shut-off of *de novo* host cell protein synthesis within 30–60 min of infection, a gene under the control of an appropriate vaccinia 'early' promoter can be processed and associate with MHC class I. It remains to be established whether such immunity is long-lived in the absence of antigenic re-stimulation, although in the case of natural infection Lau et al,[6] have suggested that, once established, virus specific CTL precursor numbers remain constant. This implies that if an adequate immunisation schedule with a live vector is used then the CTL response may be long-lasting.

Attention has often focused on the CD8 CTL response, but vaccinia also induces a range of TH1 and TH2 CD4 responses, including CTL. Cytokine release from such T cells is crucial for the efficient generation of antibody and DTH responses; as well as for its direct role in non-specific immunity, such as interferon production.

Vaccinia recombinants and vaccination programmes

Vaccinia recombinants are now being used in experimental human and veterinary vaccination programmes. In veterinary practice two distinct approaches have been taken. Firstly, disseminated large-scale release of vaccinia-rabies recombinants (encoding glycoprotein G) has induced widespread immunity against rabies in wild canines in South Belgium, by oral transmission of infected bait. This high uptake of the recombinant resulted in a virtual eradication of rabies within the test area with no transmission to man.[7] Secondly, advantage may be taken of the large number of inserts that can be made in vaccinia without inhibiting vector replication. In veterinary practice economic consideration and efficient generation of short-term immunity is of major importance. Several diseases, especially in developing countries, are under investigation. Of particular interest is the development of a rinderpest vaccine which was re-introduced into cattle with development of effective immunity against rinderpest in the absence of poxvirus pathology.[8] As these studies are a deliberate environmental release they will have to be closely scrutinised especially with regard to transmission by rodents into domestic animals and consequently to man. To date this has not been a problem.

Vaccinia and canarypox recombinants expressing HIV env have been used alone or with other immunogens in clinical trials. Both stimulate humoral and cell-mediated immunity in re-vaccinees as well as primary vaccinees, although the magnitude of T cell responses against the inserted sequence was greater in the latter group.[9] This may prove a future problem but to date numbers are small and follow-up periods short (<5 years). In addition a canarypox recombinant expressing rabies glycoprotein produced minimal reactions and induced specific antibodies.[5]

Several clinical studies are in progress using a variety of vaccinia recombinants. We are studying a vaccinia recombinant (TA-HPV) encoding a mutagenised form of the human papillomavirus 16 and 18, E6 and E7 genes as an immunotherapy for human papillomavirus associated cervical cancer. In such studies the vaccinia-induced cytopathology and lack of persistence, which reduces the value of this virus as a vector for gene therapy, is a positive future, reducing risk associated with inserted sequences which could be harmful if continually expressed.

ADENOVIRUS VECTORS

Adenoviruses are usually associated with asymptomatic or mild upper respiratory tract infections but can produce significant disease: keratoconjunctivitis, gastroenteritis, lower respiratory tract infection and disseminated infection in immunocompromised individuals. There are some 47 serotypes of human adenovirus with variable prevalence and disease-associations. Outbreaks of Acute Respiratory Disease (ARD) in US military recruits led to the introduction of a live vaccine[10] which is based on adenovirus types 4 and 7 and administered as an enteric-coated tablet. The vaccine strains are not specifically attenuated, although their virulence may have been diminished through propagation in vitro, but depend on the route of administration not to cause disease. This vaccine has proved to be safe, non-reactogenic and effective in controlling ARD in millions of recruits over 20 years. Most vectors and recombinants are, however, based on adenovirus type 5, a common serotype associated with mild infections.[11–13] In a limited human clinical trial, adenovirus 5 also generated an immune response when given as an enteric coated vaccine.[10] These observations have encouraged the use of adenovirus recombinants in vaccine development.

Adenovirus is a well-characterised virus which grows well in vitro, and is amenable to manipulation.[14] It has a double-stranded DNA genome of 35 kb and replicates in the nucleus of infected cells. Adenovirus vectors are either **replication-competent** or **replication-deficient**. While the amount of DNA that can be packaged into an adenovirus particle is limited, deletion of the non-essential E3 genes permit insertion of up 5 kb of foreign DNA (Fig. 2). Further deletions affect virus viability but vectors have been constructed based on E1 deletion mutants. This gene region is required for activating transcription from the adenovirus genome. Adenovirus E1 deletion mutants are therefore replication-deficient vectors which can only be propagated on a helper cell line expressing E1 functions (usually 293 cells). A replication-deficient adenovirus recombinant containing a transgene cloned under the control of a constitutive promoter can be propagated in 293 cells and then used to infect a target cell where only the inserted gene will be expressed (Fig. 2).

Replication-competent adenovirus vectors

Replication-competent adenovirus vectors have been used in vaccine research as an alternative to vaccinia.[12] Adenovirus recombinants have also been shown to be capable of inducing antibody, secretory[15] and cell mediated immunity which is protective against experimental pseudorabies, rabies, VSV, HSV and rotavirus infection.[16] Since recombinants expressing genes from HBV, HIV, CMV and RSV generate immune responses in animals, they are now being tested in man – 3 human volunteers have been immunised orally with a single dose of enteric coated adenovirus 7 encoding HBV surface antigen.[17]

Replication-deficient adenovirus vectors

Replication-deficient adenovirus vectors have come to prominence because of their application in gene therapy.[18] Although virus-based, the vector is conceptually similar to a direct DNA transfer system as the adenovirus is only used as a delivery vehicle for the transgene to the target cell. Ideally, the recombinant gene product is expressed in the absence of any adenovirus-specific transcription or cytotoxicity. Adenovirus $E1^-$ recombinants promote transgene expression in a wide range of cells (respiratory endothelium, hepatocytes, skeletal and cardiac muscle, neurones and astrocytes) making them a flexible gene delivery

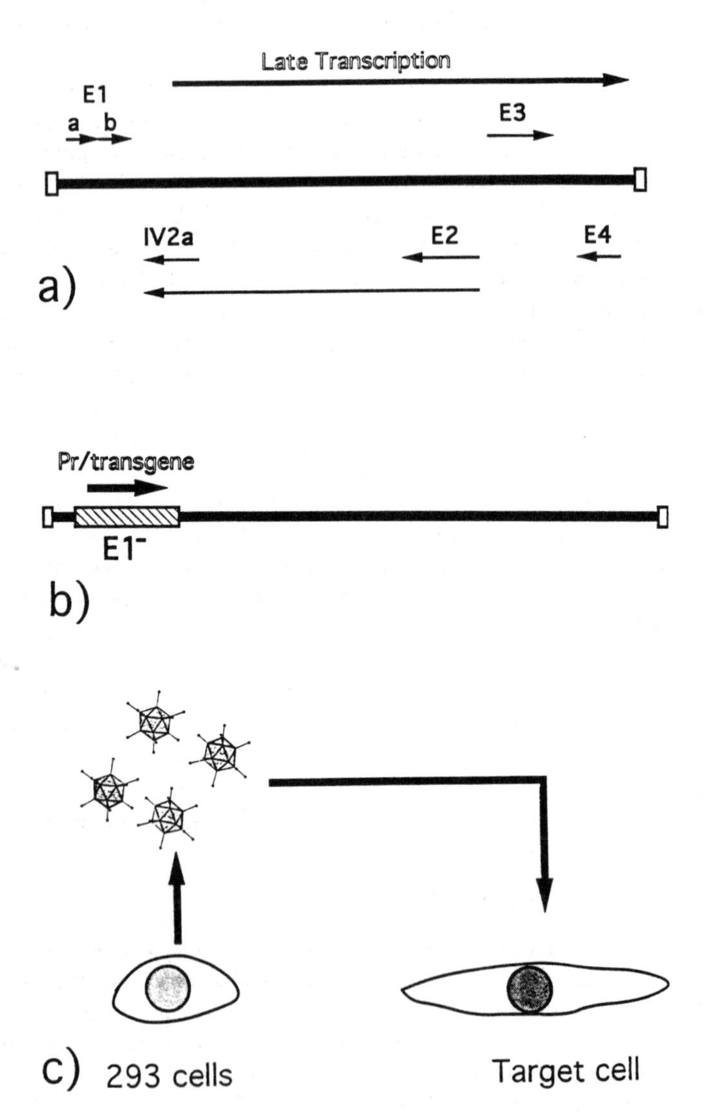

Fig. 2 **(a)** Simplified transcriptional map of adenovirus gene showing locations of early and late transcriptional units. Genes are **usually** inserted at either the E1 or E3 gene regions. **(b)** To generate a replication-deficient Ad recombinant transgenes are usually inserted into the E1 gene region under the control of a constitutive promoter (e.g. the CMV IE promoter or RSV LTR). **(c)**Adenovirus E1⁻ recombinants can be propagated in a cell line (e.g. 293 cells) expressing E1 helper functions and then used to infect the target cell (in vitro or in vivo) where there is efficient expression of the transgene only.

vehicle. Since there is no specific mechanism for maintaining the virus genome, expression is transient; nevertheless transgene expression can persist for >6 months in some cells.[16,18]

Although this replication-defective vector should not allow the expression of adenovirus proteins, when adenovirus *cftr* recombinants have been used to treat cystic fibrosis, an inflammatory response with **high** doses of adenovirus has been observed.[19] Recently it has been shown that in mice this vector can induce CD8+ CTLs to a breakthrough of early and late genes from the vector.[20,21] However, if an adenovirus with additional mutations in the E2a gene was used, the inflammatory response was diminished. These studies underline the importance of not inducing cellular immunity to the vector or transgene in gene therapy. In contrast, for vaccination, it may be important to produce an effective CTL response to the transgene. Thus these CTL responses to an adenovirus E1 deleted vector when administered to a mucosal surface is encouraging for their use in vaccine delivery.

High level expression of recombinant antigens is possible with replication-deficient adenovirus vectors.[16] This provides for biological containment, anatomically localised delivery to mucosal surfaces with low reactogenicity, yet effective immunity. There is no need for cell-to-cell spread of the vaccinating agent and a single immunisation has been sufficient to elicit protection in an animal model. Adenovirus recombinants can still promote transgene expression after multiple exposures to the vector. Encouraging results, with replication-defective adenovirus recombinants expressing a pseudorabies glycoprotein, a flavivirus non-structural protein, EBV gp220/360 and the measles virus nucleocapsid eliciting protection against virus challenge,[16] suggest further applications of this approach in man.

RETROVIRAL VECTORS

Retroviruses have been widely used in gene therapy protocols as a replication-deficient transducing vector capable of promoting stable chromosomal integration of a transgene into a target cell population. The transgene is passed to all daughter cells and provides long-term expression. While retroviral recombinants can stimulate an immune response,[22] they are not ideally suited as vehicles for ‘conventional’ recombinant vaccine delivery. Characteristically, retroviruses produce modest levels of expression, grow to relatively low titre, are relatively labile, can be inactivated by complement, are potentially oncogenic and theoretically could be rescued by endogenous retroviruses.[16] It is possible that further development of the vector as a packaging and delivery system may allow their use as a vaccine vector. Already retroviral vectors have been extensively used for ex vivo gene therapy into lineages of dividing cells where efficient gene transfer and subsequent expression has been found. They may also find a direct role in adoptive immunotherapy with ex vivo CTL. Studies from Seattle[23] with such cells allow a marker to be incorporated into the cell lines used as well as inserting a gene to block their effect should immunopathology arise.

OTHER VECTORS

Many other viruses have been considered and studied in experimental models as vectors for vaccine delivery. Oka strain varicella zoster virus, currently used as a chickenpox vaccine, has been engineered as a vector[24] as has herpes simplex virus.[25] Almond and colleagues have successfully induced anti-viral antibodies to short linear epitopes using poliovirus, but packaging constraints mitigate against widespread application of this system.[26] Although adeno-associated virus (AAV) vectors have many potential advantages as transducing vectors[27] for gene therapy, their application is currently restricted by technical constraints and they bestow no obvious advantage as agents for vaccination. Other vectors may also provide a suitable vehicle for vaccine delivery, notably bacterial expression vectors. However, as these are not being developed for gene therapy they will not be considered further.

Gene therapy may itself be applied to virus infection. Virus infections require intracellular replication and virus gene expression and this can be directly targeted by gene therapy. Introduction into cells of genetic elements designed to interfere with the virus replicative cycle - e.g. antisense RNA, ribozymes or a trans-dominant repressor[28] can be used. This has been used to inhibit virus replication in cell culture and human studies with a retrovirus encoding antisense RNA to block HIV replication may soon start.

DIRECT DNA TRANSFER

Considerable excitement was generated in vaccine research by the observation that direct inoculation muscle cells with naked plasmid DNA encoding the influenza A nucleoprotein could induce antigen expression, a specific antibody response, a specific CTL response and protection against virus challenge.[29] This direct approach is being vigorously investigated for many viral systems for vaccination as well as gene therapy, e.g. Duchenne's muscular dystrophy. A further recent advance has been the development of 'Gene Gun' in which DNA coated on minute gold beads are fired directly into the skin with in vivo gene expression is achieved when beads directly enter cells of the epidermis. This innovative technology can be used to generate a comprehensive, protective immune response using relative small amounts of DNA. Other systems for the enhanced in vivo intracellular delivery of naked DNA (e.g. receptor-mediated endocytosis, adenovirus particles, and lipofection) also have the potential to be applied to vaccination.

DISCUSSION

Vaccination has played a major role in controlling infectious disease, as exemplified by the eradication of smallpox and the successful programmes in the UK against polio, measles, mumps and rubella. Considerable scope remains, however, to develop both existing and novel vaccine strategies. Measles is still responsible for more than 1 million deaths annually, respiratory syncytial virus is a major cause of infant mortality, more than 1 million deaths annually are caused by rotavirus infections, viruses cause an estimated 20% of all cancers world-wide[30] and no effective strategy has yet been developed to control the HIV pandemic.

Vaccines that are administered to healthy individuals must be developed with caution ensuring that the use of new technologies does not produce unacceptable complications. However, this must not be used as an excuse for not studying the huge potential benefit that these technologies offer for diseases identified above. Advances in vector technology must be coupled with a greater understanding of protective immunity against viruses: the role of cellular immune response; antigen processing and presentation; antigen recognition etc. A detailed understanding of virus pathogenesis is essential, since the induction of immunopathology can aggravate disease. Gene therapy is constrained by current technology for in vivo gene delivery and provides impetus for the development of new, safe, and efficient systems. Enhanced technologies for in vivo gene delivery can be exploited to develop a new generation of safe, economical and effective vaccines.

REFERENCES

1 Morgan RA, Anderson WF. Human Gene Therapy. Annu Rev Biochem 1993: 191–217.
2 Henderson DA, Fenner F. 'Smallpox and vaccinia' In: Plotkin SA, Mortimer EA, eds. Vaccines, 2nd edn. Philadelphia: Saunders 1994.
3 Moss B. Vaccinia virus vectors. In Ellis RW, ed. Vaccines: new approaches to immunological problems. Biotechnology 1992; 20: 345–362.
4 Lane JM, Ruben FL, Neff JM, Millar JD. Complications of smallpox vaccination, 1968. National surveillance in the United States. N Engl J Med 1969; 281: 1201–1208.
5 Cadoz M, Strady A, Meignier B, et al. Immunisation with canarypox expressing rabies glycoprotein. Lancet 1992; 339: 1429–1432.
6 Lau LL, Jamieson BD, Somasundarum T, Ahmed R. Cytotoxic T-cell memory without antigen. Nature 1994; 369: 648–652.
7 Brochier B, Kieny MP, Coppens P, et al. Large-scale eradiction of rabies using recombinant rabies vaccine. Nature 1991; 354: 520–522.
8 Giavedoni L, Jones L, Mebus C, Yilma T. A vaccinia virus double recombinant expressing the F and H genes of rinderpest virus protects cattle against rinderpest and causes no pock lesions. Proc Natl Acad Sci USA 1991; 88: 8011–8015.

9 Emini EA, Putnet SD. Human immunodeficiency virus. In: Ellis RW, ed. Vaccines: new approaches to immunological problems. Biotechnology 1992; 20: 309–326.
10 Rubin RA, Rorke LB. Adenovirus vaccines. In: Plotkin SA, Mortimer EA, eds. Vaccines, 2nd edn. Philadelphia: Saunders 1994.
11 Graham FL, Prevec L. Manipulation of adenovirus vectors. In: Murray EJ, ed. Methods in Molecular Biology, Vol. 7. 1991; 7: 109–128.
12 Graham FL, Prevec L. Adenovirus-based expression vectors and recombinant vaccines. In: Ellis RW, ed. Vaccines: new approaches to immunological problems. Biotechnology 1992; 20: 363–390.
13 Grunhaus A, Horwitz MS. Adenoviruses as cloning vectors. Semin Virol 1992; 2: 237–252.
14 Horwitz MS. Adenoviruses and their replication. In: Fields BN, Knipe DM eds. Virology, 2nd edn, New York: Raven Press 1990.
15 Gallichan WS, Johnson DC, Graham FL, Rosenthal KL. Mucosal immunity and protection after intranasal immunization with recombinant adenovirus expressing herpes simplex virus glycoprotein B. J Infect Dis 1993; 168: 622–629.
16 Wilkinson GWG. Gene Therapy and Viral Vaccination. Rev Med Micro 1994; 5: 97–106.
17 Tacket CO, Losonsky G, Lubeck MD et al. Initial safety and immunogenicity studies of an oral recombinant adenohepatitis B vaccine. Vaccine 1992; 10: 673–676.
18 Wilkinson GWG, Darley RL, Lowenstein PR. Viral vectors for gene therapy. In: Latchman DS, ed. From genetics to gene therapy. Oxford: Bios Scientific, 1994.
19 Crystal RG, McElvaney NG, Rosenfeld MA et al. Administration of an adenovirus containing the human CFTR cDNA to the respiratory tract of individuals with cystic fibrosis. Nature Genet 1994; 8: 42–51.
20 Yang Y, Ertl HCJ, Wilson JM. MHC class I restricted cytotoxic T lymphocytes to viral antigens destroy hepatocytes in mice infected with E1-deleted recombinant adenoviruses. Immunity 1994; 1: 433–442.
21 Yang Y, Nunes FA, Berencsi K, Gonczol E, Engelhardt JF, Wilson, JM. Inactivation of E2a in recombinant adenovirus improves the prospect for gene therapy in cystic fibrosis. Nature Genet 1994; 7: 362–369
22 Laube LS, Burrascano M, Dejesus CE et al. Cytotoxic T lymphocyte and antibody responses generated in rhesus monkeys immunized with retroviral vector-transduced fibroblasts expressing human immunodeficiency virus type-1 IIIB env/rev proteins. Hum Gene Ther 1994; 5: 853–862.
23 Riddell SR, Watanabe KS, Goodrich JM, Li CR, Agha ME, Greenberg PD. Restoration of viral immunity in immunodeficient humans by the adoptive transfer of T cell clones. Science 1992; 257: 238–241.
24 Lowe RS, Keller PM, Keech BJ et al. Varicella-zoster virus as a live vector for the expression of foreign genes. Proc Natl Acad Sci USA 1987; 84: 3896–3900.
25 Meignier B, Longnecker R, Roizman B. In vivo behaviour of genetically engineered herpes simplex viruses R7017 and R7020: construction and evaluation in rodents. J Infect Dis 1988; 158: 602–614.
26 Evans DJ, McKeating J, Meredith JM et al. An engineered poliovirus chimaera elicits broadly reactive HIV-1 neutralising antibodies. Nature 1989; 339: 385–389.
27 Muzyczka N. Use of adeno-associated virus as a general transduction vector for mammalian cells. In Muzyczka N, ed. Viral expression vectors. Curr Top Microbiol Immunol 1992; 157: 97–129.
28 Yu M, Poeschla E, Wong-Staal F. Progress towards gene therapy for HIV infection. Gene Ther 1994; 1: 13–26.
29 Ulmer JB, Donnelly JJ, Parker SE et al. Heterologous protection against influenza by injection of DNA encoding viral protein. Science 1993; 259: 1745–1749.
30 Dalgleish AG. Viruses and cancer. Br Med Bull 1991; 47: 21–46.

British Medical Bulletin (1995) Vol. 51, No. 1, pp.217–225

Therapeutic antisense and ribozymes

J J Rossi

Center for Molecular Biology and Gene Therapy, Loma Linda University School of Medicine, Loma Linda, California, USA

The regulation of expression of genetic information by complementary pairing of sense and antisense nucleic acid strands has been termed 'antisense', and is a mechanism used throughout nature to regulate gene expression. It is now possible to design antisense DNA oligonucleotides, or catalytic antisense RNAs (ribozymes) which can pair with and functionally inhibit the expression of any single stranded nucleic acid in a sequence specific fashion. This high degree of specificity has made them attractive candidates for therapeutic agents. These molecules have the potential for the treatment of a wide variety of diseases. The recent development of retroviral as well as other viral and non-viral based delivery schemes make the clinical use of these molecules a virtual certainty.

Two decades ago the discovery in micro-organisms that regulation of the flow of genetic information was accomplished by complementary RNA-RNA pairing, or 'antisense' [1] provided evidence that perhaps any gene function could be blocked by antisense inhibition. The first successful synthetic antisense DNA applications arrested translation in vitro[2,3] and inhibited replication of Rous Sarcoma virus in cell culture.[4] Artificially produced antisense RNAs were first demonstrated to functionally inhibit expression of genes when the antisense RNAs were injected into frog oocytes.[5,6] These studies were followed by experiments in which the antisense RNAs were expressed intracellulary, resulting in successful inhibition of targeted gene expression in several different systems.[7–9] The most recent developments in antisense technology involve treatment of cells or tissue with deoxyribonucleotides harboring various chemical modifications in the sugar-phosphate backbone which render the DNAs more effective in living cells,[10] or the use of catalytic, antisense RNAs or ribozymes which bind to and irreversibly cleave targeted RNA molecules.[11]

The principles underlying the use of antisense based therapies are straight forward. The antisense, either in the form of a single stranded DNA or RNA molecule, interacts via complementary base-pairing with the targeted RNA. For DNA-RNA hybrids, the RNA involved in base-pairing is a substrate for the cellular enzyme RNAseH.[10] This enzyme, which is used in DNA replication, is primarily found in the nuclear compartment of the cell. Thus, the oligonucleotides should be available in the nucleus to be most effective. Some antisense activity may occur by a simple blockage of a protein interaction or movement along the mRNA as well, although blocking translation with antisense may be more difficult due to helical unwinding activities associated with translocating ribosomes. RNA-RNA duplexes are substrates for yet another cellular enzyme, an adenosine deaminase, which covalently modifies both the antisense and target RNAs by converting adenosines to inosines.[12] This modification functionally inactivates both RNAs. As with DNA-RNA hybrids, in the absence of the deaminase, the antisense may functionally block interactions with or movement of some protein or proteins involved in RNA processing, transport, or ex pression. The third class of antisense therapeutics are RNA molecules with enzymatic activity, or ribozymes. The ability of RNA to function as an enzymatic catalyst was first described for a self-splicing reaction involving the large ribosomal RNA precursor of Tetrahymena[13] and for the RNA component of the *E. coli* RNAseP, an RNA-protein enzyme which cleaves the leader segment from precursor transfer RNA molecules.[14] Small ribozymes have been derived from a single stranded plant viroid and virusoid RNAs that replicate via a rolling circle mechanism (reviewed in[15]). Based upon a shared secondary structure and a conserved set of nucleotides, the term 'hammerhead' has been given to one group of these self-cleavage domains.[16] The simplicity of the hammerhead catalytic domain has made it a popular choice in the design of *trans*-acting ribozymes.[17,18] Utilizing Watson-Crick base pairing, the hammerhead ribozyme can be designed to cleave any target RNA. The requirements at the cleavage site are relatively simple, and virtually any UX (where X is U, C or A) can be targeted (Fig.), although the efficiency of the cleavage reaction can vary over 100 fold between the different combinations.[19]

A second plant derived self-cleavage motif thus far only identified in the negative strand of the tobacco ringspot satellite RNA, has been termed the 'hairpin' or 'paperclip'.[20,21] An engineered version of this catalytic motif has also been shown to be capable of cleaving and multiply turning over a variety of targets in *trans*.[21] A few minimal requirements for the hairpin ribozyme substrate have been discerned and most importantly include an obligatory G at the nucleotide 3′to the site of cleavage. There is otherwise a great deal of flexibility in the substrate-guide sequence combinations making this a potentially useful catalyst against a wide array of RNA targets. These relatively simple catalytic RNAs can be engineered to harbor sequences which facilitate base pairing to any desired RNA target.[22,23] Once paired to the target site, the ribozyme effects a single stranded cleavage of the target RNA, thereby functionally destroying it. An additional attribute of ribozymes is their ability to act catalytically, and functionally destroy multiple targets. This article will focus primarily upon ribozymes and their potential applications in the treatment of human disease.

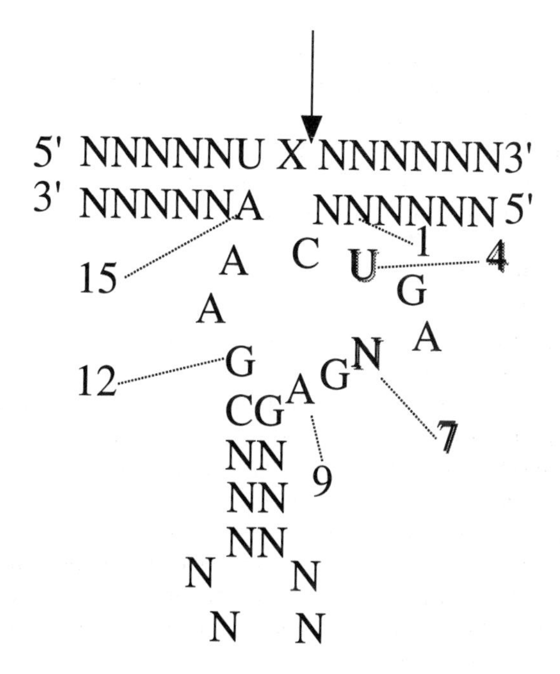

Fig Generalized depiction of a hammerhead ribozyme. The N's represent any nucleotide, and the X represents A, C, or U. The numbering of positions in the hammerhead domain is according to the recently adopted convention for hammerhead ribozymes. The site of substrate cleavage is indicated by the arrow. Once cleavage has occurred, the ribozyme can dissociate from the cleaved products and bind and cleave another substrate molecule.

Ribozymes as potential therapeutic agents

The therapeutic use of ribozymes is an attractive goal which merges the basic and applied sciences. Since all genes are expressed through RNA intermediates, the potential applications are only limited by our knowledge of the disease or diseases associated with a given RNA. In the case of viral infections, ribozymes can be tailor-made to cleave viral transcripts, thereby leaving cellular transcripts untouched. Certain oncogene transcripts also provide specific targets as a consequence of unique codon changes such as in *ras*, or chimeric transcripts generated by chromosomal rearrangements such as those associated with hematologic malignancies, including chronic myelogenous leukemia (CML) and acute lymphoblastic leukemia (ALL). Other malignancies which are characterized by elevated expression of proto-oncogenes are also targets for ribozyme action, since reductions in the levels of these elevated transcripts (and consequently their cognate proteins) can have profound effects on the transformed state.

HIV-1 is a prime target for ribozyme inactivation. As a retrovirus with an RNA genome, there are two windows of opportunity for ribozyme mediated inhibition, the first immediately following infection when all or part of the viral genome is in the form of RNA, and the second following the establishment of integrated provirus from which spliced and full length viral transcripts are produced. We began testing the concept that a ribozyme would be a useful reagent for inhibiting HIV-1 infection by carrying out a series of in vitro experiments. These studies demonstrated efficient targeting of HIV-1 transcripts in a complex RNA mixture, and led to testing of an anti-HIV-*gag* ribozyme in cell culture experiments.[24] By placing the ribozyme under the control of the human β-actin promoter, challenged cells produced sufficient amounts of the ribozyme to effect a greater than 40 fold inhibition of viral infectivity in the absence of cellular toxicity. Indirect assays utilizing RNA based PCR suggested that the inhibition was due to ribozyme mediated cleavage.

Anti-HIV-1 studies with a hairpin ribozyme targeted to a highly conserved GUC in the viral LTR have resulted in several important observations and have provided encouraging results for those interested in ribozymes as therapeutic agents.[25,26] Cells co-transfected with a ribozyme gene, an HIV-1 proviral DNA, and a Tat dependent CAT reporter construct showed an 80% reduction in Tat dependent CAT activity, and up to 95% inhibition of p24 antigen production relative to non-ribozyme producing control cells. A mutant ribozyme, which could still bind the target RNA sequence, but was unable to cleave it resulted in only a small reduction in Tat dependent CAT expression as well as p24 antigen production. When the functional ribozyme was expressed from a strong Pol III promoter (tRNA ^{Val}) 15 to 25% more inhibition was observed compared with the same ribozyme expressed from the human β-actin promoter.[26]

One of the potential attributes of ribozyme mediated inhibition of gene expression is that of target selectivity. A point mutation at the cleavage site is sufficient to abolish ribozyme mediated cleavage in vitro, and presumably should function similarly in an intracellular environment. The mutation at codon 12 in c-H-*ras* from GGU to GUU creates a site for hammerhead ribozyme mediated cleavage. An endogenously expressed ribozyme targeted to this site was effective in preventing focus formation in about 50% of NIH3T3 cells transfected with this activated *ras* gene. In contrast, cells expressing this same ribozyme, but transfected with an activated *ras* in which the codon change was at position 61 instead of 12, were not protected from foci formation by the ribozyme.[27] Although some 'antisense' effect from pairing of the ribozyme to the target RNA cannot be excluded, functional inactivation of only the cleavable *ras* mutation provided strong evidence for ribozyme mediated cleavage in these cells.

Delivery of antisense/ribozymes for therapeutic applications

The effective use of ribozymes as therapeutic agents is dependent upon effective means of delivering antisense and ribozyme gene constructs or pre-formed, chemically synthesized molecules to the appropriate target cells. Presently, retroviral vector delivery of ribozyme gene constructs looks most promising for ex vivo gene transfer protocols. These vectors can be engineered to harbor either Pol II or Pol III transcriptional cassettes for ribozyme expression. Highly engineered and well defined ribozyme transcripts are desirable over longer, poorly characterized transcripts which could impede ribozyme function. Retroviral vectors can be used for the effective expression of tRNA based Pol III transcriptional units when the transcriptional cassette is inserted within the non-transcribed region of the 5′LTR. It is also quite likely that other well defined RNA polymerase II and III transcriptional units such as those encoding the small nuclear RNAs can also be expressed using a similar strategy, expanding the potential for gene expression in a variety of cell types.

Long-term resistance to HIV-1 infection in cells transfected with Moloney murine leukemia virus vectors carrying anti-HIV-1 ribozyme genes targeted to either a common leader segment in the 5′LTR,[26,28] or to a cleavage site in the *tat* transcript[29,30] have been demonstrated. One ribozyme targeted to *tat*, which was expressed as part of the 3′untranslated region of the neomycin phosphotransferase resistance mRNA delayed expression of viral antigens in cell culture, but was less effective than a non-enzymatic antisense targeted to the same sequences.[29] The reason for this difference was not evident from the data presented, but could reflect cis-effects of transcript sequences on ribozyme folding.

There are some restrictions for expressing a well defined ribozyme transcript from a retroviral vector. If a strong promoter is inserted downstream of the viral LTR, there is the possibility of promoter interference. A ribozyme construct placed under control of the viral LTR will usually be included within a very long transcript. If a strong terminator is placed downstream of the ribozyme, it will prematurely terminate full length viral transcripts and in turn reduce the titer of virus produced in the packaging cell line.

Other viral vectors are being developed for gene therapy uses. Any vector which has applications for other forms of gene therapy should be suitable for the delivery of ribozyme encoding genes. One such vector is adeno-associated virus (AAV). Although there are not published reports of AAV delivery of ribozyme encoding genes, it has been used successfully to transduce human cells with an antisense construct which effectively blocked HIV replication in cell culture.[31] Many of the constraints imposed by genome organization in retroviral vectors will not occur in AAV, but it remains to be determined how generally useful it will be for delivering genes expressed from promoters such as Pol III (*see* also Kremer, this issue).

Liposomes are effective vehicles for macromoleclar delivery into some cell types. They may not yet be suitable for systemic delivery of antisense or ribozyme oligonucleotides, but there are certain clinical settings where liposome delivery of oligonucleotides or even gene constructs are feasible. One such setting is autologous bone marrow transplantation for treatment of chronic myelogenous leukemia. The use of ex vivo purging techniques in which the leukemic cells are selectively eliminated from the marrow populations are being explored with both antisense oligos and ribozymes. The unique *bcr-abl* fusion transcript which is present in greater than 95% of chronic myelogenous leukemia cells has been targeted by a ribozyme which hybridizes across the unique splice junction fusion joining exons from *bcr* and *abl.* [32] Synthetic DNA-RNA chimeric ribozymes in which the base pairing regions are DNA, but the catalytic center is RNA, have been delivered via cationic liposomes into an EM2 leukemic cell line. Anti-*bcr-abl* ribozyme administration via cationic liposomes specifically reduced the level of *bcr-abl* message and the p210 protein product of this oncogene, as well as inhibiting growth of these cells. An unrelated control ribozyme had no inhibitory activity. In this same study, an antisense DNA delivered by liposomes also blocked p210 protein synthesis and elicited a growth inhibitory effect which was not as strong as the ribozyme. Interestingly, the protein reduction by the ribozyme and antisense DNA was similar despite a markedly greater reduction of the *bcr-abl* transcript mediated by the ribozyme versus the antisense DNA. The liposome encapsulation was responsible for at least a three-fold increase in the amount of ribozyme entering the cells. The liposome delivery method for ribozymes is potentially applicable in a clinical setting for ex vivo purging of leukemic cells from bone marrow.

General considerations for therapeutic efficacy of antisense and ribozymes

One of the goals of antisense/ribozyme therapy should be the eradication of a virus or malignant cell population from a patient. This can only be done if the transduction or transfection of the antisense/ribozyme, as well as the biological activities of these reagents are highly efficient. On the other hand, if the antisense/ribozyme delivery is not 100% efficient, but can indirectly lead to some secondary response in the patient, it is possible to achieve a desired therapeutic effect without high efficiency transductions. 'Bystander' effects have been observed in several cancer directed gene therapy protocols. In these instances only a small fraction of the targeted cells have been transduced or transfected with the therapeutic gene, but the entire tumor regresses. This can be due to a number of factors, such as intracellular channelling of toxic substances, or to a heightened immune response rendering the entire tumor susceptible to cell-mediated immunity. The type of situation is very desirable if antisense/ribozyme approaches are to be clinically useful. An example of an enhanced immune response as a consequence of an antisense inhibition of an important growth factor has been reported.[33] Antisense RNA targeted to the IGF 1 mRNA blocked proliferation of rat glioblastoma cells in culture as well as their ability to form tumors in rats. Rats which were injected with glioblastoma cells expressing the antisense to IGF1, as well as untreated cells injected into another site in the animal, had no tumor formation, or a greatly reduced incidence of tumor formation. The antisense blockage of IGF1 may have lead to a blockade in an autocrine or paracrine pathway required for cell proliferation, but the reason why antisense and non-antisense treated cells injected into the same animal were both blocked in their tumor forming ability is not known, but appears to have involved an enhanced T-cell mediated killing of the tumor cells.

CONCLUSIONS

The therapeutic applications of antisense nucleic acids and ribozymes are expanding as a consequence of stabilizing chemical modifications and marked improvements in the technologies required to deliver these agents to cells. There are currently several clinical trials involving antisense oligodeoxynucletides, and at least one for a ribozyme. These trials range from treatment of cancer to viral inhibition. The first human clinical trials involving a retrovirally delivered ribozyme for the treatment of HIV infection will be initiated by the end of 1994. The use of these 'genetic' therapeutics is the beginning of a new era in medicine in which the drugs selectively block the flow of genetic information for only the targeted nucleic acid sequence, thereby greatly minimizing toxicity. The clinical trials currently in progress should provide the necessary 'safety' information for subsequent efficacy trials using both chemically synthesized genetic agents as well as delivery of therapeutic ribozyme and antisense genes in a gene therapy setting.

ACKNOWLEDGMENTS

Supported by grants from NIH AI29329, AI25959 and the Pediatric AIDS Foundation/American Foundation for AIDS Research 500331-14-PG.

REFERENCES

1 Eguchi Y, Itoh T, Tomizawa J. Antisense RNA. Annu Rev Biochem 1991; 60: 631–652.
2 Hastie ND, Held WA. Analysis of mRNA populations by cDNA-mRNA hybrid-mediated inhibition of cell-free protein synthesis. Proc Natl Acad Sci USA 1978; 75: 1217–1221.
3 Paterson BM, Roberts BE, Kuff EL. Structural gene identification and mapping by DNA-mRNA hybrid-arrested cell-free translation. Proc Natl Acad Sci USA 1977; 74: 4370–4374.
4 Zamecnik PC, Stephenson ML. Inhibition of Rous sarcoma virus replication by a specific oligonucleotide. Proc Natl Acad Sci USA 1978; 75: 280–284.
5 Izant JG, Weintraub H. Inhibition of thymidine kinase gene expression by antisense RNA: A molecular approach to genetic analysis. Cell 1984; 36: 1007–1010.
6 Melton DA. Injected antisense RNAs specifically block messenger RNA translation in vivo. Proc Nat Acad Sci USA 1985; 82: 144–148.
7 McGarry TJ, Lindquist S. Inhibition of heat shock protein synthesis by heat-inducible antisense RNA. Proc Nat Acad Sci USA 1986; 83: 399–403.
8 Katsuki M, Sato M, Kimura M, Yokoyama M, Kobayashi K, Nomura T. Conversion of normal behavior to shiverer by myelin basic protein antisense cDNA in transgenic mice. Science 1988; 241: 593–595.
9 van der Krol AR, Mol JNM, Stuitje AR. Modulation of eukaryotic gene expression by complementary RNA or DNA sequences. BioTechniques 1988; 6: 958–976.
10 Crooke ST. Progress toward oligonucleotide therapeutics: pharmacodynamic properties. FASEB J 1993; 7: 533–539.
11 Castanotto D, Rossi JJ, Sarver, N. Antisense catalytic RNAs as therapeutic agents. Adv Pharmacol 1994; 25: 289–317.
12 Bass BL, Weintraub H. An unwinding activity that covalently modifies its double-stranded RNA substrate. Cell 1988; 1089–1098.
13 Kruger K, Grabowski PJ, Zaug AJ, Sands J, Gottschling DE, Cech TR. Self-splicing RNA: autoexcision and autocyclization of the ribosomal RNA intervening sequence of Tetrahymena. Cell 1982; 31: 147–157.
14 Guerrier-Takada C, Gardiner K, Marsh T, Pace N, Altman S. The RNA moiety of ribonuclease P is the catalytic subunit of the enzyme. Cell 1983; 35: 849–857.

15 Diener TO. Subviral pathogens of plants: viroids and viroid like satellite RNAs. FASEB J. 1991; 5: 2808–2813.
16 Forster AC, Symons RH. Self-cleavage of plus and minus RNAs of a virusoid and a structural model for the active sites. Cell 1987; 49: 211–220.
17 Uhlenbeck OC. A small catalytic oligoribonucleotide. Nature 1987; 328: 596–600.
18 Haseloff J, Gerlach WL. Simple RNA enzymes with new and highly specific endoribonuclease activities. Nature 1988; 334: 585–591.
19 Ruffner DE. Stormo GD, Uhlenbeck OC. Sequence requirements of the hammerhead RNA self-cleavage reaction. Biochemistry 1990; 29: 10695–10702.
20 Buzayan JM, Gerlach WL, Bruening G. Non-enzymatic cleavage and ligation of RNAs commplementary to a plant virus satellite RNA. Nature 1986; 323: 349–352.
21 Hampel A, Tritz, R. RNA catalytic properties of the minimum (-) sTRSV sequence. Biochemistry 1989; 28: 4929–4933.
22 Cech TR. Ribozyme engineering. Curr Opin Struct Biol 1992; 2: 605–609.
23 Rossi JJ. Ribozymes. Curr Opin Biotechnol 1992; 3: 3–7.
24 Sarver N, Cantin EM, Chang P et al. Ribozymes as potential anti-HIV-1 therapeutic agents. Science 1990; 247: 1222–1225.
25 Ojwang JO, Hampel A, Looney DJ, Wong-Staal F. Inhibition of human immunodeficiency virus type 1 expression by a hairpin ribozyme. Proc Natl Acad Sci USA 1992; 89: 10802–10806.
26 Yu M, Poeschla E, Wong-Staal F. Progress towards gene therapy for HIV infection. Gene Ther 1994; 1: 13–26.
27 Kiozumi M, Hayase Y, Iwai S, Kamiya H, Inoue H, Ohtsuka E. Ribozymes designed to inhibit transformation of NIH3T3 cells by the activated c-Ha-ras gene. Gene 1992; 117: 179–184.
28 Weerasinghe M, Liem SE, Asad S, Read SE, Joshi S. Resistance to human immunodeficiency virus type 1 (HIV-1) infection in human CD4+ lymphocyte-derived cell lines conferred by using retroviral vectors expressing an HIV-1 RNA-specific ribozyme. J Virol 1991; 65: 5531–5534.
29 Lo KMS, Biasolo, MA, Dehni G, Palu G, Haseltine WA. Inhibition of replication of HIV-1 by retroviral vectors expressing tat-Antisense and Anti-tat ribozyme RNA. Virology 1992; 190: 176–183.
30 Zhou C, Bahner I, Larson GP, Zaia J, Rossi J. Kohn D. Inhibition of HIV-1 in human T-lymphocytes by retrovirally transduced anti-tat and rev hammerhead ribozymes. Gene 1994; (In press).
31 Chatterjee S, Johnson PR, Wong Jr, KK. Dual target inhibition of HIV by means an adeno-associated virus antisense vector. Science 1992; 258: 1485–1489.
32 Snyder DA, Wu Y, Wang JL et al. Ribozyme-mediated inhibition of bcr-abl gene expression in a Philadelphia chromosome-positive cell line. Blood 1993; 82: 600–605.
33 Trojan J, Johnson TR, Rudin SD, Ilan J, Tykocinski ML, Ilan J, Treatment and prevention of rat glioblastoma by immunogenic C6 cells expressing antisense insulin-like growth factor I RNA. Science 1993; 259: 94–97.

British Medical Bulletin 1995 Vol. 51, No. 1, pp.226–234

Gene therapy – future prospects and the consequences

M Evans
Wellcome/CRC Institute of Cancer and Developmental Biology and Department of Genetics, Cambridge, UK

N Affara
Department of Pathology, University of Cambridge, Cambridge, UK

A M L Lever
Department of Medicine, Addenbrooke's Hosptial, Cambridge, UK

The potential range and versatility of gene therapy has been outlined in the preceding chapters of this volume. It is a new form of therapeutic intervention at a molecular level with applications in many areas of medical treatment ranging from specific correction of single locus inherited genetic defects through immunisation, treatment of infectious disease, cancer and ersatz ablation surgery. It is also a new pharmacology. While most current pharmacologies seek to modify endogenous processes by the application of novel, artificial chemical compounds, gene therapy delivers a very specific biologically active agent at a particular place and time with the possibility of permanent, transient or inducible expression. As a new pharmacology it must be assessed in the context of heredity. Heredity requires two functions. Firstly, the transmission of the information from generation to generation and secondly, the expression of the inheritance.

Transmission and expression are separated at the molecular level and, in multicellular organisms, at the cellular level. Cell determination followed by differentiation at an early stage irreversibly separates the somatic lineages from the potential carriers of information to the next generation – the germ-line cells. Therapeutic gene expression may be effected transiently by the use of non-integrating vectors or by targeting cells with a strictly limited biological life. If, as is commonly the case, long-term expression is required, integrating or self-replicating vectors will be used. The latter are less easy to distribute and to control.

Genetic material in a chromosome is under direct *cis* and *trans* acting influences from near and distant parts of the genome. It is not surprising that one of the major problems with gene transfer as currently practised is that of reliable long-term expression of the transduced gene when transferred with the minimal contextual sequence. The globin gene family illustrates this well. Control of expression is dependent on 4 distant upstream regions recognised by their DNAse1 hypersensitivity and named Locus Control Regions (LCRs).[1] Until some or all of this genetic material was included in vectors globin expression in transduced cells was poor or unreliable.[2,3] Even with these regions included, globin gene transfer was unpredictable with multiple gene rearrangements commonly seen. What can be done to overcome this problem, which is likely to recur with many if not all eucaryotic gene transfers? Firstly, attempts have been made to 'clean' the construct of extraneous interfering motifs by scanning the sequence in the vector constructs for *cis* acting signals which might be responsible for rearrangements (cryptic splice sites, polyadenylation signals etc) and systematically to eliminate them by deletion or site directed mutagenesis. This empirical and painstaking process in the case of βglobin has led to more reliable gene transfer.[4]

Substituting a normal gene in place of the abnormally or non-functioning gene by homologous recombination is a second possibility and, theoretically, the ideal form of gene therapy. As yet this is practised successfully only in cell lines or animal embryonic stem cells. Reliance on the endogenous cellular processes for recombination gives an unsatisfactorily low success rate. However, enzymes have been known for a number of years (site specific recombinases) which will catalyse excision and insertion of genetic material by recognition of a particular nucleotide sequence and these have recently been used in eucaryotic gene transfer. The best understood is the bacteriophage cre/loxP system.[5,6] The cre enzyme recognises a particular oligonucleotide sequence and will excise a piece of genetic material between two of these sequences then rejoin the ends. If two DNA strands are provided each with two loxP sites the enzyme can exchange the genetic material between the sequences from one strand to the other. Introducing loxP sites into targeting constructs for homologous recombination has already been used to create site specific insertions and deletions in embryonic stem cells[7] in transgenic mice.[8,9] By putting the inserted gene under control of a tissue specific promoter a transgene can then be inserted at a specific site and made to express in a tissue specific manner.[10]

A third possibility is to attempt transfer of a large genetic unit containing the gene and all its associated control regions together perhaps with accessory genes in a self replicating format, an artificial chromosome. These would overcome limitations on the length of DNA that can be carried by the (primarily viral) based vectors currently in use. The ability to deliver large DNA segments carrying a complete gene and its regulatory sequences has obvious advantages with respect to achieving stable and tissue specific expression and has been demonstrated recently using Yeast Artificial Chromosome (YAC) vectors to create transgenic mice.[11,12] Artificial chromosomes also avoid the worries over control of the site of integration of exogenous DNA. Yeast centromeres and telomeres do not appear to function in mammalian cells[13] so the current aim is the production of a mammalian artificial chromosome vector carrying telomeres and a centromere that combines the ability to carry large pieces of DNA (several hundreds of kilobases) with the capability to segregate as an independent chromosome in dividing cells in synchrony with the host genome (for reviews see[14,15]). Two approaches have been adopted in determining the basic elements necessary to produce a functional MAC, both focussing on the use of the human Y centromere the most completely understood of the human centromeres.[16–18]

In the first, telomere mediated chromosome breakage has been used to seed the creation of internal telomeres, leading to fragmentation at the site of telomere formation[19,20] (see Fig. 1). This has been used successfully to produce functional truncated X chromosomes[19] and significantly reduced Y chromosomes.[21] More directed fragmentation may be achieved through the use of site specific recombinases. Eventually, the goal is to produce a sufficiently small chromosome which can be cloned and manipulated in a large capacity vector.

In the second approach, assembly of a MAC vector is being attempted through the progressive modification of YAC clones carrying mammalian centromere and telomere sequences.[22,23] Whilst circumventing many of the problems of current small capacity vectors, MACs have their own potential drawbacks not least the method by which such large units can be efficiently introduced to large numbers of cells.

THE CONSEQUENCES OF GENE THERAPY

Modification of the genetic material in a particular cell may affect both that cell and its descendants. The extent of the effect of a genetic alteration upon an individual will therefore depend upon the biology of the cell in question. How large a proportion of the organism will it or its descendants occupy and for how long?

The ideas for useful somatic genetic intervention are running ahead of present realities not only because their novelty needs testing but also because design and the means of delivery are still relatively rudimentary. There has been great concern about the potential dangers of using a treatment which is designed deliberately to create genetic changes as some of the vectors and also the transformed human cells are potentially propagable.

Both irrational and reasonable fears surround the potential for deliberate genetic alteration of the germ-line and this is at present forbidden by statutory codes of practice. Protocols designed for somatic

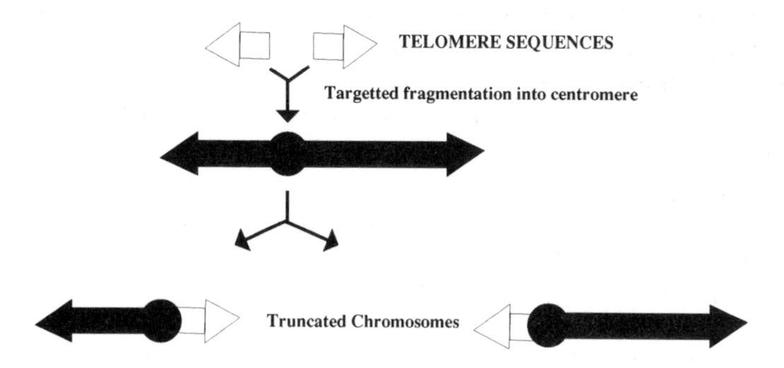

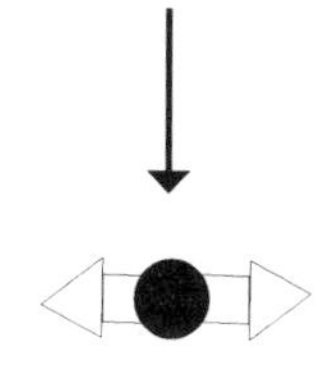

Fig. 1 Telomere mediated chromosome breakage used to seed creation of internal telomeres, leading to fragmentation at the site of telomere formation.

therapy may, however, carry with them the risk of inadvertent germ-line transformation. The risk of this event will necessarily vary with each protocol and all reasonable precautions against unwanted spread of the genetic transformation should be taken. What, though, are the risks?

Mutagenesis

All chromosomal integration apart from homologous replacement carries the potential for alteration of random endogenous loci and hence mutagenesis. Somatic mutagenesis can result in oncogenesis. Germ-line mutagenesis will potentially introduce new deleterious mutations into the human gene pool. It is clear that neither of these events is currently regarded as a complete contra-indication for therapeutic treatment, as known mutagenic agents are in daily medical use.

The genetic population

Our anthropocentric view of life considers primarily the importance of the individual and neglects the population. In biological terms the individual is merely the genetic vector for maintenance and evolution of the population genome. The individual is expendable and it is the population genome which evolves. There are several implications of a population genetics view for consideration in gene therapy.

SOMATIC INTERVENTION

Does somatic gene therapy have implications for population genetic structure and does population genetic structure have implications for somatic gene therapy?

If we carry out somatic gene therapy we do not transmit the manipulated genes in the somatic cells to future generations but we do alter the genetic 'fitness' of the individual. If gene therapy is successful in treating life-threatening disease the individual may live and reproduce and potentially pass on otherwise disadvantageous or lethal genes. Conventional medical therapy already reduces considerably the effects of some selection pressures although it imposes its own in the form of favouring individuals who are 'good responders'. This must have some effects on population genetic structure quite apart from its contribution to the population explosion. But it is unclear how large an effect this may have on the human genome. Direct somatic-cell genetic intervention differs from conventional medical treatment only in that there is a clearer direct connection between therapy and genetic selection. If the fraction of a particular allele in the population as a whole is p there should be 2 $(p–p^2)$ heterozygote individuals and p^2 homozygotes. As p is $<< 1$ in recessive conditions, the vast majority of the gene pool of a particular allele will reside in essentially asymptomatic heterozygote individuals. If at present, the affected individuals do not reproduce, the population loses a fraction p^2/p of the allele each generation. Conversely if the affected individuals are treated and have an equal chance of reproduction as those with an allele with a neutral phenotype there is no change in the proportion of the allele. Thus changes which may be caused by gene therapy are likely to be much less important than those resulting from other medical and social intervention.

In the case of syndromes caused by dominant-acting loci the full gene pool is represented by the affected individuals. Their reproductive success therefore directly influences the size of this pool in the next generation. If individuals carrying the allele do not reproduce, the frequency of the gene in the population is maintained by the occurrence of new mutations. Successful gene therapy would allow maintenance by reproduction as well as mutation and the gene frequency would rise. The syndromes are however extremely rare, (p is very small). If normal reproduction is restored this low ratio will be maintained and only very slowly increased by new mutation.

With sex linked genetic disease – effectively recessive in the female and dominant in the male – the intermediate position holds with respect to the influence of reproduction on the gene frequency. As the numbers affected are much greater (all males carrying the allele will be affected) the influence of successful therapy on gene frequency is also greater.

Could screening and avoidance of conception or birth of affected individuals remove the need for gene therapy in these types of disease?

As genetic knowledge improves, the practicalities of pre-screening for monoallelic genetic disease becomes greater. Dominant and sex-linked disease-causing alleles should be known to occur in any particular pedigree and therefore in principle the offspring may be screened ante-natally. For severe dominant conditions a high proportion of cases may represent new mutations which could not have been predicted. Pre-screening in the case of sex-linked alleles is, however, a useful exercise. Useful population or ante-natal screening for recessive alleles is only really practicable for those of high frequency. Once a family has been ascertained as a double heterozygote mating by the occurrence of the first affected child, screening of later conceptions is possible. It is therefore likely that sporadic occurrence of individuals affected either by homozygosity for a rare recessive syndrome or heterozygous for a severe dominantly inherited syndrome will not be able to be prevented by any pre-screening programme. These individuals will therefore remain and be in need of treatment.

GERM-LINE INTERVENTION

Here it is much clearer that there is direct interference with the popu lation genome because it is intended that alterations are inherited. Genetic engineering of the human species has been occurring throughout history and almost undoubtedly through pre-history by stone, sword, bullet, bomb and even biological warfare. Organised extinction of people and in particular aboriginal populations, has taken place and it is questionable whether a minor application of modern gene therapy would have any serious impact in comparison with these processes.

Genetic engineering and genetic selection of human populations on a wide scale has already been a normal event of our recent evolution.

That is not to say however that it is in any way desirable to use the latest tools of modern molecular genetics for deliberate tampering with the human population genome. In biological terms it would presently be an inefficient and uneconomic attempt. If malign and deliberate intervention in human genetics were to be envisaged direct selective breeding would undoubtedly deliver much greater initial results.

Would deliberate germ-line modification have an effect upon population genetic structure?

Clearly this would only happen with a very large scale genetic transformation or alternatively where the mutated genome has some highly selective advantage. One worrying scenario could be the introduction of a specific disease resistance possibly together with the disease pathogen. If only 'The Chosen' are protected from the disease this could have the possibility of a very large genetic change in the population. Not only by the introduction of the new allele or locus but also inadvertently by fixing adjacent alleles and by the potentially deleterious founder effects of a small population base. Removal of a mutant locus from the population genome either by genetic screening or by deliberate genetic engineering is conceivable but would have very little effect on the population distribution of alleles at other loci.

In the case of much rarer alleles any effect on the population gene frequency would be even less and the potential for population screening becomes diminishingly small.

WOULD GERM LINE GENE THERAPY EVER REALLY BE NEEDED?

Somatic gene therapy will have a direct effect upon the individual patient but any germ-line gene transformation can only have effects upon as yet unborn offspring. It is not therefore the patient who is being treated. With the possibilities of ante-natal and even preimplantational screening as well as both sperm or egg donation and adoption it is very difficult to see how deliberate germ-line intervention might be ethically justified. An untreatable, dominantly inherited disease for which there are such a multitude of possible mutations responsible that screening becomes impracticable, or one which increases in chance with each generation such as some of the triplet repeat diseases are possible cases for debate.

RISKS OF GERM-LINE TREATMENT

Is inadvertent germ-line transformation a serious problem?

In the main, risk benefit analysis has been used to assess the likelihood and extent of adverse effects of a procedure. The benefit is often measured in collective economic terms and the risks are often measured as the likelihood of injury or death. In the case of gene therapy, the parameters are reversed; the advantage is therapeutic for an individual and the risk is communal. Public risk perception is not necessarily related to actual risk, more often there is a strong component of fear of lack of control. Thus flying is feared more than car travel despite the latter being a more likely source of personal accident. In this context the apparent risk from inadvertent germ-line contamination by human gene therapy may appear to be much greater than it really is. Possibly the best approach is to be fully aware both of the best estimates of likelihood of germ-line transformation in any particular therapy and, cognisant of the enhanced public anxiety, to have a screening assay designed into the vector so that any subsequent suggestion of germ-line transmission is readily detected. For somatic cell therapy conditional lethal passenger genes are sometimes included in vectors, e.g. the thymidine kinase gene, such that treatment of the individual with Ganciclovir will specifically ablate transduced cells. In these instances it is felt that there is then a final safety brake so that disasters, such as vector mediated cell transformation can be controlled.

The real risk is pollution of the human genome

The real risk is pollution of the human genome with an accretion of non-specific effects similar to the risks of general pollution and alteration of our ecological environment. Awareness that the risks are for the population and the future and not just for the individual patient should temper any cavalier enthusiasm for poorly-controlled treatment.

REFERENCES

1. Grosveld F, Blom van Assendelft, Greaves DR, Kollias G. Position-independent, high level expression of the human β-globin gene in transgenic mice. Cell 1987; 51: 975–985.
2. Plavec I, Papayannopoulou T, Maury C, Meyer F. A human β-globin gene fused to the human β-globin locus control region is expressed at high levels in erythroid cell of mice engrafted with retrovirus-transduced hematopoietic stem cells. Blood 1993; 81: 1384–1392.
3. Chang JC, Liu D, Kan YW. A 36-base-pair core sequence of locus control region enhances retrovirally transferred human β-globin gene expression. Proc Natl Acad Sci USA 1992; 89: 3107–3010.
4. Leboulch P, Huang GMS, Humphries RK et al. Mutagenesis of retroviral vectors transducing human β-globin gene and β-globin locus control region derivatives results in stable transmission of an active transcriptional structure. EMBO 1994; 13: 3065–3076.

5 Sternberg N, Hamilton D. Bacteriophage P1 site-specific recombination. J Mol Biol 1981; 150: 467–486.
6 Sauer B, Henderson N. Site-specific DNA recombination in mammalian cells by the Cre recombinase of bacteriophage P1. Proc Natl Acad Sci USA 1988; 85: 5166–5170.
7 Gu H, Zou Y-R, Rajewsky K. Independent control of immunoglobulin switch recombination at individual switch regions evidenced through Cre-*IoxP*-mediated gene targeting. Cell 1993; 73: 1155–1164.
8 Lakso M et al. Targeted oncogene activation by site-specific recombination in transgenic mice. Proc Natl Acad Sci USA 1992; 89: 6232–6236.
9 Orban PC, Chui D, Marth JD. Tissue and site-specific DNA recombination in transgenic mice. Proc Natl Acad Sci USA 1992; 89: 6861–6865.
10 Gu H, Marth JD, Orban PC, Mossmann H, Rajewsky K. Deletion of a DNA polymerase β gene segment in T cells using cell type-specific gene targeting. Science 1994; 265: 103–106.
11 Jakobovits A, Moore AL, Green LL, Vergara GJ, Maynard-Currie CE, Austin HA, Klapholz S. Germ line transmission and expression of a human-derived yeast artificial chromosome. Nature 1993; 362: 255–258.
12 Strauss WM, Dausman J, Beard C, Johnson C, Lawrence JB, Jaenisch R. Germ line transmission of a yeast artificial chromosome spanning the murine a1(I) collagen locus. Science 1993; 259: 1904–1907.
13 Featherstone T, Huxley C. Extrachromosomal maintenance and amplification of yeast artificial chromosome DNA in mouse cells. Genomics 1993; 17: 267–278.
14 Brown WRA. Mammalian artificial chromosomes. Curr Opin Gene Dev 1992; 2: 479–486.
15 Huxley C. Mammalian artificial chromosomes: A New Tool for gene therapy. Gene Therapy 1994; 1: 7–12.
16 Cooper KF, Fisher RB, Tyler-Smith C. Structure of the pericentric long arm region of the human Y chromosome. J Mol Biol 1992; 228: 421–432.
17 Cooper KF, Fiisher RB, Tyler-Smith C. Structure of the sequences adjacent to the centromeric alphoid satellite DNA on the human Y chromosome. J Mol Biol 1993a; 230: 787–799.
18 Cooper KF, Fisher RB, Tyler-Smith C. The major centromeric array of alphoid satellite DNA on the human Y chromosome is non-palindromic. Hum. Mol. Genetics 1993b; 2: 1267–1270.
19 Farr C, Fantes J, Goodfellow PN, Cooke H. Functional reintroduction of functional human telomeres into mammalian cells. Proc Natl Acad Sci USA 1991; 88: 7006–7110.
20 Barnett MA, Buckle VJ, Evans EP et al. Telomere directed fragmentation of mammalian chromosomes. Nucl Acids Res 1993; 21: 27–36.
21 Brown KE, Barnett MA, Burgtorf C et al. Dissecting the centromere of the human Y chromosome with cloned telomeric DNA. Hum Mol Genetic 1994; 3: 1227–1237.
22 Larin Z, Fricker MD, Tyler-Smith C. *De Novo* formation of several features of a centromere by introduction of a Y alphoid YAC into mammalian cells. Hum Mol Genetics 1994; 3: 689–695.
23 Taylor SS, Larin Z, Tyler-Smith C. Addition of functional telomeres to YACs. Hum Mol Genetics 1994; 3: 1383–1386.

Index

G

H